THE
68000
MICROPROCESSOR

THE 68000 MICROPROCESSOR

Andrew M. Veronis, Ph.D.
Professor
Department of Electrical Engineering
Howard University
Washington, D.C.

VAN NOSTRAND REINHOLD COMPANY
_____ New York

Copyright ©1988 by Van Nostrand Reinhold Company Inc.
Library of Congress Catalog Card Number 87-13297
ISBN 0-442-28842-5

All rights reserved. No part of this work covered by the copyright hereon may be reproduced or used in any form or by an means—graphic, electronic, or mechanical, including photocopying, recording, taping, or information storage and retrieval systems—without written permission of the publisher.

Printed in the United States of America

Van Nostrand Reinhold Company Inc.
115 Fifth Avenue
New York, New York 10003

Van Nostrand Reinhold Company Limited
Molly Millars Lane
Wokingham, Berkshire RG11 2PY, England

Van Nostrand Reinhold
480 La Trobe Street
Melbourne, Victoria 3000, Australia

Macmillan of Canada
Division of Canada Publishing Corporation
164 Commander Boulevard
Agincourt, Ontario M1S 3C7, Canada

16 15 14 13 12 11 10 9 8 7 6 5 4 3 2 1

Library of Congress Cataloging-in-Publication Data

Veronis, Andrew.
 The 68000 microprocessor.

 Includes index.
 1. Motorola 68000 (Microprocessor) I. Title.
QA76.8.M672V47 1988   004.165   87-13297
ISBN 0-442-28842-5

This book is dedicated to my dear mother-in-law Eleanor Hough Buckler, for all the love and kindness she has shown me.

Preface

The Motorola MC68000 family of microprocessors is undoubtedly a revolutionary set of devices. The MC68000 is the first advanced 16-bit microprocessor with a 32-bit internal architecture and the first with 16-megabyte, nonsegmented, direct memory addressing. The processor's six basic addressing modes are equivalent to 14, when one considers all of the variations among these modes. Combined with the device's data and instruction types, the modes provide more than 1000 useful instructions.

The book you are about to study has been developed as an aid to the hardware designer and as a supplement to the Motorola seminars on the 68000 microprocessor. The text includes a detailed description of the MC68000 and two complete systems that show how this processor can be interfaced to the outside world.

The book follows a "top-down" approach. A brief history of microprocessors is provided first. Chapter 2 details the MC68000 by describing its registers, control lines, and capabilities.

Chapter 3 introduces a small MC68000-based system. Although this system is characterized in the book as hypothetical, it is indeed the Educational Computer Board, used in the various Motorola seminars.

The addressing modes and instructions are explained in Chapter 4, which includes helpful hints on how instructions can be used. Chapter 5 provides an in-depth description of additional instructions and numerous examples.

Chapter 6 discusses exception handling and interrupts.

Chapter 7 describes how the MC68000 processor can be connected to eight-bit and 16-bit peripheral devices. This Chapter also covers the interfacing of the Motorola Educational Computer Board to a terminal, a modem, a printer, and a cassette interface. Various interfacing programs are listed in this Chapter.

Chapter 8 provides full description of a second MC68000-based system, the VU68K. This system was built initially by students of the Computer Science Department of Vanderbilt University, and subsequently has been constructed by some of the author's students. The most interesting part of this Chapter is the detailed description of an operating system monitor, the VUBUG. Study of the VUBUG provides the reader with valuable experience in the use of the MC68000 instructions, as well as in the design of a basic, but fully functional, operating system monitor.

The writing and production of a book really involves many people, such as reviewers, copy editors, and artists. Perhaps the only chance that an author has to thank these people is through the preface of the book.

I wish to thank everyone who participated in the production of this book. I particularly wish to thank my friend Joe Gordon for helping me with the illustrations.

Most authors use the preface of their book to thank their loved ones for their patience. I wish to do the same, to thank my dear wife Elizabeth Veronis not only for her tremendous patience but also for her active participation in the typing and editing of the manuscript. Her help has been invaluable.

Appendices B and D are the copyrighted property of Motorola Semiconductors, Inc. and are included in this book by written permission.

Andrew M. Veronis
Annapolis, Maryland

Contents

Preface **vii**

Chapter **1.** **BASIC CONCEPTS 1**

BRIEF HISTORY OF MICROPROCESSORS **1**
DESIGN OF A MICROPROCESSOR **2**
   Design Considerations **2**
   Registers **3**
   Addressing Modes **3**
   Prefetch **4**
   Multiple Arithmetic-Logic Unit **5**
   Microprogramming **5**
   Peripheral Devices **5**

DATA REPRESENTATION **6**
   Terminology **6**
   Data Types **6**

Chapter **2.** **INTRODUCTION TO THE MC68000 9**

GENERAL LAYOUT **9**
DATA BUS **10**
ADDRESS BUS **10**
ASYNCHRONOUS BUS CONTROL **10**
FUNCTION CONTROL **13**
SYNCHRONOUS BUS CONTROL **14**
SYSTEM CONTROL **15**
DIRECT MEMORY ACCESS CONTROL **15**
INTERRUPT CONTROL **16**
REGISTERS **17**
   Data Registers **17**
   Address Registers **17**
   Program Counter **17**
   Status Register **17**

Chapter **3.** **A SMALL MC68000 SYSTEM 19**

INTRODUCTION **19**
BLOCK DIAGRAM AND MEMORY MAP **19**
   Block Diagram **19**
   Memory Map **21**

BUSES **22**
ADDRESS MULTIPLEXING **22**
RESET/HALT AND SYSTEM CLOCK **23**
    Reset/Halt Circuit **23**
    System Clock **28**

TIMING **28**
BUS TIMEOUT LOGIC **34**
DESIGN OF RAM AND ROM INTERFACE **34**
    ROM Circuit **34**
    RAM Circuit **35**

Chapter 4. ADDRESSING MODES; INSTRUCTION SET **42**

ADDRESSING MODES **42**
    Memory Accessing Rules **42**
    Effective Address and Extension Word **42**
    Register Direct Modes **45**
        General **45**
        Data Register Direct **45**
        Address Register Direct **47**
    Memory Address Modes **47**
        General **47**
        Address Register Indirect **47**
        Address Register Indirect with Postincrement **48**
        Address Register Indirect with Predecrement **49**
        Address Register Indirect with Displacement **49**
        Address Register Indirect with Index and Displacement **50**
    Special Address Modes **51**
        Absolute Short **51**
        Absolute Long **51**
        Immediate Mode **51**
    Program Control Modes **52**
        General **52**
        Program Counter with Displacement **52**
        Program Counter with Index **52**
    Inherent Mode **52**
    Summary **52**

INSTRUCTIONS **53**

Chapter 5. INSTRUCTION SET – A MORE INTENSIVE EVALUATION **54**

DATA MANIPULATION INSTRUCTIONS **54**
    Arithmetic Operations **54**
    Logical and Shifting Instructions **60**
        Logical Instructions **60**
        Shifting Instructions **63**
    Bit Manipulation Instructions **65**

DATA MOVEMENT INSTRUCTIONS **66**
PROGRAM CONTROL INSTRUCTIONS **69**
   Unconditional Branch **69**
   Conditional Branch **69**
POSITION INDEPENDENCE INSTRUCTIONS **70**
HIGH-LEVEL LANGUAGE AIDS **70**
PROGRAMMING HINTS **73**

Chapter **6.** **EXCEPTION HANDLING 76**

GENERAL **76**
INTERRUPTS **83**

Chapter **7.** **PERIPHERAL DEVICES 92**

INTRODUCTION **92**
MEMORY MAPPING OF I/O SPACE **92**
MC6850 ACIA **92**
MEMORY MAPPING OF ACIA **97**
GENERATING INTERRUPT REQUEST SIGNALS **97**
PARALLEL INTERFACE/TIMER **104**
DESIGNING THE PRINTER INTERFACE **106**
PROGRAMMING THE INTERFACE **108**
DESIGN OF THE CASSETTE INTERFACE **110**

Chapter **8.** **ANOTHER 68000-BASED SYSTEM 114**

HARDWARE DESCRIPTION **114**
THE OPERATING SYSTEM MONITOR **118**
MONITOR COMMANDS **119**
   The "b" Command: Set/Remove Breakpoints **120**
   The "c" Command: Copy Memory Blocks **120**
   The "d" Command: Display Data to Terminal **120**
   The "e" Command: Enter Terminal Emulator Mode **120**
   The "g" Command: Execute a User Program **121**
   The "l" Command: Load Program from Host (S-format) **121**
   The "m" Command: Examine/Modify Memory **121**
   The "p" Command: Load/Execute a Prototype Command **122**
   The "r" Command: Examine/Modify Registers **122**
   The "s" Command: Single-Step Mode **122**
   The "t" Command: Trace Program Execution **123**
TRAPS **123**
EXCEPTION PROCESSING **124**
THE MONITOR **124**

Appendix **A.** **S-RECORD OUTPUT FORMAT 153**

Appendix **B.** **INSTRUCTION SET DETAILS 159**

Appendix C. **INSTRUCTION FORMAT SUMMARY 271**
Appendix D. **MC68000 INSTRUCTION EXECUTION TIMES 293**
Appendix E. **MC68000 INSTRUCTION EXECUTION TIMES 301**
Index   313

THE 68000 MICROPROCESSOR

Chapter 1
Basic Concepts

BRIEF HISTORY OF MICROPROCESSORS

The first two microprocessors—the 4004 (a four-bit set of devices) and the 8008 (an eight-bit device on a single chip)—were produced in the early 1970s by a newly formed company, Intel Corporation. The 4004, also known as the MCS-4, was designed to replace six custom chips in a desktop calculator and was therefore programmed for serial, binary-coded, decimal arithmetic (a very common practice in handheld and desktop calculators). Although the client, a Japanese manufacturer named Busicomp, went out of business before it could put the 4004 to work, this set of devices was soon adapted for numerous other applications.

A U.S. company named Computer Terminal Corporation (also known as Datapoint) similarly requested Intel to design a push-down stack chip for a processor to be used in a CRT terminal. Datapoint intended to build a bit-serial processor in TTL logic with a shift-register memory—a design that would require a fair number of devices. Intel suggested that the entire design could be implemented in one chip. This new processor was the 8008. Although Datapoint eventually did not use the chip because of the long lead time Intel required, the device was quickly adopted by other logic design engineers, who saw the advantages to be derived from microprocessors.

At about the same time, Motorola, Texas Instruments, Zilog, and other semiconductor manufacturers were gearing up to capture a share of what was to become the largest semiconductor market. Improved devices such as the Intel 8080 (second-sourced by other manufacturers, including Texas Instruments and National Semiconductors), the Zilog Z80 (the most popular eight-bit processor ever marketed), and the Motorola 6800 (also an extremely popular eight-bit microprocessor) have dominated the market for more than a decade.

As the benefits of microprocessors became more apparent, design engineers and, more particularly, programmers increasingly demanded better performance. Eight-bit microprocessors are designed to replace logic circuits and, consequently, emphasize controller-type capabilities rather than ease-of-programming elegance. Compare, for example, the instruction format of an eight-bit processor to that of a 16-bit device, as shown in Fig. 1-1.

Clearly, an eight-bit processor lags behind in the available number of registers, instructions, and addressing modes, as well as the memory addressing range. All

2   THE 68000 MICROPROCESSOR

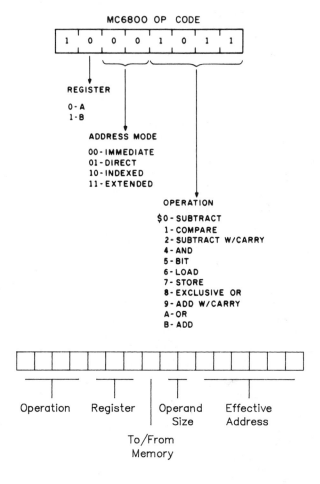

Fig. 1-1. Formats of 8-bit and 16-bit instructions.

of these features are needed for efficient programming. Thus, eight-bit processors gradually are giving way to 16-bit and 32-bit processors.

DESIGN OF A MICROPROCESSOR

Design Considerations

Numerous factors affect the overall performance of a microprocessor system, including internal organization, speed, instruction set, addressing modes, memory-handling capacity, interfacing ease, and availability of compatible peripheral devices. The system designer must consider them all.

Some of these factors will be described in the following pages. To facilitate this description, a powerful 16-bit processor—the Motorola MC68000—will be referred to from time to time. This device will not be examined in detail, however, until Chap. 2.

Registers

One significant advantage of a 16-bit microprocessor over an eight-bit device is that the former has twice the word width; as a result, a 16-bit device can handle twice as much information, thus increasing the processing speed of a system. Another advantage is the increased number of internal registers this device provides the programmer. The MC68000 excels in both of these areas.

As shown in Fig. 1-2, the Motorola MC68000 has eight 32-bit data registers, nine 32-bit address registers (registers A7 and A7' are the user and supervisor stack pointers), and a 32-bit program counter (although the maximum address range is 24 bits). Since most of its data and address registers are undedicated, the MC68000 thus provides greater flexibility.

Addressing Modes

Having a good number of addressing modes is likewise an advantage for a microprocessor. The MC68000 has 15 addressing modes. With few exceptions, each instruction operates on bytes, words (16 bits), and longwords (32 bits), and most instructions can use all 15 modes.

One weakness of an eight-bit microprocessor is its limited memory-accessing capacity. With a 16-bit address bus, this device can directly address only 65,536 addresses. Some schemes increase the address range of an eight-bit processor, or so it seems. For example, Fig. 1-3 illustrates a method called *paging*. In this scheme, the total memory area is divided into pages. Although the 16-bit address range remains unaltered, bits in another register, such as the program counter, are used to designate the number of the page. Theoretically, this practice

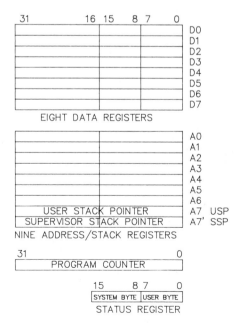

Fig. 1-2. MC68000 registers.

4 THE 68000 MICROPROCESSOR

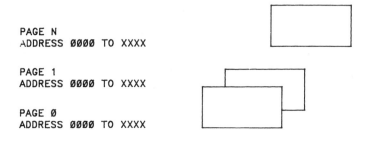

PAGE N
ADDRESS 0000 TO XXXX

PAGE 1
ADDRESS 0000 TO XXXX

PAGE 0
ADDRESS 0000 TO XXXX

Fig. 1-3. Memory paging.

increases memory capacity, but it is dependent on the bits allocated to designate page numbers. Although the addition of several page registers will eliminate the problem of page bits, paging is still limited by the fact that only a single page can be accessed at a time. This method is tricky, moreover, and time-consuming.

To overcome the deficiencies of paging, some 16-bit microprocessors use a method called *memory segmentation*. Since the memory spectrum is divided into segments, this method is similar to paging, as Fig. 1-4 shows. A segment number added to the 16-bit address identifies each segment. Segmentation allows some possibility of address relocation, but the size of each segment is a limiting factor (it cannot exceed 64 kilobytes), and the desired segment must be loaded as well.

The most straightforward method of memory accessing is called *linear accessing*. Simply speaking, a processor with linear addressing capabilities has adequate address lines to access memory directly. For example, the 23 external address lines of the MC68000 allow direct access of 8.4 million words of memory. Since programmers are always hungry for more memory, however, provisions have been made to carry out a type of paging with some control lines furnished by the MC68000. This method will be explained later. Furthermore, memory management devices can be used with the MC68000 to provide additional memory capacity.

Prefetch

A significant factor in the selection of a microprocessor is the manner in which a particular device fetches instructions from memory. After an eight-bit microprocessor fetches an instruction, the address- and data-fetching circuits and buses of

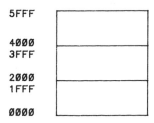

5FFF

4000
3FFF

2000
1FFF

0000

Fig. 1-4. Memory segmentation.

the device remain idle while the instruction is being executed. Needless to say, this represents a loss of time. The MC68000, in contrast, has a *prefetch queue*. During the execution of one instruction, the device fetches a number of other instructions and aligns them in the prefetch queue. Consequently, the microprocessor nearly always has an instruction available for processing. This instruction is stored in close proximity to the arithmetic-logic unit (ALU).

Multiple Arithmetic-Logic Unit

A system designer also must consider features that will increase the processing speed of a microprocessor. All eight-bit microprocessors feature only a single arithmetic-logic unit, and this is used both for data processing and for calculation of addresses. In a processor that uses indexed addressing, the offset value must be added to an address via this single ALU at a time when data could otherwise be processed.

In contrast, the MC68000 uses not only a 16-bit-wide ALU as the main data-processing mechanism but also two other 16-bit ALU to function in parallel as a 32-bit ALU for the calculation of addresses. Thus, at the same time a 16-bit datum is being processed, the address ALU can be calculating an effective address (this term will be described later). The 16-bit data ALU also is used to process 32-bit values by taking two passes at 16-bit data, one for the lower word and one for the upper.

Microprogramming

All eight-bit and most 16- and 32-bit microprocessors are designed as **hardwired logic** units—i.e., the control unit is built of logic gates permanently wired to each other. This design eliminates excessive use of components and improves speed on the one hand, but, on the other, not only reduces the flexibility of the control unit but also overcomplicates the design of a complex unit.

Microprogramming of a complex control unit simplifies design by making the unit modular; that is, each section of the unit may be modeled, built, and tested independently. Additionally, a microprogrammed design permits a customer to make design changes (although the MC68000 uses a microprogrammed design, Motorola is rather reluctant to implement a customer's microcode into this design).

Peripheral Devices

To compete successfully, a manufacturer embarking on the design of a microprocessor must provide an entire family of peripheral devices. Design and production of such devices are frequently very expensive and time-consuming. Concerned with the possible loss of their share of the microprocessor market, several manufacturers have introduced microprocessors without peripheral devices. Motorola chose to add several control lines to the MC68000 to make it directly compatible with the readily available peripheral devices from the MC6800 family. This

6 THE 68000 MICROPROCESSOR

approach afforded Motorola ample time to develop 16-bit peripheral devices and also gave customers the benefit of using low-priced eight-bit peripheral devices.

DATA REPRESENTATION

Terminology

The smallest unit of data stored in the memory of a computer is called a *bit*, an abbreviation of the words "binary digit." A bit has the value of zero (0) or one (1).

Bits are combined to make *nibbles* (four bits, useful for representing one binary-coded decimal digit (the equivalent of decimal zero to nine)) and *bytes* (eight bits). A byte may denote a single character (usually encoded in ASCII), a number from 0 to 255, or two BCD numbers (0 to 99).

The term *word* varies among computers. In all cases, a word is made up of bytes. In 16-bit computers, a word consists of two bytes; in 32-bit computers, a word consists of four bytes; and so on. Simply defined, a word is the maximum length of information that the data bus of a computer can transfer. The memory area of a computer usually has the length of the computer's word; that is, a computer is equipped with a memory 8 bits wide, 16 bits wide, etc.

A collection of words ordinarily is called a *block*.

All of these terms refer to units of storage inside a computer or memory. Distinctions must be made, however, between what various strings of bits indicate, since they may signify a character or a positive number or a false/true condition. In other words, data must be identified by "type."

Data Types

A bit is used to denote a "logical" state of "true" or "false." In this sense, the logical bit is called a *flag* and is used for comparison of two values, for branching, or for other purposes. Thus, single bits are "logical data types."

Inside a computer, a number may be represented in various ways. The number can be, for instance, an unsigned number, starting from zero, called an *ordinal*. For example, in eight-bit microprocessors, an ordinal number can be any number from 0 to 255 (00000000 to 11111111); as the data-bus width of a microprocessor increases, so does the representation of ordinal numbers.

A whole number, whether positive or negative, is called an *integer*. In all microprocessors, integers are represented in *two's complement form;* that is, the leftmost bit of an integer constitutes both the maximum value of the integer and its sign (0, for positive; 1, for negative). Various clever methods have been devised to represent numbers in two's complement form easily.

One method is shown by Dr. Christopher Morgan and Mr. Mitchell Waite in their book entitled *8086/8088 16-bit Microprocessor Primer.* Ordinal numbers from 0 to $2n^{-1}$ can be shown around a wheel, as in Fig. 1-5, so that the last number is before the first. If the wheel is separated halfway around and negative integers are assigned to positions on the separated wheel—counting backwards from zero—the two's complement representation is derived. The wheel must be separated precisely at the point where the most significant bit *(msb)*, or leftmost digit, changes sign; that is, all nonnegative numbers have a 0 as their msb, and all negative numbers have a 1 as their msb. This bit is called the *sign bit.* Thus, in 16-bit computers, integers ranging from −32,768 to +32,767 are represented; in 32-bit computers, numbers from −2,147,483,648 to +2,147,483,647 are represented.

Characters are depicted inside computers by various *codes.* The most frequently used code is the eight-bit ASCII (it is now an eight-bit code). An eight-

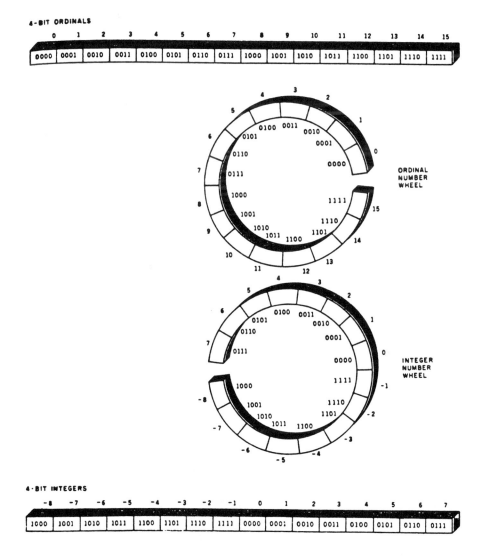

Fig. 1-5. Ordinal number representation.

bit number represents the characters of the alphabet (A through Z), numerals (0 through 9), and special characters. Most microprocessors use a subset of this eight-bit ASCII code. If, for example, a six-bit ASCII code is used, then lower-case letters cannot be represented.

A series of characters is called a *string.* In programming languages, strings are used to display a message.

Decimal numbers are denoted inside a computer in *Binary-Coded Decimal* notation (BCD). Each decimal digit, from 0 through 9, is represented by a four-bit number.

The preceding survey provides an overview of data types but is by no means complete. The reader is encouraged to study the topic of number systems in other specialized texts.

Chapter 2
Introduction to the MC68000

GENERAL LAYOUT

The MC68000 is a bulky integrated circuit that is 1.2 inches longer and 0.4 inches wider than a 40-pin package. The fact that it is equipped with numerous pins, however, makes it easier to interface.

As Fig. 2-1 shows, the MC68000 has 64 external pins that function within one of the following groups (the numbers in parentheses denote the number of pins allocated to each function):

Power supply (4)
Clock (1)
Address Bus (23)
Data Bus (16)
Function Control (3)
Synchronous Bus Control (3)
System Control (3)
Asynchronous Bus Control (5)
Direct Memory Access Control (3)
Interrupt Control (3)

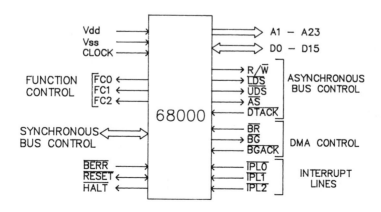

Fig. 2-1. Pin configuration of MC68000.

The orientation of the arrows shows whether a group is bidirectional or unidirectional. Each signal associated with these categories is described in this chapter. The verbs "assert" and "negate" are used throughout this text solely to dispel any doubts about the electrical status of a signal. Regardless of actual voltage level, "asserted" indicates an active signal and "negated," an inactive signal.

DATA BUS

In the MC68000, the 16 lines of the data bus are, as in any other microprocessor, bidirectional. Their function is straightforward, requiring no further description.

ADDRESS BUS

Although the MC68000 displays 23 address lines, the device is actually equipped with 24. Address A0 is encoded internally with the length of the operand to form the *Upper Data Strobe* ($\overline{UDS}$) and *Lower Data Strobe* ($\overline{LDS}$) signals. With 24 effective address lines, the total address space can be computed as 16,777,216 physical locations. Since the MC68000 memory space is organized as 16-bit words, however, the total number of physical locations is reduced to 8,388,608 words.

The address bus takes up the largest number of pins because Motorola does not use bus multiplexing (a feature that saves pins but requires the use of external latches for demultiplexing).

ASYNCHRONOUS BUS CONTROL

Although the address bus is not multiplexed, the MC68000 has an *Address Strobe* ($\overline{AS}$). Frequently, this signal can be negated by connection to a positive power supply via a pull-up resistor. There are, however, peripheral devices that function properly when $\overline{AS}$ is used to assert them.

The $\overline{AS}$ signal defines the time interval during which the address lines (A1 to A23) and the function code lines (FC0 to FC2) are valid. When a MC68000-based system uses dynamic memory, it is the $\overline{AS}$ signal that notifies the memory controller of the beginning of a cycle. The same signal also provides the lock-out mechanism for read–modify–write cycles during a Test-and-Set (TAS) instruction.

The MC68000 has the capability of dividing its memory range into eight-bit sections.* The $\overline{UDS}$ and the $\overline{LDS}$ delineate the time during which data are transferred over the data bus. When either (or both) of these signals is asserted, the Read/Write (R/$\overline{W}$) line also is asserted, and the address on the address bus is valid.

---

*This includes peripheral devices, since the MC68000 uses memory-mapped input/output (I/O) devices.

The $\overline{\text{UDS}}$ and $\overline{\text{LDS}}$ are used to permit byte operands as well as word and longword data. Both signals are asserted for word transfers. For byte transfers, $\overline{\text{UDS}}$ is asserted only on an even address (D8 to D15) and $\overline{\text{LDS}}$ only on an odd address (D0 to D7). Thus, to move byte data, all devices on the upper half of the data bus must be strobed with $\overline{\text{UDS}}$ and all devices on the lower half with $\overline{\text{LDS}}$.

The R/$\overline{\text{W}}$ line dictates the direction of data transfer. This single line is timed so that it can control the direction of data-bus buffers on multiprocessor systems. Since this single line accomplishes the functions of both read and write (a feature inherited from MC6800 devices), it is worth noting that data are read when the line is active–high and written when the line is active–low. Once an address is valid during a write cycle, placing the R/$\overline{\text{W}}$ line low and combining it with an active strobe enable the transfer of data to static memories.

The MC68000 must be notified of the termination of a bus cycle. There are three ways by which a bus cycle is terminated. One of them belongs to the asynchronous bus control group, and the other two will be discussed later. The normal termination signal to the MC68000 is the Data Acknowledge line ($\overline{\text{DTACK}}$), which informs the processor that the data to be processed are valid on the data bus. Since this line is one of the most significant inputs to the device, a designer must be careful about how and when $\overline{\text{DTACK}}$ is supplied. If a $\overline{\text{DTACK}}$ signal is not received, the MC68000 will remain idle indefinitely, waiting all the while for the $\overline{\text{DTACK}}$ to indicate that data are available. The $\overline{\text{DTACK}}$ and several other signals will be described at greater length in Chap. 3.

Now that all of the asynchronous bus control signals have been identified, it is appropriate to examine the timing diagram of a read cycle, as shown in Fig. 2-2, and of a write cycle, as shown in Fig. 2-3. An interesting point, shown in both diagrams, is that the R/$\overline{\text{W}}$ line, whether on initiation of a read or a write cycle, is always asserted in the read mode. This safety feature eliminates the possibility of accidental destruction of data in memory.

Let us examine the read cycle first. At the leading edge of S2, the $\overline{\text{AS}}$, $\overline{\text{LDS}}$, and $\overline{\text{UDS}}$ lines are all asserted until the trailing edge of S6, when data are latched onto the data bus, and $\overline{\text{DTACK}}$ has been asserted. In other words, in the asynchronous bus mode, the MC68000 initiates a read or write cycle by asserting the address strobe and waiting for a $\overline{\text{DTACK}}$ before assuming that data on the bus are valid. If the MC68000 does not receive a $\overline{\text{DTACK}}$ at the trailing edge of S4, the device

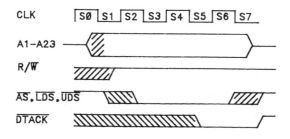

Fig. 2-2. Read cycle of MC68000.

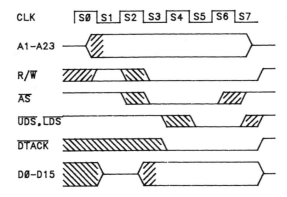

Fig. 2-3. Write cycle of MC68000.

enters S5 and S6 and performs an internal synchronization process. Then, the MC68000 introduces wait states and remains in this condition until the $\overline{\text{DTACK}}$ is received.

Delay in the arrival of $\overline{\text{DTACK}}$, mind you, may be either intentional or unintentional. It is the latter that should be of more concern to a system user. For example, an intentional $\overline{\text{DTACK}}$ delay may be generated for devices that require additional access time (because of slow memories or peripherals). In this case, a shift register or delay line is used, to allow cycles to be lengthened in one-clock-cycle increments. Thus, the asynchronous action of $\overline{\text{DTACK}}$ allows the construction of systems with variable cycles, from 500 nsec @ 8MHz all the way up to the maximum delay required.

The write cycle presents several variations in timing. The $\overline{\text{LDS}}$ and $\overline{\text{UDS}}$ assertion takes place in S4 rather than simultaneously with $\overline{\text{AS}}$. The R/$\overline{\text{W}}$ line changes to the write mode in S2, when $\overline{\text{AS}}$ is asserted.

Figure 2-4 shows a minimum configuration of an MC68000-based system with all of the asynchronous bus signals, excluding $\overline{\text{AS}}$, in place. The system is designed for byte addressing, as explained earlier.

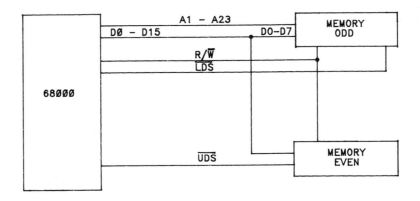

Fig. 2-4. Minimum configuration of MC68000 system.

Table 2-1. Status of Function Lines.

STATE	MODE	FC2	FC1	FC0
Reserved — Motorola	User	0	0	0
Data space	User	0	0	1
Program space	User	0	1	0
Reserved — user	User	0	1	1
Reserved — Motorola	Supervisor	1	0	0
Data space	Supervisor	1	0	1
Program space	Supervisor	1	1	0
Interrupt Acknowledge	Supervisor	1	1	1

FUNCTION CONTROL

Three lines (FC0 to FC2) indicate the state of the processor. The MC68000 can be in one of two modes—the user or the supervisor mode. Table 2-1 provides a summary of the processor state as indicated by the function code lines. In this table, FC2 indicates whether the MC68000 is in the user or supervisor mode. Assertion of all three lines indicates that the MC68000 has acknowledged an interrupt. Table 2-1 may be put into practice by the use of a 74LS138 decoder, as Fig. 2-5 shows.

The function lines are decoded to separate memory into four sections. Data memory is defined as the area that contains variables, vectors, stacks, queues, strings, tables, lists, or any other type of data found separate from the instructions, and fixed operands, which are found with the instructions that use the operands. The watchdog timer circuit, discussed in Chap. 3, signals a bus error if a DTACK is not asserted on time (about 10 microseconds). Such an error may be caused by the failure of a memory access to remain within the allocated memory space. As described later, the function control lines can also be used for further expansion of the memory capacity of the MC68000.

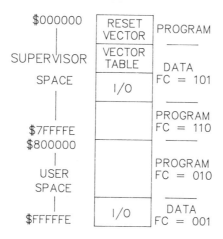

Fig. 2-5. Decoding of function lines.

14 THE 68000 MICROPROCESSOR

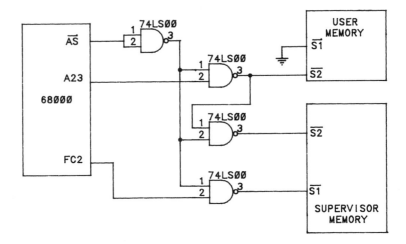

Fig. 2-6. Use of function line FC2 to distinguish between supervisor and user memory areas.

Since line FC2 indicates at all times whether the MC68000 is in user or supervisor mode, this line can be effectively used, with simple gating, to prevent accidental access of supervisor memory by a user. Figure 2-6 shows just such a scheme. When both the $\overline{AS}$ and FC2 lines are asserted, the inputs to the NAND gate are high; thus, the NAND gate asserts the S1 chip select of the supervisor memory. When an address in the user area is accessed, the NAND gate asserting the user S2 prevents the access of the supervisor S2.

SYNCHRONOUS BUS CONTROL

The three synchronous bus control signals are used to interface the MC68000 with MC6800 peripheral devices. The *Enable* signal (E) is the phase-two clock that the latter require and that defines the periods of data to and from the processor. The second signal, the *Valid Memory Address* ($\overline{VMA}$), is used in the chip-select circuitry of a MC68000 system using MC6800 peripheral devices. During reference to a peripheral, $\overline{VMA}$ meets all timing requirements for a chip-select input. The $\overline{VMA}$ signals on both the MC6800 and the MC68000 are identical in function but opposite in voltage levels; the MC6800 $\overline{VMA}$ is active–high, whereas the MC68000 $\overline{VMA}$ is active–low. The reason for this difference is that the MC68000 $\overline{VMA}$ prevents accidental addressing of peripherals when the bus is three-stated.

The third synchronous bus signal, called the *Valid Peripheral Address* ($\overline{VPA}$), is one of the signals that can be used to terminate a bus cycle. For each system application of the MC68000, bus cycles are likely to have different durations. Thus, if a constant-frequency clock is used to drive the Enable signal (E) on the peripherals, there must be a guarantee that data are transferred with respect to the clock, a requirement not often met in asynchronous-bus systems. The $\overline{VPA}$

INTRODUCTION TO THE MC68000 15

line on the MC68000, however, accomplishes this task easily. When a peripheral address is decoded, the $\overline{VPA}$ signal, rather than $\overline{DTACK}$, is asserted. This approach notifies the processor to become compatible with the MC6800 family by waiting for the proper phase of E and then asserting $\overline{VMA}$. At this point, the address lines and R/W signal are already valid. If the sequence begins too late during the E phase, all address and control signals remain stable until the next cycle, when compatible transfer can be ensured.

SYSTEM CONTROL

The third signal used to terminate a bus cycle is part of the three lines that comprise the system control group. The *Bus Error line* ($\overline{BERR}$) terminates a bus cycle in the MC68000 system whenever an abnormal condition is sensed. This line operates in conjunction with the *Halt* ($\overline{HLT}$) line, which also belongs to the system control group. When both $\overline{BERR}$ and $\overline{HLT}$ are asserted, a bus error is signaled, and the processor enters a rerun cycle.

The flowchart in Fig. 2-7 shows the steps that the MC68000 takes during a rerun cycle. Whenever the $\overline{BERR}$ and $\overline{HLT}$ lines are asserted (both active–low) during the initiation of a bus cycle, the processor completes the cycle and asserts its three-state outputs, thus preventing any information from reaching the buses. Shortly thereafter, the $\overline{BERR}$ line is negated, and, after a period of more than one clock cycle, the $\overline{HLT}$ line is also negated. At this point, the processor must determine whether a read–modify–write cycle is in progress for a Test-And-Set instruction. If so, the processor enters a bus exception-processing routine; that is, a rerun cycle routine is not executed. If a TAS instruction is not present, the MC68000 reruns the cycle during which the bus error line was asserted.

The $\overline{HLT}$ line also may be used in conjunction with the third line of the system control group—the RESET line. The MC68000 can be reset in two ways—i.e., during power-on or by a manual switch. The MC68000 also has a RESET instruction, which asserts the reset line and causes the reset of all external devices connected to the processor's reset line. During the execution of this instruction, the state of the processor, other than the program counter, is unaffected, and execution continues with the next instruction.

When the RESET and $\overline{HLT}$ lines are asserted simultaneously, either a power-on or a manual switch reset occurs. When the $\overline{HLT}$ line alone is asserted, however, a double bus fault occurs, and the processor must be reset to recover from this fatal error.

DIRECT MEMORY ACCESS CONTROL

The three lines in the direct memory access (DMA) control group are the *Bus Request* ($\overline{BR}$), which the DMA controller provides to the processor, the *Bus Grant* ($\overline{BG}$), which the processor sends to the controller, and the *Bus Grant Acknowledge* ($\overline{BGACK}$), which the controller sends to the processor.

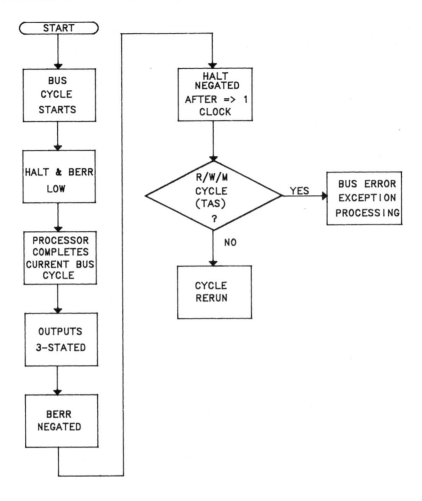

Fig. 2-7. Rerun cycle of MC68000.

INTERRUPT CONTROL

The interrupt control is the last of the control line groups. This control consists of lines IPL0 to IPL2 (Interrupt Priority Lines). Although interrupts will be described in detail in a later section, it would be of benefit to say a few words about the MC68000 interrupt system.

The MC68000 is capable of handling both vectored and autovectored interrupts. In a vectored interrupt system, the interrupting device transmits a vector number, which, multiplied by four, provides an interrupt routine address in a table of interrupts residing in memory. Some devices, including most MC6800 devices, however, cannot provide a vector number and must be autovectored. In an autovectored interrupt system, the processor examines the priority status of an interrupt to determine which vector number should be used. The interrupting device generates an interrupt request by asserting the $\overline{\text{IPL}}$ lines.

When a peripheral device is recognized as an autovector device by asserting $\overline{\text{VPA}}$ instead of $\overline{\text{DTACK}}$, the processor translates the interrupt priority into one of eight locations in the vector table, fetches the vector, and branches to the interrupt service routine. Other signals are also involved during the autovector process, but this involvement will be explained later.

REGISTERS

The number of registers in the MC68000 already has been discussed. The reader must become familiar, however, with the idiosyncracies that some registers display.

Data Registers

Any data register in the MC68000 may be used for handling byte, word, or longword operand. The length of the operand to be handled is stated in an instruction. None of the MC68000 data registers is dedicated to a specific task; that is, any data register may be used as an index register, a temporary storage area for an operand, or an accumulator.

Address Registers

The nine address registers are restricted slightly in the size of operand that the registers may contain; they can contain only a word or longword. Furthermore, although any of the address registers may be used as user "stack pointers," two registers—A7 and A7'—are dedicated as stack pointers.

At the supervisor level, the operating system program can use both the supervisor stack pointer and the user stack pointer. Consequently, the user stack location can be changed in the course of switching from task to task.

Program Counter

The program counter is 32 bits long, but only 24 bits are used for effective addressing. This counter functions as it would in any other digital computer having the same organization; that is, the program counter always is automatically incremented to point to the next instruction to be executed.

Status Register

The 16-bit status register, shown in Fig. 2-8, is divided into two sections—the supervisor section and the user section. The latter is also called the *Condition Code Register,* simply to preserve some relation with the MC6800 register bearing the same name.

18 THE 68000 MICROPROCESSOR

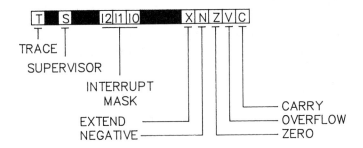

Fig. 2-8. Status register of MC68000.

The user portion of the status register is almost identical to that of the MC6800, with the added flag of Extend. This flag is asserted when a value is to be sign-extended for alignment purposes. The N flag is set when the result of an operation produces a negative value. The Z flag is set when the result of an operation produces a zero value (it is important to know when a division must use this value). The overflow flag, V, is set when an overflow results. The carry flag, C, is set when a carry occurs.

When the processor enters the Trace mode (as in a single-step operation, described later), the T flag is set. When the processor enters the supervisor mode because of a bus error or other condition, the S flag is set.

The three interrupt bits act as interrupt mask bits for the $\overline{IPL}$ lines. The interrupt flags are always set to a value lower than the one present on the $\overline{IPL}$ lines.

Chapter 3
A Small MC68000 System

INTRODUCTION

This chapter explains the design of a small 68000-based system, beginning with the design of reset/halt circuits and the basic RAM and ROM system. Since the operation of most peripheral devices requires programming, peripheral devices will be examined after some exposure to the programming of the MC68000. This chapter will show how different signals are applied and provide various ways of interfacing them.

Since expansion of this system is contemplated, various features present in larger systems, such as buffering of the buses, will also be considered.

BLOCK DIAGRAM AND MEMORY MAP

The two main steps in the design of any microprocessor system are its definition both in words and block diagram form and the design of its memory map.

The MC68000 can be interfaced to other devices very easily. Any type of memory device can be used, from bytewide RAM to dynamic RAM. Since bytewide RAM is more expensive and physically larger than dynamic RAM, however, the latter will be used here. Some read-only memory is also needed to store the operating system program. Finally, serial circuits (for terminal and modem interface), parallel circuits (for printing), and audio cassette input-output circuits are needed.

Block Diagram

Figure 3-1 depicts a small, yet fully functional, system that fits our description. One of the slower versions of the MC68000 — the MC68000L4 (4 MHz) — is used.

The RAM is the popular 4116, 16K × 1 bit dynamic device. The system is equipped with 16 of these RAMs arranged as 16 kilowords (16K × 16). The ROM, which consists of two MC68A364, 8K × 8 bit devices, is also arranged as 16 kilowords. The ROM is read on a byte or word basis. Provision must be made for the system not to waste time trying to write into ROM space if a user attempts to do so.

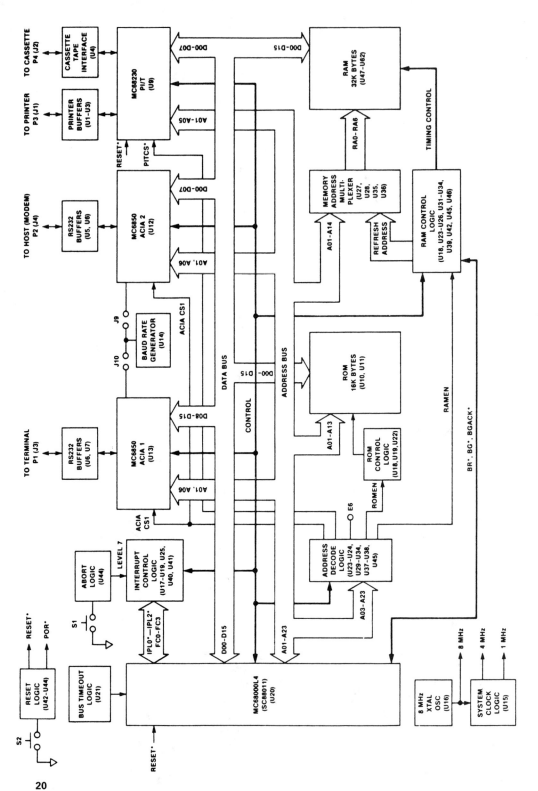

Fig. 3-1. Our MC68000-based system.

Two MC6850 (eight-bit) Asynchronous Communications Interface Adapters (ACIA) provide serial communication. One of these devices is used to interface with an external terminal and the other with a modem. A baud rate generator is included to provide variable clock rates for these devices.

A MC68230 Parallel Interface/Timer (PI/T) furnishes the parallel interface and audio cassette functions.

Memory Map

Figure 3-2 sets out the memory map of the system. Two requirements, set by Motorola, are that the table with the interrupt and trap vectors (256 in all) must be positioned at the bottom of the memory map of any MC68000 system (0000000 to 0003FF) and that the reset and stack pointer vectors must occupy the first eight locations. Since the system, whether on power-on or manual reset, must always load the same address into the program counter and system stack pointer without reloading the RAM each time, a small but clever trick is played—that is, overlapping the first eight locations of ROM and RAM. Thus, the contents that the program counter and system stack pointer require must be stored in the

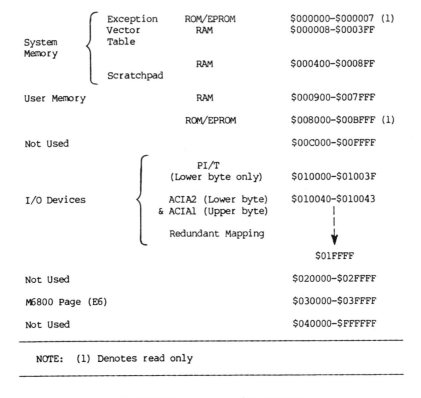

Fig. 3-2. Memory map of our system.

ROM permanently. Whether on power-on or manual reset, these eight locations can be loaded into RAM and thus become part of a vector table occupying 256 contiguous locations.

The remaining RAM area can be divided into two sections—one (from 000008 to 0008FF) to be used as a scratchpad for the operating system firmware; the other (from 000900 to 007FFF), to serve as the user memory area.

The ROM will reside in the area from 008000 to 00BFFF. The area from 00C000 to 00FFFF will be left open for future expansion or as a work area. The area from 010000 to 01FFFF will be occupied by the MC68230 and the two ACIA. Another unused area will be from 01FFFF to 02FFFF. The area from 030000 to 03FFFF will be left for the addition of any other MC6800 peripheral devices. One more unused area will be between 04000 and FFFFFF. All addresses are shown in hexadecimal notation.

BUSES

Although this system would function without address and data buffer devices, good design practice dictates that buffers be used whenever future expansion is contemplated. The schematic in Fig. 3-3 shows the buffering of the 23 address lines. Here, the 74LS373 latch is used as a buffer, but its latching input is disabled by its connection to the positive power supply via a pull-up resistor. Provision is made, however, for asserting the latching input by its connection to the $\overline{AS}$ line via a jumper wire. An 8T97 buffer is used to buffer the $\overline{AS}$ and other control lines. Some of the buffered lines are shown in Fig. 3-3.

Buffering of the data bus requires more thought. This bus is bidirectional, and the direction-enable signals of the buffers must be connected to the control signals of the MC68000.

The 74LS245 is an octal (eight-input, eight-output), noninverting, bidirectional buffer. In the schematic shown in Fig. 3-4, this device is asserted continuously by connecting the $\overline{Chip}$ $\overline{Enable}$ (Pin 19) to ground. The direction of the buffers can be controlled by the combination of gates shown.

When Pin 1 is asserted (active–low), direction is towards the MC68000. When Pin 1 is negated (high), direction is from the processor to the external devices. Thus, during a read operation, data are transferred to the MC68000 from either the low or high data byte. During a write operation, the $R/\overline{W}$ line negates the direction-enable pin of the buffer, allowing transfer of data to the data bus.

ADDRESS MULTIPLEXING

Since high-density dynamic RAMs are used, address lines A1 to A14 must be multiplexed in order to generate the row and column addresses required during read and write cycles. The multiplexers also provide refresh addresses to the RAM. The circuit in Fig. 3-5 shows the use of dual four-line to one-line 74LS153 multiplexers. The enable signals—Pins 1 and 15, respectively—are connected to ground so that the device may remain asserted at all times. Additional circuits associated with the decoding of the memory will be discussed in later sections.

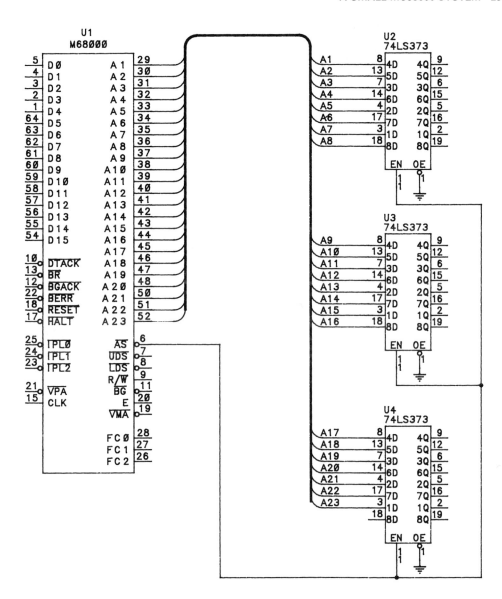

Fig. 3-3. Buffering of 23 address lines.

Two circuits that can be designed at this stage are the reset/halt circuit and the system clock circuit.

RESET/HALT AND SYSTEM CLOCK

Reset/Halt Circuit

Several specifications must be taken into account before design of a reset/halt circuit is possible. The reset circuit must be able to serve the system both during

24 THE 68000 MICROPROCESSOR

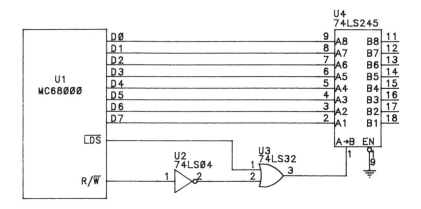

Fig. 3-4. Buffering using the 74LS245 octal noninverting bidirectional buffers.

the initial power-on and whenever a manual switch is pressed. The latter would function, for example, to release the system from a fatal error.

Motorola provides the following specifications for a reset/halt circuit: During power-on, the reset and halt signals should be asserted for slightly longer than 100 msec to allow for the stabilization of various internal circuits. When a manual switch is used, the reset and halt signals should be asserted for about ten clock cycles.

A reset-exception (a term to be discussed later) processing routine is executed after the reset signal is negated on the leading edge of a clock cycle. The flow chart in Fig. 3-6 shows the sequence of events that occurs during a reset.

During initiation of a reset, the (S)upervisor flag in the status register is set, the (T)race flag is reset, and the interrupt mask flags in the status register are set to seven. The next two steps set the system stack pointer; that is, vector

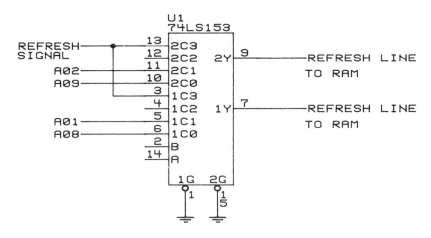

Fig. 3-5. MC68000 address multiplexing.

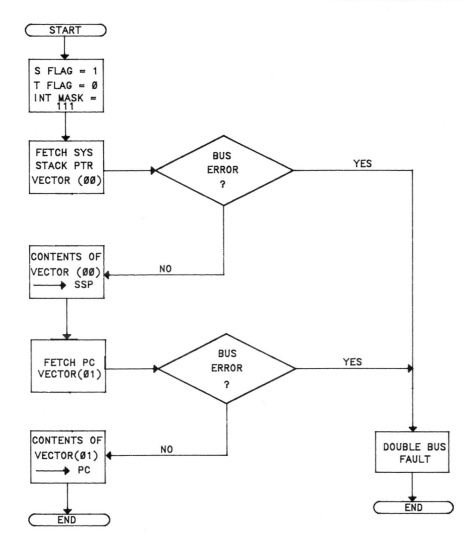

Fig. 3-6. Flowchart of the MC68000 reset activity.

number 00 is fetched from the vector table. At this point, the processor determines whether a bus error has occurred. If it hasn't, the contents of vector number 00 are transferred to the stack pointer. Vector number 01 is fetched next, and the bus-error possibility is re-examined. If two bus errors have occurred, the system enters a double bus fault condition, which normally is fatal and requires system reset. If not, the contents of vector number 01 are transferred to the program counter.

A combined reset/halt circuit is shown in Fig. 3-7. The circuit uses the MC3456 timer device, whose time-constant requirements are set by the resistor–capacitor combinations shown to satisfy the reset/halt, power-on timing specifications.

26 THE 68000 MICROPROCESSOR

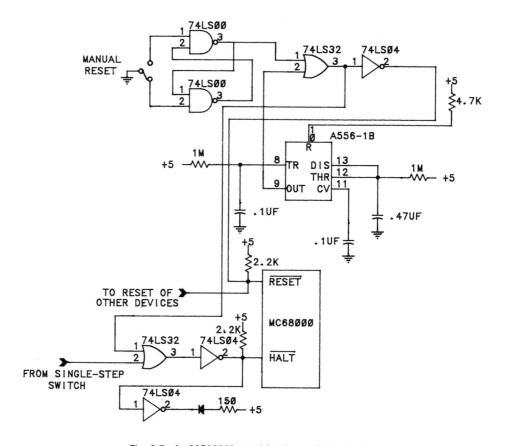

Fig. 3-7. An MC68000 combined reset/halt circuit.

The manual reset switch is debounced by a NAND flip-flop and is combined, through an OR gate, with the power-on reset signal from the timer and connected to the reset pin of the MC68000. The open-collector inverter satisfies the active-low input requirements of the MC68000 pin. The 2.2-kΩ pull-up resistor negates the reset input when the latter is not used.

The same OR-inverter arrangement is used on the halt input. A light-emitting diode is turned on when the halt signal is asserted. The halt signal may also be used as a single-instruction execution mechanism. In this case, a manual switch arrangement, similar to the reset, is connected to the signal through the OR and inverter gates.

The circuit shown in Fig. 3-8 — a slight modification of the previous one — is the circuit to be used in our small system. It produces a $\overline{POR}$ (Power On Reset) signal used in the ROM $\overline{DTACK}$ generation circuit (to be described later).

Although the small system does not include a single-step circuit, the design in Fig. 3-9 may be used for this purpose. Each time the $\overline{AS}$ line is asserted, the flip-flop is reset. If the upper switch is in the single-step position, the processor

A SMALL MC68000 SYSTEM 27

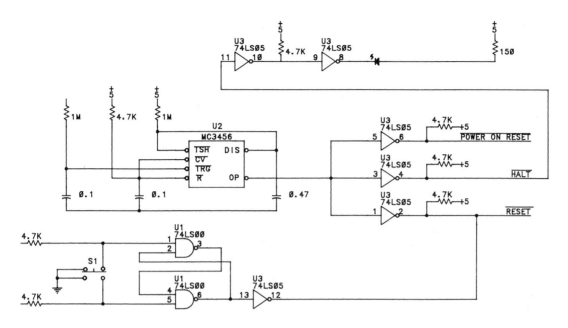

Fig. 3-8. Modified reset circuit used in our system.

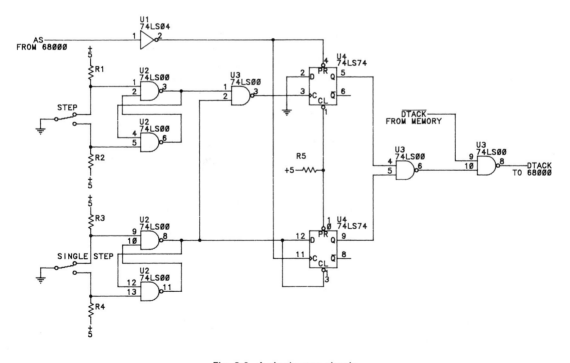

Fig. 3-9. A single-step circuit.

halts and remains halted until the lower switch is toggled. In this way, the asynchronous buses can be controlled manually.

System Clock

The small system uses a readily available, 8-MHz crystal oscillator, as shown in Fig. 3-10. A four-bit, ripple binary counter reduces this frequency to produce the 4-MHz clock frequency that the MC68000 needs and the 1-MHz frequency required by some peripheral devices. The system uses all three of the clock frequencies.

TIMING

The speed with which a microprocessor executes instructions is of major concern to a design engineer. The small system includes components that permit appropriate future expansion, but the effect of these devices on the overall speed of the system have not been discussed.

In Chap. 2, the MC68000 was shown as being an asynchronous device, and the behavior of the $\overline{DTACK}$ lines supports this description. Synchronous operation of the MC68000 should not be excluded, however, since even its asynchronous lines are timed on a synchronous system clock.

Figure 3-11 shows that all data and control lines are sensed on the leading edge and latched on the trailing edge of the system clock (shown in states, each full clock cycle being two S states). For example, the $\overline{DTACK}$ line is sensed, and asserted, one set-up time period before the trailing edge of state S4. If assertion occurs earlier than the set-up time of the trailing edge, a wait state of one full clock cycle is added to the timing. When $\overline{DTACK}$ becomes asserted on the trailing edge of the clock state, data are latched during the trailing edge of the next full clock cycle.

Thus, unless the $\overline{DTACK}$ signal is low for one set-up time, as required, the processor introduces wait states. Addition of these wait states, coupled with the presence of other devices, such as buffers or the gates used to generate the row address signal ($\overline{RAS}$) in dynamic memories, may slow down a system.

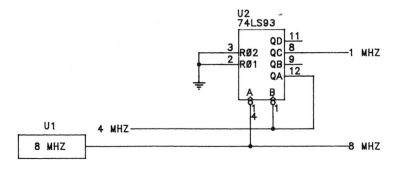

Fig. 3-10. The oscillator circuit used in our system.

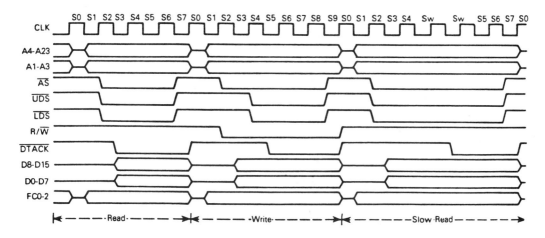

Fig. 3-11. Timing activity of the MC68000.

Table 3-1 indicates the operation, at nominal clock frequency, of an MC68000-based system using RAM of various access times and Low-power Schottky (LS) or Schottky (S) devices. For example, consider using RAM with an access time of 150 nsec and LS buffers with a propagation delay of 56 nsec. The MC68000 at 8 MHz provides a total internal delay of 70 nsec; the $\overline{AS}$ to $\overline{RAS}$ delay is 22 nsec. Thus, the total bus latency is 298 nsec (sum of the above delays), and the system can operate (with no wait states) at a nominal frequency of 8 MHz.

The significant point, which Table 3-1 stresses, is cost of a system versus performance. For example, consider the last column of the table, showing the use of 450-nsec RAM and LS buffers. The critical path of $\overline{AS}$ to $\overline{RAS}$ is constant throughout the table. Thus, if slower and consequently cheaper RAM is used, it is seen that the lower clock speed (4-MHz) MC68000 must be used to avoid wait states. If a faster clock speed is chosen, then wait states must be introduced for the speeds of the processor and the RAM to be matched.

The factor of speed must be re-evaluated from the standpoint of instruction cycle time. The MC68000 requires a nominal read time of four clock periods—of which 2.5 are allocated to bus latency—and a nominal write cycle of five clock periods—of which 3.5 are allocated to bus latency. Thus, referring once more to Table 3-1, to avoid wait states but still afford the 348 nseconds of bus latency, a designer who uses 200-nsec RAMs and LS buffers must use either a 7.18-MHz clock or faster (Schottky) buffers.

Table 3-2 shows the operation of an MC68000 with 200-nsec RAMs and LS buffers. As shown, an ideal instruction of one read and one write consumes 17 clock cycles; with a system clock of 8 MHz (125 nsec), this represents 2125 nsec. In this case, a system provides 100-percent performance. The table also shows that, in nonideal (actual) operation, the system loses 15 percent of its performance, a percentage 3 percent higher than if a designer had decided to operate the system at a reduced clock frequency. The reason is simple: the MC68000 uses full cycles

Table 3-1. Operating Frequency for Various Operating Times *(Courtesy, Motorola, Inc.).*

RAM ACCESS SPEC (NANOSECONDS)	50	100	150	50	100	150	200	200	250	200	250	300	350	400	450
Buffers 'S240 (4 × 7 ns) 'LS240, 8T26	28	28	28	28	28	28	28	28	28	56	56	56	56	56	56
AS − RAS	7	7	7	7	7	7	7	7	7	22	22	22	22	22	22
MC68000 Delay (Data Setup and AS Delay)															
12.5 MHz (10 + 50)				60											
10 MHz (10 + 50)	60	60	60	60	60	60									
8 MHz (15 + 55)						70	70	70	70						
6 MHz (25 + 65)										90	90	90			
4 MHz (30 + 75)													105	105	105
Bus Latency	145	195	245	145	195	245	298	305	355	368	418	468	533	583	633
Max. Operating Frequency (no waits)	17.2	12.8	10.2	17.2	12.8	10.2	8.3	8.19	7.04	6.7	5.98	5.34	4.69	4.2	3.94
Nominal Operating Frequency (no waits)*	12.5	12.5	10.2	10.0	10.0	8.0	8.0	7.18	7.04	6.7	5.98	5.34	4.0	4.0	3.94

*Allowable within maximum clock frequency specified for MPU

Table 3-2. Operation with LS Buffers and 200-nsec RAMs (*Courtesy*, Motorola, Inc.).

RAM ACCESS SPEC (NANOSECONDS)	50	100	150	50	100	150	150	200	200	250	200	250	300	350	400	450
Buffers 'S240 (4 × 7 ns) 'LS240, 8T26	28	28	28	28	28	28	56	28	56	28	56	56	56	56	56	56
AS – RAS	7	7	7	7	7	7	22	7	22	7	22	22	22	22	22	22
MC68000 Delay (Data Setup and AS Delay) 12.5 MHz (10 + 50) 10 MHz (10 + 50) 8 MHz (15 + 55) 6 MHz (25 + 65) 4 MHz (30 + 75)	60	60	60	60	60	60	70	70	70	70	90	90	90	105	105	105
Bus Latency	145	195	245	145	195	245	298	305	348	355	368	418	468	533	583	633
Max. Operating Frequency (no waits)	17.2	12.8	10.2	17.2	12.8	10.2	8.3	8.19	7.18	7.04	6.7	5.98	5.34	4.69	4.2	3.94
Nominal Operating Frequency (no waits)*	12.5	12.5	10.2	10.0	10.0	10.0	8.0	8.0	7.18	7.04	6.7	5.98	5.34	4.0	4.0	3.94

*Allowable within maximum clock frequency specified for MPU

32 THE 68000 MICROPROCESSOR

as wait states. Thus, a cost savings can be effected here by using 250-nsec RAMs with Schottky buffers. The overall performance remains the same.

As the last line in Table 3-2 indicates, performance may be improved further if the full cycle of wait states can be reduced by, say, 50 percent. Doing so is not impossible if flip-flops are used, as shown in Fig. 3-12. The clock-stretching circuit shown here will extend S4 (the $\overline{\text{DTACK}}$ latching cycle) by unit periods of the oscillator input to the flip-flop. This circuit, however, will not stretch S2 since data strobes are not output until S3 of a write cycle.

A useful chart by which the performance of a system can be evaluated appears in Fig. 3-13. The left-hand side of the chart denotes, in microseconds, the average execution time of a single two-bus-cycle instruction. The nominal clock frequencies are the lines sloping downward from right to left. Memory access times are the lines sloping upward from right to left. In the case of 200-nsec and 250-nsec RAM, two curves are given—one for RAM buffered with Schottky devices and the other for RAM buffered with Low-power Schottky devices. Values such as wait states and cycle time are given at the bottom of the chart; these are used in conjunction with the other sections.

Let us use some values in Table 3-2 derived from this chart. The 8-MHz clock line crosses the 0-wait-state line between the area of the 200 LS RAM and the 200 S RAM. Using Schottky buffers and excluding wait states, the bottom of the chart shows that a two-instruction sequence can be executed in 17 cycles, or 2.12 μsec (i.e., two times the 1.06-μsec point on the chart).

The use of LS buffers and 200-nsec RAM would require one wait state, and the execution time would increase to 2.5 μsec. With a circuit similar to that in Fig. 3-12, however, the execution time will drop to 2.32 μsec.

The chart also allows comparison of performance in speed at various clock frequencies, RAM access time, and LS or S buffers. For example, the execution time does not vary significantly at 6-MHz/250-nsec RAM (1.42 μsec), 6.41-MHz/300-

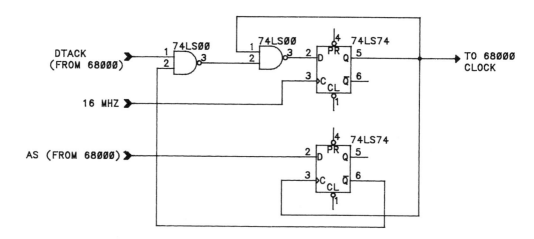

Fig. 3-12. Clock stretching circuit using flip-flops.

A SMALL MC68000 SYSTEM 33

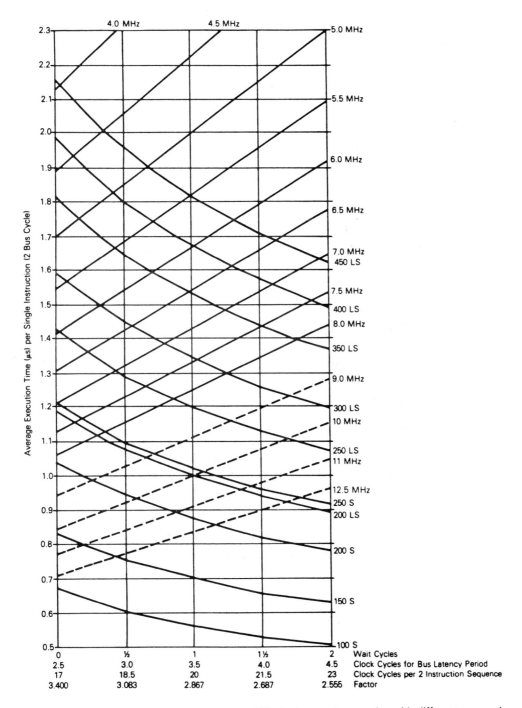

Fig. 3-13. Performance of a MC68000 using various TTL devices and memories with different access times.

nsec RAM (1.44 μsec) or 7-MHz/300-nsec RAM (1.43 μsec).

The bottom line of the chart provides values ("factors") that can be used to plot a memory system—that is, when a factor is multiplied by the total required bus latency, the product is the average execution time per simple instruction for the indicated occurrence of wait states for the particular two-instruction sequence.

BUS TIMEOUT LOGIC

It was mentioned earlier that some provision must be made to avoid wasting time if, for instance, writing into ROM memory space should be attempted. Addressing of an unused location in a memory area or failure of a circuit to respond will also waste time.

The circuit in Fig. 3-14—usually called a "watchdog timer"—consists of a 74LS175, quad D-type flip-flop, which is connected as a four-bit serial shift register. After the circuit is cleared via the $\overline{AS}$ line, four clock cycles taken from the E clock of the MC68000* are "walked" through it. A total delay, or bus timeout, of 10 μsec is produced.

DESIGN OF RAM AND ROM INTERFACE

Several circuit groups must be used for the interface of the RAM and ROM. The first circuit must be a general decoding circuit for the RAM, ROM, and some MC6800 peripheral devices (the latter are also part of a memory-mapped scheme). Since use of these peripheral devices is planned, a $\overline{VPA}$ bus termination signal must also be generated. The circuit in Fig. 3-15 demonstrates a general decoding scheme for the small system under study here.

Gates U1, U2, U3, U4, U5, U6, U7, U8, U9, U10, and U11 decode address lines A3 to A15. These gates are combined with the output of the 74LS138 decoder (U30) to generate a ROM enable signal (ROMEN) in the address area from 008000 to 00BFFF and a RAM enable signal (RAMEN) in the area from 000008 to 007FFF. The address range selected is shown at the output of the corresponding gate in Fig. 3-15.

Gate U4 performs an interesting task. As mentioned earlier, the first eight memory locations are overlapped by RAM and ROM. The output of this gate is used to assert the ROMEN and RAMEN signals in this memory area.

The 74LS138 decoder also selects the memory areas for ACIA (010040 to 010043) and the parallel interface/timer device (01000 to 0103F). Several outputs of this decoder are not connected and can be used for future expansion within the unused memory-map areas.

ROM Circuit

Two MC68A364 ROM are used, as shown in Fig. 3-16. Each has a storage capacity of 8 kilobytes times 8 bits (8 kilowords). When the ROMEN enable signal

---

*E = MPU clock/10; in this case, E = 400 kHz. Each stage provides a delay of 2.5 μsec (total of 10 μsec).

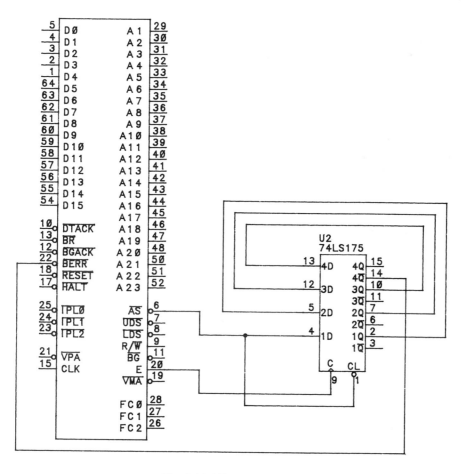

Fig. 3-14. Watchdog timer.

selects both devices simultaneously, the total ROM space is 16 kilobytes (or 8 kilowords) times 16 bits (16 kilowords).

The MC68A364 has various access-time speeds. For economy, we will select the slow (350-nsec) version.

The function of the $\overline{\text{DTACK}}$ generation circuit with respect to the ROM is illustrated by the timing diagram in Fig. 3-16. The $\overline{\text{AS}}$ and $\overline{\text{ROMEN}}$ signals are asserted on the leading edge of S2, and $\overline{\text{DTACK}}$ is sensed on the leading edge of S4. Since a slow memory has been chosen, however, the timer must assert $\overline{\text{DTACK}}$ later than S4 (in about 500 to 625 nsec). When the system senses that $\overline{\text{DTACK}}$ is not present, it introduces wait states. When $\overline{\text{DTACK}}$ is finally asserted, data are sensed (S5) and latched (S6).

RAM Circuit

The choice of a slow dynamic RAM (450-nsec) for our system means that a timer circuit must be designed for the $\overline{\text{DTACK}}$. A circuit must also refresh the DRAM,

36 THE 68000 MICROPROCESSOR

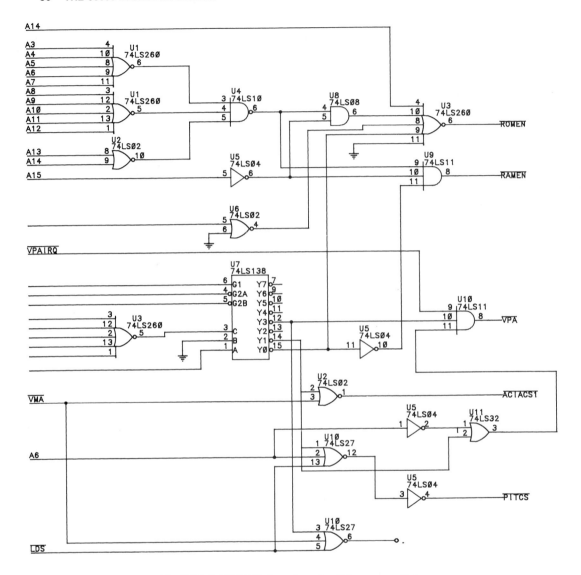

Fig. 3-15. RAM-ROM decoding circuit for our system.

usually once every 1.5 msec, and preferably while the processor is not busy with the buses. The direct-memory access signals are prime candidates for this circuit. Furthermore, a technique called *RAS refresh only* can be used. This dynamic, memory-refresh technique is appropriate with asynchronous systems since it is not possible to accomplish a memory refresh in such systems without interfering with the processor cycles. When a high-priority RAS refresh request is generated, a refresh cycle is initiated at the completion of a processor cycle in progress.

This technique is called *cycle stealing.* The memory-cycle requests from the processor are interrupted and a refresh cycle inserted in their place; thus, a normal cycle is stolen from the processor to carry out refreshing of the memory.

A SMALL MC68000 SYSTEM   37

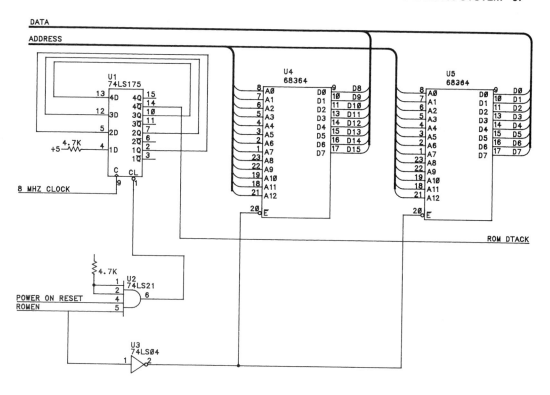

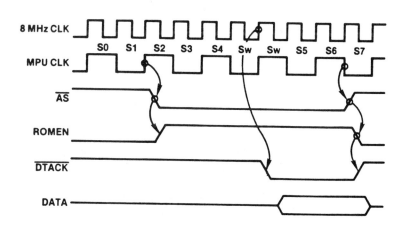

Fig. 3-16A. ROM devices used in our system and timing diagram of $\overline{\text{DTACK}}$ with respect to operation of the devices.

In large systems, arbitration circuits are used to accommodate the cycle-stealing technique. In our small system, however, a simple handshake approach of a request ($\overline{\text{BR}}$), grant ($\overline{\text{BG}}$), and acknowledge ($\overline{\text{BGACK}}$) is sufficient.

The timer circuit for our system is shown in Fig. 3-17. This circuit provides the following control signals:

38 THE 68000 MICROPROCESSOR

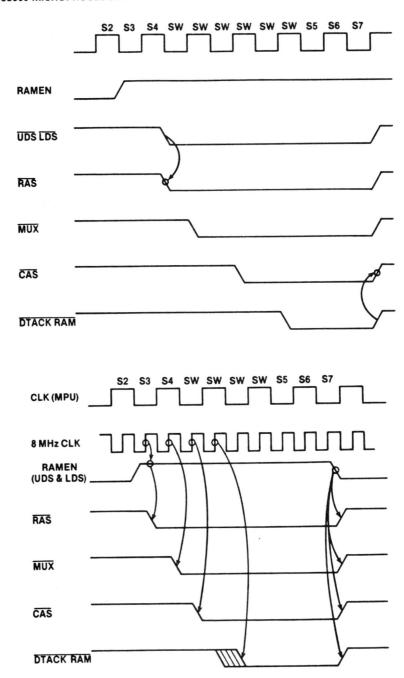

Fig. 3-16B. ROM devices used in our system and timing diagram of $\overline{\text{DTACK}}$ with respect to operation of the devices.

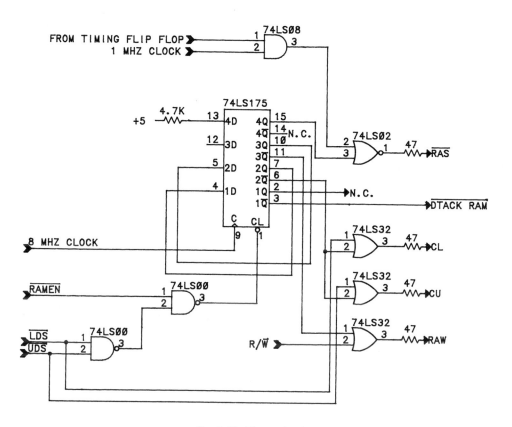

Fig. 3-17. Timer circuit.

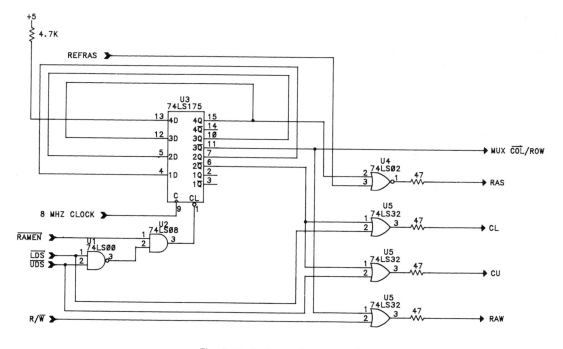

Fig. 3-18. Cycle stealing method.

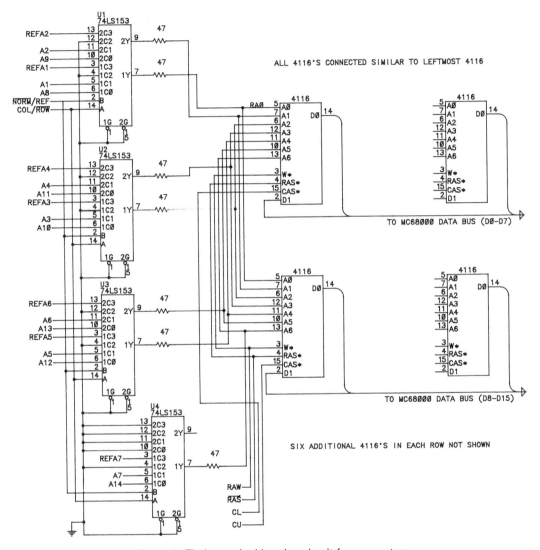

Fig. 3-19. Timing and addressing circuit for our system.

1. $\overline{\text{Column/Row}}$ multiplex signal—used to select the 74LS153 multiplexers
2. $\overline{\text{DTACK RAM}}$—used to signal $\overline{\text{DTACK}}$ to the MC68000
3. $\overline{\text{RAS}}$—used to refresh the row addresses of the DRAM
4. CU, CL (Upper Column, Lower Column)—used to select either the upper or lower columns of the DRAM
5. RAW—used as a read/write signal

A second circuit, depicted in Fig. 3-18, carries out the cycle-stealing technique. This circuit is, essentially, a timing circuit, controlled by the handshake signals mentioned earlier. It generates the signals to assert the 74LS153 multiplexers.

Combined with the circuit in Fig. 3-17, it forms the timing and addressing circuit for the DRAM. The complete memory circuit is shown in Fig. 3-19.

Completion of the memory circuit temporarily suspends discussion of the MC68000 hardware features. This discussion will be resumed when the programming features necessary for the design of input–output and interrupt circuits have been described.

Chapter 4
Addressing Modes; Instruction Set

ADDRESSING MODES

The MC68000 has six addressing categories, each of which has variations that provide a total of 15 addressing modes, as shown in Table 4-1. Closer examination of these addressing modes reveals that they can be classified in four major groups, as follows: (1) Register Direct modes, (2) Memory Address modes, (3) Special Address modes, and (4) Program Control modes.

Memory Accessing Rules

To avoid address errors, which will result in the interruption of a program, three rules must be observed:
1. Sixteen-bit (word) and 32-bit (longword) data must be accessed from an even address.

   Correct: MOVE.W. (A1)+,DO if A1 initially contains 00001000.
   Wrong: MOVE.W. (A1)+,DO if A1 initially contains 00011133.

   The latter access generates an address trap error.

2. Bytes can be accessed from either an odd or even address.
3. Opwords must be on an even address.

Boundaries for the various sizes of data are represented on page 44, where N is the address, an even number.

In the case of the longword, since the default value of the MC68000 is the 16-bit word, a 32-bit word is formed by "joining" two 16-bit words.

Effective Address and Extension Word

An *effective address* is an address that contains an operand and is part of the operation word. As shown in Fig. 4-1, this address consists of two three-bit subfields—i.e., the mode and the register.

ADDRESSING MODES; INSTRUCTION SET

Table 4-1. Addressing Modes.

REGISTER DIRECT ADDRESSING:
A. Data register direct $EA = D_n$
B. Address register direct $EA = A_n$
C. Status register direct $EA = SR$

ABSOLUTE DIRECT ADDRESSING:
A. Absolute short $EA = \text{(Next word)}$
B. Absolute long $EA = \text{(Next two words)}$

PROGRAM COUNTER RELATIVE ADDRESSING:
A. Relative with offset $EA = (PC) + d_{16}$
B. Relative with index and offset $EA = (PC) + (X_n) + d_8$

REGISTER INDIRECT ADDRESSING:
A. Register indirect $EA = A_n$
B. Postincrement register indirect $EA = A_n$
$A \leftarrow A_n + N$
C. Predecrement register indirect $A_n \leftarrow A_n - N$
$EA = (A_n)$
D. Register indirect with offset $EA = (A_n) + d_{16}$
E. Indexed register indirect with offset $EA = (A_n) + (X_n) + d_8$

IMMEDIATE ADDRESSING:
A. Immediate Data = Next word or words
B. Quick immediate Inherent data

IMPLIED ADDRESSING:
A. Implied register $EA = SR, USP, SP, PC$

KEY:
A_n, D_n: Address register and data register, respectively, with subscript to denote number of register
d_n: Displacement, with subscript to denote the number of bits
EA: Effective address
N: Value ($N = 1, 2,$ or 4)
PC: Program counter
SP: System stack pointer
SR: Status register
USP: User stack pointer
X_n: Address or data register used as index register
( ): Contents of

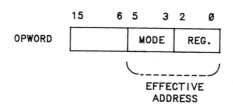

Fig. 4-1. Effective address.

44 THE 68000 MICROPROCESSOR

		7 6 5 4 3 2 1 0 7 6 5 4 3 2 1 0	
1 bit	N	Byte 0 / Byte 1	N + 1

		15 8 7 0	
1 byte	N	(7) Byte 0 (0)/ Byte 1	N + 1
		Byte 2 Byte 3	N + 3

		15 0	
1 word	N	Word 0	N + 1
	N + 2	Word 1	N + 3
	N + 4	Word 2	N + 5

		15 0	
1 longword	N	(31) Longword 0 (High-order word)	N + 1
	N + 2	Longword 0 (Low-order word) (0)	N + 3
	N + 4	Longword 1 (High-order word)	N + 5
	N + 6	Longword 1 (Low-order word)	N + 6

The mode bits define the addressing mode of the instruction, and the register bits designate the register involved (0 to 7). For absolute and immediate addressing, the mode bits remain the same (111), while the register bits contain a code that, in absolute addressing, distinguishes between long and short and, in immediate addressing, denotes that particular mode.

As Fig. 4-2 shows, to specify an operand completely, an effective address may need additional information, ranging in length from one to several words; that is, depending on the addressing mode selected, additional 16-bit extension words may follow the op code. These words provide additional addressing information and may extend the total length of an instruction by as much as ten bytes.

Table 4-2 lists the various combinations for compilation of an effective address. The $ symbol indicates a hexadecimal address; the # symbol indicates a number that is interpreted as a value rather than as an address.

15	14	13	12	11	10	9	8	7	6	5	4	3	2	1	0
Operation Word																
(First word specifies operation and modes)																
One- or two-word immediate operand, if any																
Source effective address extension, if any																
(One or two words)																
Destination effective address extension, if any																

Fig. 4-2. Instruction format of the MC68000.

Table 4-2. Effective-Address Combinations.

EA MODE	REG.	ADDRESSING MODE	NOTATION
000	Reg.#	Data Register Direct	D_n
001	Reg.#	Address Register Direct	A_n
010	Reg.#	Address Register Indirect	(A_n)
011	Reg.#	Address Register Indirect with Postincrement	$(A_n)+$
100	Reg.#	Address Register Indirect with Predecrement	$-(A_n)$
101	Reg.#	Address Register Indirect with Displacement	$d(A_n)$
110	Reg.#	Address Register Indirect with Index	$d(A_n, R_x)$
111	000	Absolute Short	\$XXXX
111	001	Absolute Long	\$XXXXXXXX
111	100	Immediate	#XXXX

The MC68000 manipulates single effective-address or double effective-address instructions. In a single effective-address instruction, as shown in Fig. 4-3, the 16-bit operation word contains the opcode, the data size, and the six-bit effective address.

In the double effective-address instruction, the operation word contains the opcode, a six-bit destination effective-address, and a six-bit source effective-address.

OPWORD	DATA SIZE	MODE	REGISTER

Fig. 4-3. Single effective-address instruction.

Register Direct Modes

General. In two of the register direct modes, an operand is held in either a data register or an address register.

Data Register Direct. This mode is used to access a data register; that is, the effective address holds the mode code and the number of the register involved in the operation.

EXAMPLE 4-1: CLR.W D0

This is a single effective-address instruction; its format is shown in Fig. 4-4. The first two nibbles designate the opcode (0100 0010). The next two bits represent the size of the data to be manipulated. In this case, the code for designation of the 16-bit operand is 01. The last six bits of the instruction format indicate the effective address.

The format in Fig. 4-4 should not be considered as representative of all single effective-address instructions of the MC68000. Contents of registers in the 6800 before and after execution of a particular instruction are as follows:

46 THE 68000 MICROPROCESSOR

```
 15        8  7 6     5       3  2    0
 Opcode    Data size  Mode    Reg. #
 0100 0010 /    01    /  000  /  000
```

Fig. 4-4. Instruction format of CLR.W D0 instruction.

Before:

```
PC=00000000 SR=2700=.S7..... US=FFFFFFFF SS=00000786
D0=00001000 D1=FFFF4D4D D2=FFFF3352 D3=00000000
D4=FFFF4E71 D5=00000000 D6=00000001 D7=000001FD
A0=000080B6 A1=0000077C A2=00003006 A3=00000554
A4=00023352 A5=00000540 A6=0000054A A7=00000786
```

After:

```
PC=00003006 SR=2704=.S7..Z.. US=FFFFFFFF SS=0000078A
D0=00000000 D1=FFFF4D4D D2=FFFF3352 D3=00000000
D4=FFFF4E71 D5=00000000 D6=00000001 D7=000001FD
A0=000080B6 A1=0000077C A2=00003006 A3=00000554
A4=00023352 A5=00000540 A6=0000054A A7=0000078A
```

Let us try a double effective-address instruction.

EXAMPLE 4-2: MOVE.W D0, D1

In this case, we wish to move 16 bits of data from data register D0 to data register D1. Since this instruction handles data, we can select one of the three data sizes— (B)yte (eight bits), (W)ord (16 bits), or (L)ongword (32 bits).

Before:

```
PC=00003002 SR=2704=.S7..Z.. US=FFFFFFFF SS=00000786
D0=00123456 D1=FFFFFFFF D2=FFFFF77D D3=FFFFFFFF
D4=F7F77FFF D5=FFFFFFFF D6=DFFF7FFF D7=FFFFFFFF
A0=FF7FFFFF A1=FFFFFFFF A2=FFFF7FFF A3=FFFFFFFF
A4=FFFFFFF7 A5=BFDFFFFF A6=FFFE7F7F A7=00000786
```

After:

```
PC=00003002 SR=2700=.S7..... US=FFFFFFFF SS=00000786
D0=00123456 D1=FFFF3456 D2=FFFFF77D D3=FFFFFFFF
D4=F7F77FFF D5=FFFFFFFF D6=DFFF7FFF D7=FFFFFFFF
A0=FF7FFFFF A1=FFFFFFFF A2=FFFF7FFF A3=FFFFFFFF
A4=FFFFFFF7 A5=BFDFFFFF A6=FFFE7F7F A7=00000786
```

The operation word for this instruction is shown in Fig. 4-5. An observant reader may notice that the instruction format in this figure differs from the arrangement

ADDRESSING MODES; INSTRUCTION SET 47

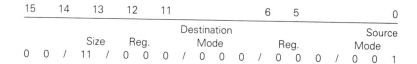

Fig. 4-5. Instruction format of MOVE W . D0, D1.

of the mnemonics in the instruction. The mnemonics show the source register (D0) first and the destination register (D1) second, while the instruction format reverses this order. Internally, the processor encodes the instruction as shown in the instruction format in Fig. 4-5. A programmer should not be concerned, however, with the encoding of the instruction and must follow the order of the mnemonics (source first; destination second).

Address Register Direct. In this type of addressing mode, the operand is located in an address register specified by the effective-address register.

EXAMPLE 4-3: MOVE.L A0,D0

Before:

```
PC=00003002 SR=2700=.S7..... US=FFFFFFFF SS=00000786
D0=00123456 D1=FFFF3456 D2=FFFFF77D D3=FFFFFFFF
D4=F7F77FFF D5=FFFFFFFF D6=DFFF7FFF D7=FFFFFFFF
A0=00002000 A1=FFFFFFFF A2=FFFF7FFF A3=FFFFFFFF
A4=FFFFFFF7 A5=BFDFFFFF A6=FFFE7F7F A7=00000786
```

After:

```
PC=00003006 SR=2700=.S7..... US=FFFFFFFF SS=0000078A
D0=00002000 D1=FFFF3456 D2=FFFFF77D D3=FFFFFFFF
D4=F7F77FFF D5=FFFFFFFF D6=DFFF7FFF D7=FFFFFFFF
A0=00002000 A1=FFFFFFFF A2=FFFF7FFF A3=FFFFFFFF
A4=FFFFFFF7 A5=BFDFFFFF A6=FFFE7F7F A7=0000078A
```

Memory Address Modes

General. Memory address modes are used to access an operand in a memory location. All modes in this category are variations of indirect addressing and can be used as reference pointers to memory, to process sequential data, to perform stacking operations, to move blocks of data, and to manipulate elements within an array.

Address Register Indirect. This mode can be used as a variable reference pointer to memory. The address of the operand is held in an address register specified in the effective address register subfield.

EXAMPLE 4-4: MOVE.W (A0), D1

Before:

```
PC=00000032 SR=2708=.S7.N... US=FFFFFFFF SS=0000078E
D0=000020FE D1=FFFF1223 D2=FFFFF77D D3=FFFFFFFF
D4=F7F77FFF D5=FFFFFFFF D6=DFFF7FFF D7=FFFFFFFF
A0=00002000 A1=FFFFFFFF A2=FFFF7FFF A3=FFFFFFFF
A4=FFFFFFF7 A5=BFDFFFFF A6=FFFE7F7F A7=0000078E
           002000    12
           002001    23
           002002    34
```

After:

```
PC=00000032 SR=2708=.S7.N... US=FFFFFFFF SS=0000078E
D0=000020FE D1=FFFF1223 D2=FFFFF77D D3=FFFFFFFF
D4=F7F77FFF D5=FFFFFFFF D6=DFFF7FFF D7=FFFFFFFF
A0=00002000 A1=00002010 A2=FFFF7FFF A3=FFFFFFFF
A4=FFFFFFF7 A5=BFDFFFFF A6=FFFE7F7F A7=0000078E
```

Address Register Indirect with Postincrement. In this mode, the address of an operand is held in an address register specified in the effective-address register subfield. After use of the address, it is incremented by one, two, or four, depending on whether the accessed operand is a byte, word, or longword. If, however, the address register is the stack pointer and the operand is a byte, the address is incremented by two in order to keep the stack pointer on a word boundary (an even address).

EXAMPLE 4-5: MOVE.W (A1)+, D0

Before:

```
PC=00000000 SR=2700=.S7..... US=FFFFFFFF SS=00000786
D0=123678AA D1=FFFFFFFF D2=FFFFFFFF D3=FFFFFFFF      002000   20
D4=FFFFFFFF D5=FFFFFFFF D6=FFFFFFFF D7=FFFFFFFF      002001   30
A0=00002000 A1=00002000 A2=FFFFFFFF A3=FFFFFFFF      002002   44
A4=FFFFFFFF A5=FFFFFFFF A6=FFFFFFFF A7=00000786      002003   AA
```

After:

```
PC=00003006 SR=2700=.S7..... US=FFFFFFFF SS=0000078A
D0=12362030 D1=FFFFFFFF D2=FFFFFFFF D3=FFFFFFFF
D4=FFFFFFFF D5=FFFFFFFF D6=FFFFFFFF D7=FFFFFFFF
A0=00002000 A1=00002002 A2=FFFFFFFF A3=FFFFFFFF
A4=FFFFFFFF A5=FFFFFFFF A6=FFFFFFFF A7=0000078A
```

This mode is useful for handling sequential data, such as tables, for moving blocks of data, and for stack unloading operations.

ADDRESSING MODES; INSTRUCTION SET

EXAMPLE 4-6: MOVE.W (A0)+,(A2)+

This instruction will move one word, starting at the address contained in A0, to the address contained in A2. After execution of the instruction, both addresses are incremented by two. Thus, this instruction can be used repeatedly to move a block of data from A0 through A0 + N, where N is an ascending multiple of two, to A1 through A1 + N. Naturally, after this instruction, a second instruction must be added, to keep count of the words to be moved.

Before:

```
PC=00000000 SR=2700=.S7..... US=FFFFFFFF SS=00000786
D0=0030FF46 D1=FFFF4D4D D2=FFFFFFFF D3=00000000
D4=FFFF4E75 D5=00000000 D6=00000001 D7=000001FF
A0=00001000 A1=FFFFFFFF A2=00002004 A3=00000554
A4=0000FFFF A5=00000540 A6=0000054A A7=00000786
```

After:

```
PC=00000404 SR=2708=.S7.N... US=FFFFFFFF SS=0000078E
D0=0030FFFE D1=FFFF4D4D D2=FFFFFFFF D3=00000000
D4=FFFF4E75 D5=00000000 D6=00000001 D7=000001FF
A0=00001002 A1=FFFFFFFF A2=00002006 A3=00000554
A4=0000FFFF A5=00000540 A6=0000054A A7=0000078E
```

Address Register Indirect with Predecrement. This mode works in a manner opposite to the address register indirect mode with postincrement; that is, this mode decrements an address before use. Therefore, this mode is suitable for stack loading operations (first-in, last-out) and also for processing of sequential data in a descending order.

EXAMPLE 4-7: MOVE.W-(A0),-(A1).

This instruction first decrements each address by two and then moves one data word from (A0)-2 to (A1)-2.

Address Register Indirect with Displacement. When this mode is used, the address of the operand is the sum of the address held in an address register and a sign-extended 16-bit displacement.

EXAMPLE 4-8: CLR.L $06(A0).

Before:

```
PC=00000404 SR=2708=.S7.N... US=FFFFFFFF SS=00000796
D0=0030FFFE D1=FFFF4D4D D2=FFFFFFFF D3=00000000
D4=FFFF4E75 D5=00000000 D6=00000001 D7=000001FF
A0=00001000 A1=FFFFFFFF A2=00002008 A3=00000554
A4=0000FFFF A5=00000540 A6=0000054A A7=00000796
```

50   THE 68000 MICROPROCESSOR

```
001000   31
001001   31
001002   31
001003   31
001004   FF
001005   FF
001006   FF
001007   FF
```

After:

```
PC=00003008  SR=2704=.S7..Z..  US=FFFFFFFF  SS=000007A2
D0=0030FFFE  D1=FFFF4D4D  D2=FFFFFFFF  D3=00000000
D4=FFFF4E75  D5=00000000  D6=00000001  D7=000001FF
A0=00001000  A1=FFFFFFFF  A2=00002008  A3=00000554
A4=0000FFFF  A5=00000540  A6=0000054A  A7=000007A2
```

```
001006   00
001007   00
001008   00
001009   00
00100A   89
00100B   CB
```

This addressing mode is suitable for accessing elements within an array or for accessing input–output locations within a memory range assigned to I/O devices. By using positive or negative displacement values, locations forward or behind a base address can be accessed. The address register indirect with displacement mode is also suitable for accessing individual variables in the stack. For example, one area in the stack may be used to store local variables, while another area stores data passed to subroutines. By use of the positive–negative displacement technique, the two stack areas may be accessed at will.

Address Register Indirect with Index and Displacement. In this mode, the address of the operand is the sum of the address held in an address register; the sign-extended, low-order, eight-bit displacement; and the contents of an index register. The latter can be either a data register or an address register.

EXAMPLE 4-9: CLR.W $2(A1, A3.W)

Before:

```
PC=00003008  SR=2704=.S7..Z..  US=FFFFFFFF  SS=000007A6
D0=0030FFFE  D1=FFFF4D4D  D2=FFFFFFFF  D3=00000000
D4=FFFF4E75  D5=00000000  D6=00000001  D7=000001FF
A0=00001000  A1=00001050  A2=00002008  A3=00001300
A4=0000FFFF  A5=00000540  A6=0000054A  A7=000007A6
```

After:

```
PC=00003008  SR=2704=.S7..Z..  US=FFFFFFFF  SS=000007AE
D0=0030FFFE  D1=FFFF4D4D  D2=FFFFFFFF  D3=00000000
```

```
D4=FFFF4E75 D5=00000000 D6=00000001 D7=000001FF           002352  00
A0=00001000 A1=00001050 A2=00002008 A3=00001300           002353  00
A4=0000FFFF A5=00000540 A6=0000054A A7=000007AE           002354  FF
                                                          002355  FF
                                                          002356  FF
                                                          002357  FF
```

The address register indirect mode with index and displacement can be used to access data within a multiple record array.

Special Address Modes

A code, rather than a register number in the effective address, designates one of the three special addressing modes.

Absolute Short. In this mode, an extension word holds the address of the operand; that is, before use, the 16-bit address is sign-extended. Thus, the absolute short mode can define a permanent address within a 64-kilobyte range.

Absolute Long. Unlike the absolute short mode, which operates within the low or high 64 kilobytes of memory, the absolute long mode can be used within the entire 16-megabyte memory area. This mode requires two words of extension. These two 16-bit words are "joined" (first word: Address High; second word: Address Low) to form the address of the operand.

Immediate Mode. In the immediate mode, any value following the opcode is the operand.

EXAMPLE 4-10: MOVE.L #$1000,D0

Before:

```
PC=000093C6 SR=2709=.S7.N..C US=FFFFFFFF SS=00000782
D0=00323332 D1=FFFF4D4D D2=FFFF3352 D3=00000000
D4=FFFF4E71 D5=00000000 D6=00000001 D7=000001FD
A0=000080B6 A1=00008354 A2=00000414 A3=00000554
A4=00023352 A5=00000540 A6=0000054A A7=00000782
```

After:

```
PC=00000000 SR=2700=.S7..... US=FFFFFFFF SS=00000786
D0=00001000 D1=FFFF4D4D D2=FFFF3352 D3=00000000
D4=FFFF4E71 D5=00000000 D6=00000001 D7=000001FD
A0=000080B6 A1=0000077C A2=00003006 A3=00000554
A4=00023352 A5=00000540 A6=0000054A A7=00000786
```

A variation of the immediate mode is the *Quick Immediate mode.* In this mode, the data are contained in an eight-bit field within the operation word. This eight-bit value is sign-extended, and the entire 32-bit value is transferred to the data register involved.

The Quick Immediate mode, although described here, could be categorized as an independent mode. It is found, for example, with arithmetic instructions. Its advantage? When operand values are between 1 and 8, use of this mode saves execution time.

Program Control Modes

General. The modes in this category load a new address to the program counter and transfer execution of the program starting at the new address.

Program Counter with Displacement. One word extension is used in the program counter mode with displacement. The address of an operand is the sum of the contents of the program counter and a sign-extended, 16-bit displacement in the extension word. The content of the program counter is the address in the extension word.

Program Counter with Index. This mode requires one word of extension. The address of an operand is the sum of the program counter contents, an eight-bit displacement (low-order byte of the extension word), and the contents of the index register.

One advantage of the program counter mode is that it can be used in the manipulation of position-independent programs. Since the program counter always contains the location of the next instruction, the current instruction may refer to data or program locations for branches relative to the instruction itself.

A restriction has been placed on this mode, and for a good reason: It cannot be used to specify a destination operand. This restriction prevents a program that contains errors from destroying itself inadvertently. The restriction also prevents programmers from using the dangerous practice of writing self-modifying code.

Inherent Mode

The inherent mode is not classed with the other modes because the former contains very few instructions. Inherent instructions usually do not show an operand. The operation word itself normally indicates the location of the operand.

Summary

To recapitulate:

1. In direct or absolute addressing, the operand is specified by a 16-bit or 32-bit address that is part of the instruction.

2. The register-deferred addressing mode has several variations. In the address register indirect mode, the contents of the register are the effective address. In the

address register indirect with predecrement, the effective address first is decremented and then used. In the address register indirect with postincrement, the effective address is used and then incremented. In the address register indirect with displacement, the effective address is the sum of the contents of an address register and a 16-bit displacement. In the address register indirect with displacement and index, the effective address is the sum of the contents of an address register, an eight-bit displacement, and the contents of an index register; the latter may be another address register or a data register.

3. The program counter modes transfer control to another location in the program. The modes basically are branching modes. In the program counter relative, the effective address is the sum of a 16-bit displacement and the contents of the program counter. In the program counter with index, the effective address is the sum of an eight-bit displacement, the contents of the program counter, and the contents of an index register.

INSTRUCTIONS

The instructions of the MC68000 are divided into four main categories: (1) data transfer instructions, (2) data processing instructions, (3) program control instructions, and (4) system control instructions.

The first group—data transfer instructions—includes the MOVE instructions, the SWAP instruction, and the EXCHANGE instruction. These instructions can transfer data between the two halves of a register, between two registers, between a register and a memory location, and between two memory locations. A MOVE instruction can also read and modify the contents of a status register.

The second group—data processing instructions—includes instructions for 8-bit, 16-bit, and 32-bit addition and subtraction, 16-bit multiplication and division, and Binary-Coded Decimal operations. The same group includes logic and shifting instructions—such as AND, OR, Exclusive-OR—and shifting by one or more bits (one single shift or rotate instruction can move register data by as many as 32 bits positions left or right).

The MC68000 is able to manipulate single bits too; the processor can select, test, set, or clear individual bits. This feature is very important in input–output operations.

The program control group includes both unconditional and conditional branch instructions. There are 14 conditional branch instructions, and all of them test the various flags of the condition code register. There are four unconditional branch instructions (JMP, JSR, BRA, BSR). Naturally, the return from a branch instruction could be counted as well, but is not included here.

Finally, the various instructions in the system control group include those that can alter the contents of the status register, the RESET instruction, and the exception processing instructions.

A more detailed description of many instructions, with programming examples, is provided in Chap. 5.

Chapter 5
Instruction Set—A More Intensive Evaluation

The instruction set that the MC68000 uses truly makes this device a programmer's dream. The MC68000 is a processor for the implementation of high-level languages. The "orthogonality" of the processor provides significant assistance to compiler designers.

Orthogonality is a measure of the number and power of features implemented (the fewer and more powerful, the better) and the regularity with which groups of these features combine (the fewer special restrictions, the better). For example, the addressing modes of the MC68000 are orthogonal with respect to the address registers; there is no restriction on which address register is to be used with a given addressing mode. Consequently, all address registers are easily accessible to a compiler.

Similarly, the orthogonality of instructions crossed with the addressing modes also makes selection of an addressing mode by compilers more effective.

Finally, the orthogonality of data register usage crossed with instructions reduces restrictions on the specification of a particular data register.

DATA MANIPULATION INSTRUCTIONS

Arithmetic Operations

The most common type of arithmetic involves integers, and the instruction sets of every computer can accommodate such operations as add and subtract. Some confusion exists in the interpretation of the terms **integer** and **fixed point,** and the two are often used interchangeably. To do so, however, is not always valid. An integer is a whole number with no fractional parts—e.g., 1, 2, 3. A fixed-point number is one whose radix point is not variable.* Numbers such as 4.35 and 55.32 are fixed-point numbers, with the decimal point fixed at two. An integer is a fixed-point number with the radix point fixed at zero. Thus, integers can be

---

*The radix point is the notation that separates the whole portion of a real number from its fractional part. In general, reference to a radix point is made by the number base represented. Thus, we have the decimal point for base 10, the binary point for base 2, and the hexadecimal point for base 16.

considered as a subset of fixed-point numbers; that is, all integers are fixed-point numbers, but not all fixed-point numbers are integers.

Integer arithmetic instructions that the MC68000 uses include ADD.X, SUB.X, CMP.X, TST.X, AND CLR.X. Other arithmetic instructions will be mentioned later. In the instructions listed, the X designates the size of the operand (byte, word, or longword). There are variations of some of these instructions that are used for addressing purposes. For example, the ADD instruction may be used to change the low eight bits of an operand, whereas the ADDA (Add Address) instruction may be used to add values held in address registers.

The arithmetic and logic instructions of the MC68000 are very similar in the ways in which they function and in which the condition codes are affected as a result of the execution of an instruction and the selection of available addressing modes, registers, and operands. This feature is advantageous since only one uniform set of rules must be remembered during program design.

At this point, an important feature must be mentioned. An experienced programmer always attempts to determine (or already knows) whether an instruction will affect any of the status register flags. Flags are important in arithmetic, comparing, and other operations. For example, if the instruction ADDA.B A1, A2 is used, a 68000 assembler will signal an error, because the ADDA instruction does not affect any flags and can, therefore, be used only with word- or longword-size operands.

The ADDQ (Add Quick) instruction is a "quick immediate mode" instruction that adds a value between 1 and 8 to any alterable address. What is the need for such an instruction, however, since the MC68000 provides an ADDI (Add Immediate) instruction? The answer is faster execution. The ADDQ instruction is briefer.

EXAMPLE 5-1: ADD.W (A2)+,D0

Before:

```
PC=00003006 SR=2700=.S7..... US=FFFFFFFF SS=00000792
D0=00000001 D1=FFFF4D4D D2=FFFF3352 D3=00000000
D4=FFFF4E71 D5=00000000 D6=00000001 D7=000001FD
A0=00002000 A1=0000077C A2=00003008 A3=00000554
A4=00023352 A5=00000540 A6=0000054A A7=00000792
                  003008   4E
                  003009   71
                  00300A   4E
                  00300B   71
```

After:

```
PC=00003006 SR=2700=.S7..... US=FFFFFFFF SS=00000796
D0=00004E72 D1=FFFF4D4D D2=FFFF3352 D3=00000000
D4=FFFF4E71 D5=00000000 D6=00000001 D7=000001FD
A0=00002000 A1=0000077C A2=0000300A A3=00000554
A4=00023352 A5=00000540 A6=0000054A A7=00000796
```

EXAMPLE 5-2: ADDQ.L #2, A5

Before:

PC=00003006 SR=2700=.S..... US=FFFFFFFF SS=00000796
D0=00004E72 D1=FFFF4D4D D2=FFFF3352 D3=00000000
D4=FFFF4E71 D5=00000000 D6=00000001 D7=000001FD
A0=00002000 A1=0000077C A2=0000300A A3=00000554
A4=00023352 A5=00000540 A6=0000054A A7=00000796

After:

PC=00003006 SR=2700=.S..... US=FFFFFFFF SS=00000796
D0=00004E72 D1=FFFF4D4D D2=FFFF3352 D3=00000000
D4=FFFF4E71 D5=00000000 D6=00000001 D7=000001FD
A0=00002000 A1=0000077C A2=0000300A A3=00000554
A4=00023352 A5=00000542 A6=0000054A A7=0000079A

The ADDX (Add Extended) instruction uses the X flag in the status register in the addition operation; that is, the source operand, the destination operand, and the X flag are added together, and the sum is placed in the destination location. An interesting fact about the X flag is that it may be set or unset by an arithmetic operation that immediately precedes the ADDX instruction, and multiprecision operations may thus be performed. Although the X flag is an exact copy of the C flag, unlike the latter, the former is not affected by instructions such as some of the MOVE.

In execution of an ADDX instruction, the operands may be addressed in two ways:

1. Both operands may be located in data registers specified in the instruction.
2. Both operands may be located in memory and accessed by the predecrement mode, using address registers specified in the instruction.

Examine the flags that this instruction affects (consult the MC68000 Instruction Set in the Appendix), and it will be seen that all of them, except the Z flag, are set as they would be during an ADD instruction. The (Z)ero flag is cleared if the result is nonzero but remains unchanged rather than set, as would be the case if the result were zero. This feature can be used in multiprecision operations. The Z flag can be set before the several ADDX instructions that compose a multiprecision, arithmetic operation are executed. The Z flag will be cleared for any nonzero, intermediate values produced and at the completion of the multiprecision operation. If, however, Z is still set at the end of the operation, then all of the intermediate values produced were zero, and the final result is thus also zero.

EXAMPLE 5-3: ADDX.L D0,D1

Before:

PC=00003006 SR=2700=.S7..... US=FFFFFFFF SS=0000079A
D0=00000021 D1=00000010 D2=FFFF3352 D3=00000000

```
D4=FFFF4E71 D5=00000000 D6=00000001 D7=000001FD
A0=00002000 A1=0000077C A2=0000300A A3=00000554
A4=00023352 A5=00000542 A6=0000054A A7=0000079A
```

After:

```
PC=00003006 SR=2700=.S7..... US=FFFFFFFF SS=0000079E
D0=00000021 D1=00000031 D2=FFFF3352 D3=00000000
D4=FFFF4E71 D5=00000000 D6=00000001 D7=000001FD
A0=00002000 A1=0000077C A2=0000300A A3=00000554
A4=00023352 A5=00000542 A6=0000054A A7=0000079E
```

The subtraction category of arithmetic operations has the SUB, SUBI, SUBQ, SUBX, and SUBA instructions; all are the exact counterparts of the ADD group.

The MC68000 provides multiplication and division instructions but only for 16-bit operands. There are two multiplication instructions (MULU, or multiply unsigned; and MULS, or multiply signed) and two division instructions (DIVU; DIVS). A 32-bit destination is used to store results. For division instructions, however, the destination stores both the remainder (high-order 16 bits) and the quotient (low-order 16-bits).

EXAMPLE 5-4: MULU #$03, D2

Before:

```
PC=00000000 SR=2704=.S7..Z.. US=FFFFFFFF SS=00000786
D0=0000FF0D D1=00000000 D2=00000002 D3=00000000
D4=FFFFFFFF D5=FFFFFFFF D6=DFFFFFFF D7=FFFFFFFF
A0=00010040 A1=000000C0 A2=FFFFFFFF A3=FFFFFFFF
A4=FFFFFFFF A5=00000541 A6=0000054F A7=00000786
```

After:

```
PC=00003008 SR=2700=.S7..... US=FFFFFFFF SS=0000078A
D0=0000FF0D D1=00000000 D2=00000006 D3=00000000
D4=FFFFFFFF D5=FFFFFFFF D6=DFFFFFFF D7=FFFFFFFF
A0=00010040 A1=000000C0 A2=FFFFFFFF A3=FFFFFFFF
A4=FFFFFFFF A5=00000541 A6=0000054F A7=0000078A
```

EXAMPLE 5-5: MULS D3,D4

Before:

```
PC=00003008 SR=2700=.S7..... US=FFFFFFFF SS=0000078A
D0=0000FF0D D1=00000000 D2=00000006 D3=00000004
D4=00000010 D5=FFFFFFFF D6=DFFFFFFF D7=FFFFFFFF
A0=00010040 A1=000000C0 A2=FFFFFFFF A3=FFFFFFFF
A4=FFFFFFFF A5=00000541 A6=0000054F A7=0000078A
```

After:

```
PC=00000032 SR=2708=.S7.N... US=FFFFFFFF SS=0000078E
D0=0000FFFF D1=00000000 D2=00000006 D3=00000004
```

```
D4=00000040 D5=FFFFFFFF D6=DFFFFFFF D7=FFFFFFFF
A0=00010040 A1=000000C0 A2=FFFFFFFF A3=FFFFFFFF
A4=FFFFFFFF A5=00000541 A6=0000054F A7=0000078E
```

EXAMPLE 5-6: DIVU D1,D2

Before:

```
PC=00000032 SR=2708=.S7.N... US=FFFFFFFF SS=0000078E
D0=0000FFFF D1=00000006 D2=00000060 D3=00000004
D4=00000040 D5=FFFFFFFF D6=DFFFFFFF D7=FFFFFFFF
A0=00010040 A1=000000C0 A2=FFFFFFFF A3=FFFFFFFF
A4=FFFFFFFF A5=00000541 A6=0000054F A7=0000078E
```

After:

```
PC=00000030 SR=2708=.S7.N... US=FFFFFFFF SS=00000796
D0=0000FFFF D1=00000006 D2=00000010 D3=00000004
D4=00000040 D5=FFFFFFFF D6=DFFFFFFF D7=FFFFFFFF
A0=00010040 A1=000000C0 A2=FFFFFFFF A3=FFFFFFFF
A4=FFFFFFFF A5=00000541 A6=0000054F A7=00000796
```

The CMP (Compare) instruction is included in the arithmetic group because, in effect, a subtraction occurs during execution of the instruction. The source operand is subtracted from the destination and, although the result of this subtraction is discarded, the status register flags are affected. Thus, the CMP instruction is useful for purposes of testing and branching.

The compare group also has a CMPI (Compare Immediate) instruction and a CMPA (Compare Address) instruction. The former subtracts the value after the opcode from the contents of an address, and the condition code flags are altered according to the result. The latter instruction subtracts the contents of an address from a destination address register; the flags are altered according to the result.

A handy instruction is the CMPM (Compare Memory), which is always used in the postincrement mode and thus allows comparison of multiple memory locations.

The TST (Test an Operand) instruction is also included in the arithmetic group because a subtraction occurs. A zero is subtracted from the contents of a destination, and, although the result is discarded, the condition code flags are altered.

The NEG (Negate) instruction changes an operand to a negative value; that is, the destination is subtracted from zero. The operation affects the C, Z, N, V, and X flags.

EXAMPLE 5-7: NEG.L (A0)

Before:

```
PC=00003006 SR=2719=.S7XN..C US=FFFFFFFF SS=000007A2    002000    EF
D0=0000FFFF D1=00000FFF D2=00000010 D3=00000004         002001    EF
```

INSTRUCTION SET—A MORE INTENSIVE EVALUATION

```
D4=00000040 D5=FFFFFFFF D6=DFFFFFFF D7=FFFFFFFF    002002  00
A0=00002000 A1=000000C0 A2=FFFFFFFF A3=FFFFFFFF    002003  01
A4=FFFFFFFF A5=00000541 A6=0000054F A7=000007A2    002004  FF
                                                   002005  FF
                                                   002006  FD
```

After:

```
PC=00003006 SR=2711=.S7X...C US=FFFFFFFF SS=000007A6  002000  10
D0=0000FFFF D1=00000FFF D2=00000010 D3=00000004       002001  10
D4=00000040 D5=FFFFFFFF D6=DFFFFFFF D7=FFFFFFFF       002002  FF
A0=00002000 A1=000000C0 A2=FFFFFFFF A3=FFFFFFFF       002003  FF
A4=FFFFFFFF A5=00000541 A6=0000054F A7=000007A6       002004  FF
                                                      002005  FF
```

The NEGX negates a value and then subtracts the X bit from the negated value.

All of these arithmetic instructions are used with operands in two's complement form. The MC68000 provides instructions, however, for manipulation of decimal operands. These instructions are: ABCD (Add Binary Coded Decimal), NBCD (Negate Binary Coded Decimal), and SBCD (Subtract Binary Coded Decimal). The legal operand for any of these instructions is a byte, representing two BCD values.

The ABCD and SBCD instructions manipulate operands as follows:

1. Between two data registers specified in the instruction.
2. Between two memory locations using two address registers and the pre-decrement mode.

EXAMPLE 5-8: ABCD -(A1), -(A2)

Before:

```
PC=00003006 SR=2700=.S7..... US=FFFFFFFF SS=000007BA  001FFF  03
D0=0000FFFF D1=00000FFF D2=00000010 D3=00000004       002000  00
D4=00000040 D5=FFFFFFFF D6=DFFFFFFF D7=FFFFFFFF       002001  00
A0=00002000 A1=00002000 A2=00002100 A3=FFFFFFFF       002002  00
A4=FFFFFFFF A5=00000541 A6=0000054F A7=000007BA       0020FF  04
                                                      002100  10
                                                      002101  00
                                                      002102  00
```

After:

```
PC=00003006 SR=2700=.S7..... US=FFFFFFFF SS=000007BE  0020FF  07
D0=0000FFFF D1=00000FFF D2=00000010 D3=00000004       002100  10
D4=00000040 D5=FFFFFFFF D6=DFFFFFFF D7=FFFFFFFF       002101  00
A0=00002000 A1=00001FFF A2=000020FF A3=FFFFFFFF       002102  00
A4=FFFFFFFF A5=00000541 A6=0000054F A7=000007BE
```

Logical and Shifting Instructions

Logical Instructions. These instructions include the NOT, OR, AND, and EOR. All addressing modes previously discussed may be used with these instructions.

The simplest instruction is NOT, which is used to complement an operand.

EXAMPLE 5-9: NOT.W D1

Before:

```
PC=00003006 SR=2700=.S7..... US=FFFFFFFF SS=000007BE
D0=0000FFFF D1=00000FFF D2=00000010 D3=00000004
D4=00000040 D5=FFFFFFFF D6=DFFFFFFF D7=FFFFFFFF
A0=00002000 A1=00001FFF A2=000020FF A3=FFFFFFFF
A4=FFFFFFFF A5=00000541 A6=0000054F A7=000007BE
```

After:

```
PC=00003006 SR=2708=.S7.N... US=FFFFFFFF SS=000007C2
D0=0000FFFF D1=0000F000 D2=00000010 D3=00000004
D4=00000040 D5=FFFFFFFF D6=DFFFFFFF D7=FFFFFFFF
A0=00002000 A1=00001FFF A2=000020FF A3=FFFFFFFF
A4=FFFFFFFF A5=00000541 A6=0000054F A7=000007C2
```

Since addresses should not be complemented (although, sometimes this feature is convenient), a NOT instruction works only with data registers.

The OR instruction requires two operands since it performs the ORing of two bits—e.g., 11001 ORed with 11100 yields 11101.

EXAMPLE 5-10: OR.W D1,D2

Before:

```
PC=00003006 SR=2708=.S7.N... US=FFFFFFFF SS=000007C2
D0=0000FFFF D1=0000F000 D2=00000111 D3=00000004
D4=00000040 D5=FFFFFFFF D6=DFFFFFFF D7=FFFFFFFF
A0=00002000 A1=00001FFF A2=000020FF A3=FFFFFFFF
A4=FFFFFFFF A5=00000541 A6=0000054F A7=000007C2
```

After:

```
PC=00003006 SR=2708=.S7.N... US=FFFFFFFF SS=000007C6
D0=0000FFFF D1=0000F000 D2=0000F111 D3=00000004
D4=00000040 D5=FFFFFFFF D6=DFFFFFFF D7=FFFFFFFF
A0=00002000 A1=00001FFF A2=000020FF A3=FFFFFFFF
A4=FFFFFFFF A5=00000541 A6=0000054F A7=000007C6
```

EXAMPLE 5-11: OR.L #$00FF, D1

Before:

```
PC=00003006 SR=2708=.S7.N... US=FFFFFFFF SS=000007C6
D0=0000FFFF D1=0000F000 D2=0000F111 D3=00000004
```

INSTRUCTION SET – A MORE INTENSIVE EVALUATION

```
D4=00000040 D5=FFFFFFFF D6=DFFFFFFF D7=FFFFFFFF
A0=00002000 A1=00001FFF A2=000020FF A3=FFFFFFFF
A4=FFFFFFFF A5=00000541 A6=0000054F A7=000007C6
```

After:

```
PC=00003008 SR=2700=.S7..... US=FFFFFFFF SS=000007CA
D0=0000FFFF D1=0000F0FF D2=0000F111 D3=00000004
D4=00000040 D5=FFFFFFFF D6=DFFFFFFF D7=FFFFFFFF
A0=00002000 A1=00001FFF A2=000020FF A3=FFFFFFFF
A4=FFFFFFFF A5=00000541 A6=0000054F A7=000007CA
```

The AND instruction is used to mask a value—i.e., to drop any unwanted bits in an operand without affecting the remaining bits.

EXAMPLE 5-12: AND.L #FFFF,D0

Before:

```
PC=00003008 SR=2700=.S7..... US=FFFFFFFF SS=000007CA
D0=0000FFFF D1=0000F0FF D2=0000F111 D3=00000004
D4=00000040 D5=FFFFFFFF D6=DFFFFFFF D7=FFFFFFFF
A0=00002000 A1=00001FFF A2=000020FF A3=FFFFFFFF
A4=FFFFFFFF A5=00000541 A6=0000054F A7=000007CA
```

After:

```
PC=00003008 SR=2700=.S7..... US=FFFFFFFF SS=000007CE
D0=0000FFFF D1=0000F0FF D2=0000F111 D3=00000004
D4=00000040 D5=FFFFFFFF D6=DFFFFFFF D7=FFFFFFFF
A0=00002000 A1=00001FFF A2=000020FF A3=FFFFFFFF
A4=FFFFFFFF A5=00000541 A6=0000054F A7=000007CE
```

The EOR (Exclusive-OR) instruction provides a result of one when two bits of different value are EORed; when bits are of similar value, the EOR result is zero. This instruction is sometimes used to clear a register.

EXAMPLE 5-13: EOR.L D0,D0

Before:

```
PC=00003008 SR=2700=.S7..... US=FFFFFFFF SS=000007CE
D0=0000FFFF D1=0000F0FF D2=0000F111 D3=00000004
D4=00000040 D5=FFFFFFFF D6=DFFFFFFF D7=FFFFFFFF
A0=00002000 A1=00001FFF A2=000020FF A3=FFFFFFFF
A4=FFFFFFFF A5=00000541 A6=0000054F A7=000007CE
```

After:

```
PC=00003004 SR=2704=.S7..Z.. US=FFFFFFFF SS=000007D2
D0=00000000 D1=0000F0FF D2=0000F111 D3=00000004
D4=00000040 D5=FFFFFFFF D6=DFFFFFFF D7=FFFFFFFF
```

A0=00002000 A1=00001FFF A2=000020FF A3=FFFFFFFF
A4=FFFFFFFF A5=00000541 A6=0000054F A7=000007D2

An important point to take account of in the EOR instruction is that the source register must be a data register, whereas a data register in the AND and OR instructions can be either the source or destination.

The immediate mode of the AND, OR, and EOR instructions provides a useful function. In any of these three instructions in this mode, the destination may be the status register. Thus, any or all of the bits in the status register may be altered by using these logical instructions in the immediate mode.

EXAMPLE 5-14: AND.L #$0,SR

Before:

PC=00003004 SR=2704=.S7..Z.. US=FFFFFFFF SS=000007D2
D0=00000000 D1=0000F0FF D2=0000F111 D3=00000004
D4=00000040 D5=FFFFFFFF D6=DFFFFFFF D7=FFFFFFFF
A0=00002000 A1=00001FFF A2=000020FF A3=FFFFFFFF
A4=FFFFFFFF A5=00000541 A6=0000054F A7=000007D2

After:

PC=00003004 SR=2704=.S7..Z.. US=FFFFFFFF SS=000007D6
D0=00000000 D1=0000F0FF D2=0000F111 D3=00000004
D4=00000040 D5=FFFFFFFF D6=DFFFFFFF D7=FFFFFFFF
A0=00002000 A1=00001FFF A2=000020FF A3=FFFFFFFF
A4=FFFFFFFF A5=00000541 A6=0000054F A7=000007D6

The AND instruction cleared the status register.

EXAMPLE 5-15: OR.B #$01,SR

Before:

PC=00003004 SR=2704=.S7..Z.. US=FFFFFFFF SS=000007D6
D0=00000000 D1=0000F0FF D2=0000F111 D3=00000004
D4=00000040 D5=FFFFFFFF D6=DFFFFFFF D7=FFFFFFFF
A0=00002000 A1=00001FFF A2=000020FF A3=FFFFFFFF
A4=FFFFFFFF A5=00000541 A6=0000054F A7=000007D6

After:

PC=00003006 SR=2705=.S7..Z.C US=FFFFFFFF SS=000007DA
D0=00000000 D1=0000F0FF D2=0000F111 D3=00000004
D4=00000040 D5=FFFFFFFF D6=DFFFFFFF D7=FFFFFFFF
A0=00002000 A1=00001FFF A2=000020FF A3=FFFFFFFF
A4=FFFFFFFF A5=00000541 A6=0000054F A7=000007DA

In this case, the OR instruction sets the carry flag.

INSTRUCTION SET—A MORE INTENSIVE EVALUATION   63

Shifting Instructions. The four shifting and rotating instructions move bit patterns within a register or a memory location. These instructions are: Arithmetic Shift (Left or Right), Logical Shift (Left or Right), Rotate (Left or Right), and Rotate with Extend (Left or Right).

Figure 5-1 shows the format of the Logical Shift Left instruction. The instruction, LSL.W D0,D1, shifts the contents of D1 left by as many bits as are designated in a value held in D0. Bits shifted out of the high-order bit are copied into both the carry and extend flags; zeros are shifted into the low-order bit.

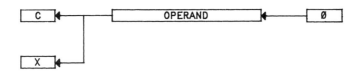

Fig. 5-1. Format of logical shift left instruction.

EXAMPLE 5-16: LSL.W D0, D1

(Observe the contents of both registers before and after execution of this instruction.)

Before:

```
PC=00003004 SR=2708=.S7.N... US=FFFFFFFF SS=000007DE
D0=00000002 D1=0000F0FF D2=0000F111 D3=00000004
D4=00000040 D5=FFFFFFFF D6=DFFFFFFF D7=FFFFFFFF
A0=00002000 A1=00001FFF A2=000020FF A3=FFFFFFFF
A4=FFFFFFFF A5=00000541 A6=0000054F A7=000007DE
```

After:

```
PC=00003004 SR=2719=.S7XN..C US=FFFFFFFF SS=000007E2
D0=00000002 D1=0000C3FC D2=0000F111 D3=00000004
D4=00000040 D5=FFFFFFFF D6=DFFFFFFF D7=FFFFFFFF
A0=00002000 A1=00001FFF A2=000020FF A3=FFFFFFFF
A4=FFFFFFFF A5=00000541 A6=0000054F A7=000007E2
```

Constants also may be used to define the number of shift positions.

EXAMPLE 5-17: LSR.W #$04,D0

Before:

```
PC=00003004 SR=2704=.S7..Z.. US=FFFFFFFF SS=000007E6
D0=00000010 D1=0000C3FC D2=0000F111 D3=00000004
D4=00000040 D5=FFFFFFFF D6=DFFFFFFF D7=FFFFFFFF
A0=00002000 A1=00001FFF A2=000020FF A3=FFFFFFFF
A4=FFFFFFFF A5=00000541 A6=0000054F A7=000007E6
```

After:

```
PC=0D0A0004 SR=2708=.S7.N... US=FFFFFFFF SS=000007EA
D0=000000FF D1=0000C3FC D2=0000F111 D3=00000004
D4=00000040 D5=FFFFFFFF D6=DFFFFFFF D7=FFFFFFFF
A0=00002000 A1=00001FFF A2=000020FF A3=FFFFFFFF
A4=FFFFFFFF A5=00000541 A6=0000054F A7=000007EA
```

When an operand in memory must be shifted, the instruction indicates the effective address. In such a case, the operand is shifted only one bit.

EXAMPLE 5-18: LSL.W (A1)

(Observe the contents of the memory location $3000 before and after execution of the instruction.)

Before:

```
PC=0D0A0004 SR=2708=.S7.N... US=FFFFFFFF SS=000007EA
D0=000000FF D1=0000C3FC D2=0000F111 D3=00000004
D4=00000040 D5=FFFFFFFF D6=DFFFFFFF D7=FFFFFFFF
A0=00002000 A1=00003000 A2=000020FF A3=FFFFFFFF     003000  E8 ? 01
A4=FFFFFFFF A5=00000541 A6=0000054F A7=000007EA     003001  48 ? 00
                                                    003002  4E ? 00
                                                    003002  4E ? 00
                                                    003003  75 ? 00
                                                    003004  4E ? .
```

After:

```
PC=00000032 SR=2708=.S7.N... US=FFFFFFFF SS=000007EE
D0=000000FF D1=0000C3FC D2=0000F111 D3=00000004
D4=00000040 D5=FFFFFFFF D6=DFFFFFFF D7=FFFFFFFF     003000  02
A0=00002000 A1=00003000 A2=000020FF A3=FFFFFFFF     003001  00
A4=FFFFFFFF A5=00000541 A6=0000054F A7=000007EE     003002  00
                                                    003003  00
                                                    003004  4E  .
```

The LSL instruction can be used in multiplication by powers of 2. In contrast, the LSR instruction does not provide correct results with negative numbers in division, since zeros are shifted from the left and reset the sign bit. The arithmetic shift instructions remedy this problem. Although similar in format to the logical shift instructions, the arithmetic shift instructions differ in their treatment of the condition code flags.

Consider the format of the ASR instruction shown in Fig. 5-2. The bits shifted from the left are copies of the sign bit, and thus, during a division, both positive and negative numbers are treated correctly; that is, in the case of a negative number, the ASR instruction shifts 1s from the left.

The rotate instructions eliminate a problem that shift instructions present; i.e., the loss of bits coming off the end of an operand.

INSTRUCTION SET – A MORE INTENSIVE EVALUATION 65

```
         ┌──────────────────────┐    ┌───┐
    ────▶│       OPERAND        ├───▶│ C │
         └──────────────────────┘ │  └───┘
                                  │  ┌───┐
                                  └─▶│ X │
                                     └───┘
                  ASR
```

Fig. 5-2. Arithmetic shift instruction.

The ROL and ROR instructions may rotate an operand by the number of bits specified in a register or by a constant; the instructions may also rotate an operand in memory by one bit. In all three of these cases, the rotate instruction copies the high-order or low-order bit of the operand into the carry flag, as shown in Fig. 5-3.

The two rotate-with-extend-instructions copy any bits shifted out of the high-order or low-order bit into both the carry and extend flags, as shown in Fig. 5-4. The previous value of the extend bit is shifted into the high-order or low-order bit, depending on the direction of the rotation. These rotate-with-extend instructions are useful for shifting operands larger than 32 bits.

EXAMPLE 5-19:

Assume that a 64-bit value, located in D0, D1, is to be shifted left. Two instructions – LSL.L#$01,D1 and ROXL.L #$01, D0 – are to accomplish this task. The first instruction shifts the low-order 32 bits of the operand and places the dropped bit in the X flag. The second instruction uses the saved bit in the X flag and rotates the high-order 32 bits.

Bit Manipulation Instructions

There are five instructions in the bit manipulation instruction group: Bit Set (BSET), Bit Test (BTST), Bit Clear (BCLR), Bit Change (BCHG), and Test and Set (TAS).

There are two means by which to specify the bit to be manipulated – i.e., either with a data register or a series of bits in the bit instruction opcode. If a register is affected, the bit number can be from 0 to 31; if a memory location is affected, the bit number can be from 0 to 7.

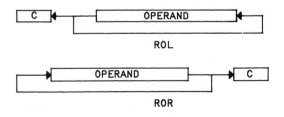

Fig. 5-3. Rotate instruction.

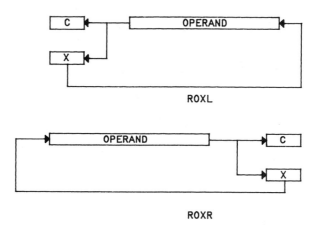

Fig. 5-4. Rotate with extend instruction.

Bits in memory are identified by the bit number of the byte at which the bits are located. An entire memory byte is read by the MC68000, a bit in that byte is manipulated, and then the entire byte is written back in its original address.

The TAS instruction deserves special attention. This is the only instruction that uses the read–modify–write (R–M–W) cycle of the MC68000. The TAS instruction is used in multiprocessor configurations of the MC68000 family and is indivisible. It locks out all accesses to the designated address until processing work at that location is completed. Its operation proceeds along the following lines.

The MC68000 selects a given byte to represent the status of a particular shared resource. This byte is commonly known as a *semaphore.* If a TAS instruction indicates that the semaphore is negative (by the presence of a 1 in its most significant bit), the querying processor knows that the resource is in use and can either continue to retest until the semaphore byte indicates a 0 in the msb, or process another task.

Since a TAS instruction immediately sets the msb of a semaphore to 1 and the instruction cannot be interrupted before completion, all processors in the shared system have accurate information about the shared resource. The msb is cleared by the microprocessor that has access to the shared resource.

Execution of a TAS instruction is associated with the read–modify–write cycle. During the TAS execution and the R–M–W cycle, the system prevents access of the semaphore byte by any other device between the time when the TAS reads the byte and when it sets the msb. Thus, two processors cannot read the semaphore byte simultaneously and be advised that a shared resource is free.

DATA MOVEMENT INSTRUCTIONS

As described in Chap. 4, the general instruction for transfers is the MOVE. Two special types in this category are the MOVEQ (Move Quick) and MOVEM (Move Multiple Registers) instructions.

INSTRUCTION SET—A MORE INTENSIVE EVALUATION

When a program segment requires a register to hold a constant of small value, the MOVEQ instruction provides a fast solution for initializing that register to the particular value. This instruction extends the sign bit of any signed eight-bit immediate value between -128 and +127, so that this value is interpreted correctly as a 32-bit operand and transfers the bit into a data register. Since the value to be manipulated is part of the instruction, the latter is executed faster. This "quick mode"—another variation of the MC68000 addressing modes—is also used by some arithmetic instructions.

More often than not, programs require stacking operations, during which the contents of a set of registers are saved, the registers are loaded with new values, and, after manipulation of these new values, the original contents of the registers are restored. The MOVEM instruction performs this task in an efficient, orderly, and expeditious manner.

EXAMPLE 5-20: MOVEM A1/A5/D3, $2000

This instruction will copy the contents of D3, A1, and A5 into memory locations $2000, $2002, and $2004, as shown in Fig. 5-5.

EXAMPLE 5-21: MOVEM D0/D5/A0 - A2, -(A4)

This instruction will copy the contents of D0, D5, A0, A1, and A2 in the order shown in Fig. 5-6 into five consecutive memory locations. The starting memory location will be predecremented value held in A0.

EXAMPLE 5-22: MOVEM (A7)+,A0 - A6/D0 - D7

The contents of D0 through D7 and A0 through A6 are copied into 15 consecutive memory locations in the order shown in Fig. 5-7. After execution of the instruction, the contents of A7 are the starting address incremented 15 times.

The MOVEA (Move Address) instruction moves the contents of an effective address to a destination address that an address register holds.

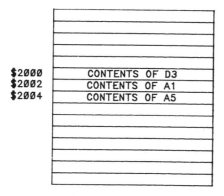

Fig. 5-5. Example 5-20.

68 THE 68000 MICROPROCESSOR

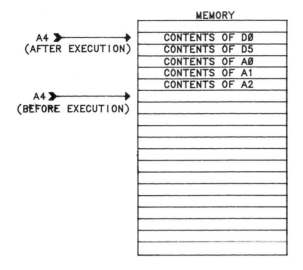

Fig. 5-6. Example 5-21.

The MC68000 uses the MOVEP (Move Peripheral Data) instruction to transfer data to 6800 peripheral devices such as the 6850 Asynchronous Communications Interface Adapter. This peripheral has two memory-mapped ports that appear as the low-order bytes of two consecutive memory words. One point to remember about the 6850 is that this device was intended for eight-bit data-bus processors. Thus, in an eight-bit data bus, the consecutive bytes are next to each other, whereas, in the 16-bit 68000 bus, they alternate.

The MOVEP instruction remedies the inconvenience in the interconnection of eight-bit peripheral devices and processors with a larger data bus. The instruction uses an address and a displacement, thus transferring data between a data

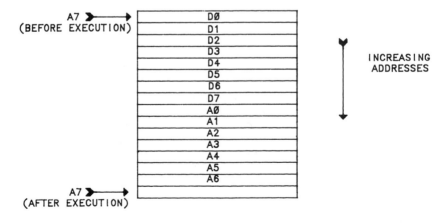

Fig. 5-7. Example 5-22.

register and the memory-mapped device, starting at the specified location and incrementing by 2.

PROGRAM CONTROL INSTRUCTIONS

The two types of program control instructions are the unconditional branch and the conditional branch.

Unconditional Branch

BRA <Label> is a relative branch instruction. The contents of the program counter (PC) are replaced by a new address that is defined by the current contents of the program counter and a displacement. The displacement is a two's complement value that counts the relative distance in bytes of the new address of program transfer. The value in the PC is the address of the current instruction plus 2. If the eight-bit displacement in the instruction is zero, then the word immediately after the instruction (16-bit displacement) is used.

Before the execution of a branch with BSR <Label>, the 32-bit address of the instruction after the branch instruction is transferred into the stack (the stack is predecremented). Program execution continues at a new address defined by the current contents of the PC plus 2. If the eight-bit displacement is zero, the word immediately after the branch instruction is used.

RTS restores the previous contents of registers. On execution, the value of the program counter before the branch is retrieved from the stack.

The MC68000 also uses the unconditional JUMP-type instruction, which transfers program execution to another address, without, however, using a displacement. The new absolute address is part of the instruction. The JMP instruction has the JSR as its counterpart.

Conditional Branch

Bcc (Branch on Condition Code) is the conditional branch form of program control instructions; it is stated as follows:

```
If cc is true
Then New PC = displacement + opword length + 2
Else no operation
```

The displacement is a 16-bit value that provides an addressing range between −32,768 and +32,767 bytes.

There are 14 different versions of the Bcc instruction, including BGT (Branch if greater than), BLT (Branch if less than), BEQ (Branch if equal), and BHI (Branch if higher).

Frequently, a programmer needs to branch to an earlier address to generate a programming loop. To do so, the MC68000 uses the DBcc (Decrement Counter and Branch on Condition Code) instruction. This instruction employs any data register as a counter and performs a branch on the basis of the evaluated condition of the code and the contents of the specified data register.

During execution of a DBcc instruction, the MC68000 first evaluates the condition for which the instruction calls. If the code condition is met, execution continues with the next instruction and the loop is terminated. If the condition is not met, the specified register is decremented by 1. If the resulting value is -1, the loop again terminates, and execution continues with the next instruction; otherwise, a branch to the top of the loop occurs.

An interesting point is that DBcc tests for -1. Most looping program segments require additional instructions to ensure that a loop can execute zero times if required **and** that it can test for the specified condition **before** the execution of an iteration. By entering a loop just before the DBcc instruction (at the end of a loop) and by having the DBcc instruction end a loop on a value of -1 instead of 0, both conditions can be met without the addition of an explicit second test. Furthermore, a simple conditional branch instruction that uses the same DBcc instruction lets a programmer determine whether a program has exited from a loop as a result of the iteration counter or the condition.

The DBcc instruction is useful in the manipulation of strings. For example, in conjunction with a MOVE instruction and predecrement/postincrement modes, a DBRA (Decrement and Branch always) instruction will fill a block of memory, copy strings, or reverse strings. A DBNE (Decrement and Branch if Not Equal) instruction used with the CMPM and predecrement mode will compare two strings.

POSITION INDEPENDENCE INSTRUCTIONS

As described previously, the MOVEA instruction can be used to move the contents of a block of memory. This address, however, may be defined in the instruction as a label, a point that imposes two requirements—i.e., the address of the label must be defined in the instruction, and the program must be loaded precisely at the location defined by the ORIGIN (ORG) directive of the assembler. These two requirements place a limitation on the MOVEA instruction in view of position independence.

The MC68000 provides the LEA (Load Effective Address) and PEA (Push Effective Address) instructions for position independence. Although the position-dependent MOVEA instruction uses a value assembled in absolute mode, the LEA instruction evaluates the value of a label using, if necessary, program counter relative addressing; that is, the LEA evaluates and places the address in the specified address register (this instruction works only with address registers as destination). The LEA does not access the value stored at the resulting address. The PEA instruction evaluates an address in the same manner as the LEA but, instead of loading it into an address register, stores it in the stack.

HIGH-LEVEL LANGUAGE AIDS

Modern programming techniques require structured and modular programming for easier design, debugging, and maintenance of programs. Modular programming implies the use of reentrant and recursive subroutines that have local variable areas and are brought together for a final product. One of the more important aspects of high-level language implementation, therefore, is efficient procedure calls and parameter passing. The MC68000 uses two instructions to meet these requirements.

The LINK and UNLNK (unlink) instructions deal with automatic manipulation of a procedure's temporary stack area, which is indicated by a "frame pointer." A frame pointer is an address register that a programmer designates for this use. Just before a procedure entry, the LINK instruction saves the calling procedure's frame pointer in the stack, updates the frame pointer for the called procedure, and then, by adding a displacement to the stack pointer, allocates local variable storage in the stack. On exiting from the procedure, the UNLNK instruction resets the stack pointer, thereby releasing the exited routine's local variable storage and then resetting the calling routine's frame pointer.

Study the example program in Fig. 5-8, the activity of which is flowcharted in Fig. 5-9.

The LEA instruction assigns A3 as the frame pointer and loads address $2000 into this register. A second LEA initializes the stack point to address $1FF0. Before Procedure A calls Procedure B, the former places parameters on top of the stack (PEA −6(A3)). After the subroutine call to Procedure B, the return address to A is pushed onto the stack (LEA 4(SP),SP).

The LINK instruction contains the name of the frame pointer (in this case, A3) and a displacement that indicates the amount of memory to be saved for local variables (#-$10). When this instruction is executed, the following activity occurs: The contents of the frame pointer (pointing to a stack location that contains the previous frame pointer) are pushed onto the stack. The frame pointer itself

```
              LEA     $2000,A3
              LEA     $1FF0,SP
PROCA         NOP
              NOP
              NOP
              PEA     -6(A3)
              JSR     PROCB(PC)
              LEA     4(SP),SP
              NOP
              NOP
              UNLK    A3
              RTS
; end of PROCA
;
PROCB         LINK    A3,#-$10
              NOP
              NOP
              NOP
              UNLK    A3
              RTS
;end of PROCB
              END
```

Fig. 5-8. Example program.

72 THE 68000 MICROPROCESSOR

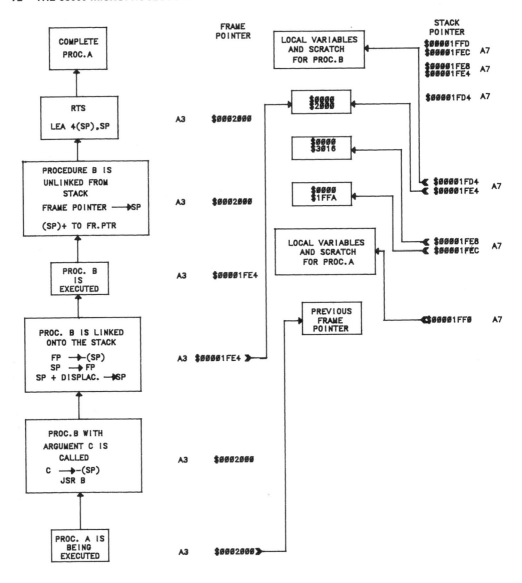

Fig. 5-9. Flowchart for example program.

is loaded with the same address as the stack pointer, and the stack pointer is changed by the displacement given in the instruction. The displacement (#-$10) has a signed value and must be negative to save local variable space; if it were positive, information would be lost from the stack.

As shown in Fig. 5-9, the stack pointer points to the top of the stack and the frame pointer to one word below the local variable area in Procedure B. When the UNLNK instruction is executed, the process is reversed, leaving Procedure B to execute an RTS instruction, returning control to Procedure A.

INSTRUCTION SET—A MORE INTENSIVE EVALUATION

Yet another class of instructions—Exception Handling—will be treated in Chap. 6.

PROGRAMMING HINTS

This section provides guidelines in the application of MC68000 instructions and addressing modes. A programmer should keep in mind some differences between the MC68000 and other processors. Although some of the guidelines have already been discussed, they will be recapitulated here.

Advice that a novice programmer should always follow is to consult the manufacturer's databook. It should be remembered that instructions work with some registers but not others; that instructions affect condition codes differently; that execution times of instructions differ. In short, use of the proper instructions in the proper place promotes faster execution of programs.

The paragraphs that follow will set forth some tricks that the MC68000 can play on a programmer unfamiliar with the device.

The MC68000 treats addresses and data differently. Instructions that affect addresses, such as MOVEA and ADDA, are only word or longword in size. Since the MC68000 address range is wider than 16 bits, word values are sign-extended to 32 bits before being used as addresses.

Unlike most data operations, address operations do not affect condition code flags.

A DBcc instruction is very efficient, but its use in loops is frequently confused. With a DBcc at its end, looping will continue until the condition code is true. Confusion results because the instruction can be thought of as decrementing and branching back if the condition is false. For example, if the MC68000 DBEQ (Decrement and Branch if Equal) were to be replaced by another instruction, most likely a BNE (Branch if Not Equal), not a BEQ, would be brought into play.

Remember also that, with DBcc instructions, a loop count stops at -1. If a loop is to be executed only once, it should be entered at the top with the counter already decremented by 1. The program listing in Fig. 5-10 searches, in a table of X bytes to which A2 points, for the first byte that contains zeros.

If a DBcc instruction is to be used, the condition codes must be initialized so that the instruction does not fall through when the loop jumps back to it.

Finally, data registers used as counters in loop operations must be decremented as word quantities. Thus, if more than 216 iterations are to be carried out, nested DBcc loops should be used.

```
              MOVE.W    #X-1,D0   ; Initialize loop by one
                                  ; less
     LOOP:    TST.B     (A2)+     ; Is byte a zero?
              DBEQ      D0,LOOP   ; If not, AND D0 is
                                  ; still >= 0, loop back
```

Fig. 5-10. Program listing.

The program listing in Fig. 5-11 uses two nested loops to checksum a list of bytes with a length specified in the longword D0.

Since a MOVE instruction cannot be used with a displacement relative to the program counter, a LEA<LABEL>(PC) instruction is substituted and the address altered through an address register.

Postincrement addressing is faster than predecrement.

The MOVEM instruction can be used efficiently for stack operations that involve a fair number of registers. If a couple of registers are to be pushed onto the stack, however, it is just as fast to move one at a time.

In light of the need to sign-extend a word value in address operations, the word-address operations can be slower than longword address operations.

When multiplication or division by a power of 2 is required, use shifting instructions rather than MUL or DIV. Remember the restriction on the use of a logic shift right (division) with negative numbers. Multiplication of an operand by a power of 2 is accomplished more quickly by repeated addition of registers to themselves rather than by shifting. Similarly, when extended-precision arithmetic is performed with the MC68000, the instruction ROXL #1, Dn can be replaced by ADDX Dn, Dn, to save two to four cycles, depending on the size of the operand.

Speed of execution is very important. In creation of address registers, the instruction MOVE.L #0, An consumes 12 cycles, whereas SUB.L An, An consumes only eight. Since the CLR (Clear) instruction does not work with address registers, it cannot be used in this case. Also, remember that CLR always reads from an operand before clearing it. Thus, never use the CLR to write a zero into a memory-mapped device address if the read will affect the device. Scc (Set condition code) and MOVE instructions also perform a read before a write but are less likely to cause problems.

It is important to know which instructions and addressing modes sign-extend an address or data. The following lists provide this information.

The addressing modes that sign-extend an address or data are as follows:

1. Absolute short: Word address extended to longword.
2. Address register direct (as destination): Word data extended to longword.

```
                MOVE        #0, D3          ; Initialize checksum
                MOVE.W      D0, D1          ; Long word of loop
                                            ; length in D1
                MOVE.L      D0,D2           ; Get high word of loop
                SWAP        D2              ; length in D2 to use
                                            ; for outer loop
                BRA.S       START           ; Enter at end of loop
LOOP:           ADD.B       (A1)+,D3        ; Add next byte into sum
START:          DBRA        D1,LOOP         ; Inner loop: loop on low
                                            ; word of D0
                DBRA        D2,LOOP         ; Outer loop: loop on
                                            ; high word
```

Fig. 5-11. Program listing.

3. Address register indirect with displacement: Word displacement extended to longword.
4. Address register indirect with index: (a) Word index extended to longword, and (b) byte displacement extended to longword.
5. Program counter with displacement: Word displacement extended to longword.
6. Program counter with index: (a) Word index extended to longword, and (b) byte displacement extended to longword.

The instructions that sign-extend data are as follows:

1. ADDA.W (ADDQ.L to An = ADDQ.L): Source data sign-extended to longword.
2. CMPA.W.: Source data sign-extended to longword.
3. EXT.W or EXT.L: Byte sign-extended to word and word to longword.
4. SUBA.W (SUBQ.W to An = SUBQ.L): Source data sign-extended to longword.
5. MOVEA.W: Destination is an address register.
6. MOVEM.: Memory to registers; destination is any register.
7. MOVEQ.L: Immediate byte sign-extended to longword; destination is a data register.

Chapter 6
Exception Handling

GENERAL

Design of an input-output circuit for our hypothetical computer was postponed until discussion of programming, but it also requires knowledge of the manner in which this processor behaves with I/O devices. This chapter provides the information about I/O handling.

Whenever a processor deviates from the orderly sequence of program execution because of an illegal instruction, a malfunction of hardware, or even a request for service from an input-output device, a condition called "exception" occurs.

The MC68000 operates, at all times, in either the supervisor mode or the user mode. The S/U flag in the status register indicates the mode in which the MC68000 is operating at any given time.

Programs other than those designed for system control execute mostly at the user level. Operation in the supervisor mode, however, affords certain privileges normally prohibited during the user mode. Table 6-1 lists the privileges granted in both modes.

Within the two modes, the MC68000 operates in one of three processing states—Normal, Halted, or Exception. The Normal state is associated with instruction execution. During this state, memory references occur for the purposes of fetching instructions and operands and storing results.

The Halted state usually indicates a serious hardware failure that will not allow further orderly execution of a program.[*] For example, if a second bus error occurs during the processing of a bus error exception, the processor assumes that the system is unusable and halts.

The Exception state is associated with interrupts, trap instructions, tracing, and other exceptional conditions. The flowchart in Fig. 6-1 shows how the MC68000 handles an exception. When confronted with an exception, the processor first copies the current contents of the status register into a temporary register, then

---

[*]In MC68000 texts, the word "catastrophic" is frequently used to identify this type of failure. Since this term is often associated with irreversible destruction, however, and a novice programmer may think that it means that a system has been permanently damaged, it is avoided in this text. Normally, a MC68000 system can be revived from this state by pressing a manual reset switch.

Table 6-1. Privilege States.

	USER MODE	SUPERVISOR MODE
Entered by	S set to 0	Recognition of a trap, reset, or interrupt
FC2 =	0	1
Other stack pointers	A0–A6	User stack pointer as well as A0–A6
Status bits available (Read) (Write)	C, V, Z, N, X, I0–I2, S, T C, V, Z, N, X	C, V, Z, N, X, I0–I2, S, T Same as above
Instructions available	All, except those on right	All, including: STOP, RESET MOVE TO SR ANDI to SR ORI to SR EORI to SR MOVE USP to <ea> MOVE to USP RTE

sets the S flag, and finally clears the T flag. If an interrupt causes the exception, the MC68000 also sets interrupt flags I0 through I2 to the corresponding masking interrupt level (more on this when interrupts are discussed).

After the flags are set, the processor vectors (branches) to a trap, i.e., to a known memory location that contains a user-supplied exception-handling subroutine. The next step saves the current program counter and the copied contents of the status register in the stack. The last step fetches and executes the contents of the exception-handling subroutine.

The order in which the status of the processor is saved before the exception routine is executed is shown in Fig. 6-2. In decreasing address value, the program counter (return address after execution of the routine) is saved first and the copied contents of the status register second. In the case of a reset, bus error, or illegal address error, additional words are stored in the stack.

Note that the system stack pointer is always used during an exception, regardless of the state of the processor when the exception is noticed.

The new contents of the status register during exception handling are as follows:

1. S = 1, so that the exception routine is always executed in the supervisor mode.
2. T = 0, so that exceptions can be handled normally even when the main program is being traced.

78   THE 68000 MICROPROCESSOR

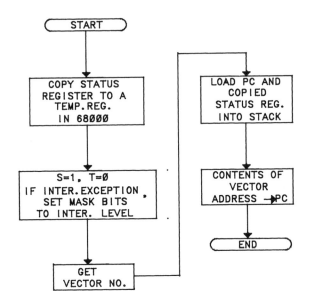

Fig. 6-1. MC68000 exception handling.

3. I0 through I2 are affected only by the reset exception and by interrupts. These bits are set to the corresponding masking interrupt value.

The MC68000 handles two types of exceptions:

1. Internal exceptions, caused by instructions (TRAP, TRAPV, CHK, DIV), address errors, and entry of the processor into a trace mode (T = 1)
2. External exceptions, caused by interrupts of various kinds, bus errors, or reset

The MC68000 provides 256 exception vectors, as shown in Table 6-2. Each vector number occupies four bytes, for a total memory space of 1024 bytes. On power-up of a system, these vectors must be loaded at the bottom (0–1K) of the memory map. Table 6-2 shows both vector numbers and vector addresses. A vector address is calculated by multiplying the vector by four. As already mentioned, a deviation from normal operation will create an exception.

EXAMPLE 6-1: MOVE.W D0, 6(A0)

In this case, the effective address is the sum of the offset (6) and the contents of the address register A0. If the contents are odd, the effective address becomes odd, and the instruction produces an exception as an illegal instruction.

EXAMPLE 6-2: MOVE.W D0, #$2001.

This instruction is illegal and will cause a branch to Vector No. 4. The address #$2001 is not at a word boundary.

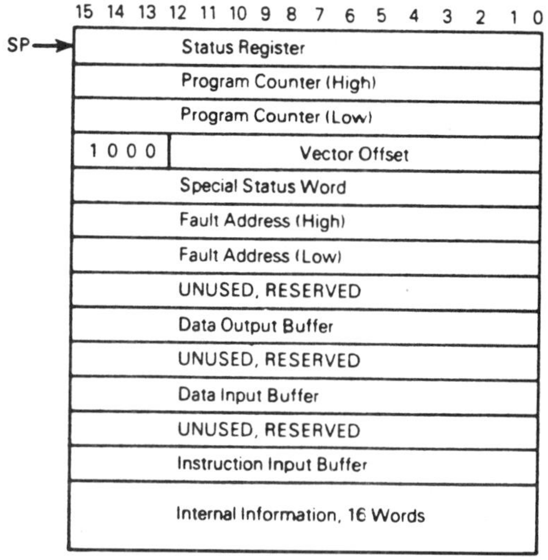

EXCEPTION HANDLING

```
       15 14 13 12 11 10 9 8 7 6 5 4 3 2 1 0
SP → ┌──────────────────────────────────────┐
     │           Status Register            │
     ├──────────────────────────────────────┤
     │        Program Counter (High)        │
     ├──────────────────────────────────────┤
     │        Program Counter (Low)         │
     ├─────────┬────────────────────────────┤
     │  1 0 0 0│        Vector Offset       │
     ├─────────┴────────────────────────────┤
     │          Special Status Word         │
     ├──────────────────────────────────────┤
     │         Fault Address (High)         │
     ├──────────────────────────────────────┤
     │         Fault Address (Low)          │
     ├──────────────────────────────────────┤
     │           UNUSED, RESERVED           │
     ├──────────────────────────────────────┤
     │          Data Output Buffer          │
     ├──────────────────────────────────────┤
     │           UNUSED, RESERVED           │
     ├──────────────────────────────────────┤
     │           Data Input Buffer          │
     ├──────────────────────────────────────┤
     │           UNUSED, RESERVED           │
     ├──────────────────────────────────────┤
     │       Instruction Input Buffer       │
     ├──────────────────────────────────────┤
     │       Internal Information, 16 Words │
     └──────────────────────────────────────┘
```

NOTE: The stack pointer is decremented by 29 words, although only 26 words of information are actually written to memory. The three additional words are reserved for future use by Motorola.

Fig. 6-2. Saving the status of the MC68000.

EXAMPLE 6-3: MOVE D0, SR

If a program supplies this instruction when the system is in the user mode, a privilege violation exception occurs because this instruction is used with the system in supervisor mode. As a result, the system branches to Vector No. 8.

Address 0 in Table 6-2 shows the vectors for an external reset. Although other vectors occupy four bytes, the vector for reset—actually, two adjacent vector locations—occupies eight bytes because these two locations contain the initial value of the system stack pointer and the new value of the program counter.

When an external reset is asserted, the MC68000 does not save any previous values on the stack since the stack pointer may not refer to a valid address.

An exception handling routine normally appears as follows:

```
EXCPTN   MOVEM.L  Da-Dx/Ab-Az, -(SP); Stack any
                  ;registers involved in the
                  ;routine
           :
           :
                  ;body of routine
           :
         MOVEM.L  (SP)+, Da-Dx/Ab-Az  ; Restore registers.
         RTE                          ; Return to main
                                      ; program
```

It is important to know which of the MC68000's several return instructions to use. The RTE must be used in this program module since this instruction always

Table 6-2. MC68000 Exception Vectors.

VECTOR NUMBER(S)	ADDRESS DEC	ADDRESS HEX	SPACE	ASSIGNMENT
0	0	000	SP	Reset: Initial SSP
–	4	004	SP	Reset: Initial PC
2	8	008	SD	Bus Error
3	12	00C	SD	Address Error
4	16	010	SD	Illegal Instruction
5	20	014	SD	Zero Divide
6	24	018	SD	CHK Instruction
7	28	01C	SD	TRAPV Instruction
8	32	020	SD	Privilege Violation
9	36	024	SD	Trace
10	40	028	SD	Line 1010 Emulator
11	44	02C	SD	Line 1111 Emulator
12*	48	030	SD	(Unassigned, reserved)
13*	52	034	SD	(Unassigned, reserved)
14*	56	038	SD	(Unassigned, reserved)
15	60	03C	SD	Uninitialized Interrupt Vector
16-23*	64	04C	SD	(Unassigned, reserved)
	95	05F		–
24	96	060	SD	Spurious Interrupt
25	100	064	SD	Level 1 Interrupt Autovector
26	104	068	SD	Level 2 Interrupt Autovector
27	108	06C	SD	Level 3 Interrupt Autovector
28	112	070	SD	Level 4 Interrupt Autovector
29	116	074	SD	Level 5 Interrupt Autovector
30	120	078	SD	Level 6 Interrupt Autovector
31	124	07C	SD	Level 7 Interrupt Autovector
32-47	128	080	SD	TRAP Instruction Vectors
	191	0BF		–
48-63*	192	0C0	SD	(Unassigned, reserved)
	255	0FF		–
64-255	256	100	SD	User Interrupt Vectors
	1023	3FF		–

*Vector numbers 12, 13, 14, 16 through 23, and 48 through 63 are reserved for future enhancements by Motorola. No user peripheral devices should be assigned these numbers.

restores the status register and program counter from the system stack. The RTS instruction restores these registers from either the system or the user stack. Thus, if a previous instruction changed the mode, RTS could be accessing the wrong stack.

The RTR (Return and Restore Condition Codes) should not be considered as an alternative. This instruction restores the program counter and stack pointer from values on the stack but sets only the eight bits of the condition code and leaves the status side of SR unaffected. Thus, in this case, RTR could not replace the RTE instruction.

Some instructions intentionally create exceptions, such as the TRAP instruction. There are 16 user-defined, trap-instruction vectors, and these always direct program control to a designated trap routine at the supervisor level. These vectors can be used as software interrupts to call the operating system, to simulate interrupts during debugging operations, to signal the completion of a task, or to indicate that an error condition has appeared in a routine.

Two other instructions—TRAPV (Trap-on-overflow) and CHK (Check-register-against-bounds)—examine operating conditions and cause a trap if certain conditions are not met.

The instruction TRAPV will cause a trap whenever the overflow bit in the status register is set. A single routine at the operating system level may then handle every overflow occurrence.

Figure 6-3 illustrates the function of the CHK instruction. This instruction determines whether the contents of a selected register are within the bounds of zero and a specified upper limit. Whenever the instruction determines that the register contents fall outside the specified bounds, CHK initiates a trap.

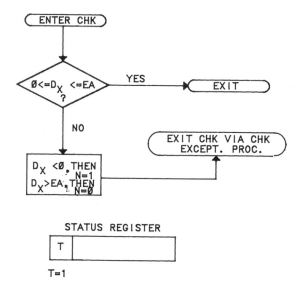

Fig. 6-3. CHK instruction.

The CHK instruction may also be used to verify that a stack does not overrun, that a string of characters fits into an allocated space, that an entry into an array is within its dimensions, or that a task does not access data outside a designated space.

An attempt to execute certain instructions not implemented in current versions of the MC68000 family can cause the processor to access one of two traps. These instructions have opcodes that begin with 1010 or 1111 and are listed, in Table 6-2, as Line 1010 Emulator and Line 1111 Emulator. Such instructions are reserved for future expansion, but, since the vector already exists, it can be used to the advantage of a programmer. That is, a programmer can design custom instructions that can be executed as exception-handling routines. These routines may serve the same function as macros.

In addition to "intentional" exception instructions, irregular use of some instructions may also cause an exception. For example, an attempt to divide by zero is detected before the operands are modified, and the system then branches to the corresponding vector. An overflow condition during a division will divert the normal execution of this operation. During a division overflow, the overflow flag is set, but the result is not copied into the destination; the operation leaves the operands unchanged. Program execution continues with the next instruction, though a succeeding TRAPV instruction could call the supervisor for special processing.

The trace vector at location 24 is of particular interest; it has been provided to assist in program development and debugging. A trace routine usually accompanies a single-step hardware circuit and is executed as shown in Fig. 6-4.

Instruction tracing is initiated by turning on the T flag in the status register. That done, the execution of each instruction is followed by a tracing operation, which might be a routine to print out register or memory contents or any other necessary debugging operation.

Branching to a trace service routine is carried out in a slightly different manner from branching to other traps. The program counter and status register of the main program are stored on the supervisor stack, the trace flag is reset to 0, and the system is set to supervisor mode (S = 1). Next, the trace vector is fetched and loaded into the program counter.

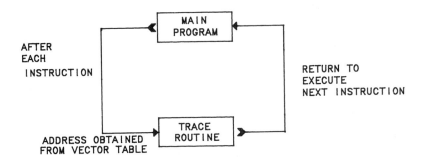

Fig. 6-4. Trace routine.

A trace routine is also terminated with an RTE instruction. To turn one off, the stack location that contains the saved status register must be modified to reset the T bit (T=0). Then, when the RTE instruction restores the program counter and status register from the supervisor stack, the trace is disabled and the system returned to normal program execution.

INTERRUPTS

Interrupts are exceptions too, but normally they are caused by an external device or an abnormal condition resulting from an external signal. The MC68000 services two types of interrupts—intentional interrupts and undesirable interrupts. The first type, called *user interrupts,* is further classified as autovectored interrupts (provided to service 68000 devices) and user-defined vectored interrupts. The second type, the undesirable interrupts, will be discussed later.

The MC68000 provides seven levels of interrupts, one of which is nonmaskable (Level 7). The interrupting device places the level of an interrupt on the three interrupt lines ($\overline{IPL0}$ through $\overline{IPL2}$), and the level is copied on address lines A1 to A3. If all of the $\overline{IPL}$ lines are at zero, no interrupt is pending.

When an interrupt is requested via the $\overline{IPL}$ lines, the MC68000 compares the interrupt request level to the interrupt mask in the status register to determine whether to process the interrupt. An interrupt will not be recognized until the following two requirements are met. First, the incoming interrupt level must be higher than the mask level set in the interrupt mask bits of the status register. Nonmaskable interrupts are assigned the highest level. Second, the three interrupt control lines must be held at the interrupt request level until the processor acknowledges the interrupt by initiating an interrupt acknowledge bus cycle (all FC lines are set to 1 and $\overline{AS}$ is asserted).

The two specified requirements guarantee recognition and execution of an interrupt, but one may still be processed even if the request level is taken away before the interrupt acknowledge bus cycle. Since the MC68000 samples the interrupt request lines once during the execution of every instruction, an interrupt that has been held for as few as two clock periods of the system clock may be recognized.

The flowchart in Fig. 6-5 shows the activity of the MC68000 during an interrupt.

EXAMPLE 6-4: I0–I2 = 0 1 0 (interrupt mask set to level No. 2)
$\overline{IPL0}$–$\overline{IPL2}$ = 0 1 1 for two clock cycles.

A level-six interrupt is requested and remains on the interrupt request lines. In this example, a level-three interrupt request may, but will not necessarily, be recognized since the $\overline{IPL}$ lines do not hold this level until an IACK cycle is initiated (remember that the level-six interrupt wiped out the level-three interrupt on the $\overline{IPL}$ lines). A level-six interrupt will be recognized if it stays on the $\overline{IPL}$ lines long enough for FC0 through FC2 to be set to high, $\overline{AS}$ to be asserted (signaling

84 THE 68000 MICROPROCESSOR

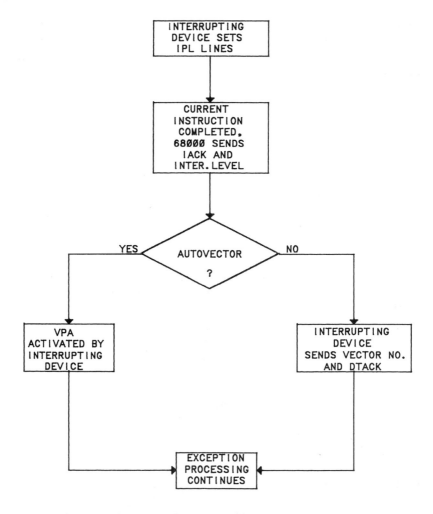

Fig. 6-5. Interrupt.

initiation of the IACK cycle), and A1, A2, and A3 lines to be set to the level of the interrupt request.

Let us discuss the activity of a user-defined vectored interrupt. If the requirements for an interrupt are met during a request and the interrupting device has an internal vector register with a vector number, this eight-bit number is transferred to data lines D0 through D7 of the MC68000. At the same time, the interrupting device asserts the $\overline{DTACK}$ line to terminate the interrupt acknowledge bus cycle. The MC68000 then uses the vector number to calculate the user-vector address to which the processor must branch in order to execute the interrupt service routine.

The MC68000 allocates 192 user interrupt vectors. These vectors are accessed sequentially (Nos. 64 to 255). Therefore, if fewer than 193 interrupts are needed, as is most commonly the case, each interrupt can be assigned a unique vector number, which also can be interpreted as a priority. Vector number 64 is assumed to be the lowest and 255 the highest priority. The vector number (an eight-bit value between 00000000 and 10111111) can be generated by encoding the interrupt level on the IPL lines and adding 64.

Figure 6-6 depicts a method for generating user vectors.

Two latches are used to ensure not only that interrupts are not lost but that the vector number transferred to D0 through D7 is the result of only one interrupt. The latter step is very important since a new interrupt request, one generated during an interrupt acknowledge bus cycle, could cause a vector number to enter a state of transition when the processor tries to latch the vector number from the data bus. Thus, latch no. 1 prohibits acceptance of new interrupts until latch no. 2 has the proper vector number. With three-state outputs, latch no. 2 isolates the vector number being held from the data bus until IACK is asserted.

After a sufficient delay to allow the vector number to propagate to latch no. 2, latch no. 1 is released to allow new interrupt requests to be latched.

Figure 6-7 shows a partial circuit for user-defined, vectored, priority interrupt handling.

The circuit can be expanded in a daisy-chain fashion to handle 24 groups of eight interrupt lines each, for a total of 192 lines. Each group of lines is fed into a latch-encoder combination, as shown in Fig. 6-7. Each stage of an encoder disables the previous stage and thus sets a priority among the groups. Within each group, interrupts are prioritized into eight levels; the levels are represented by a three-bit code on lines A0, A1, and A2 of the encoder.

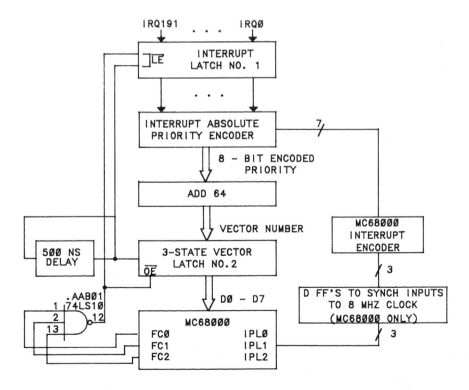

Fig. 6-6. Generating user interrupt circuit with latches.

86 THE 68000 MICROPROCESSOR

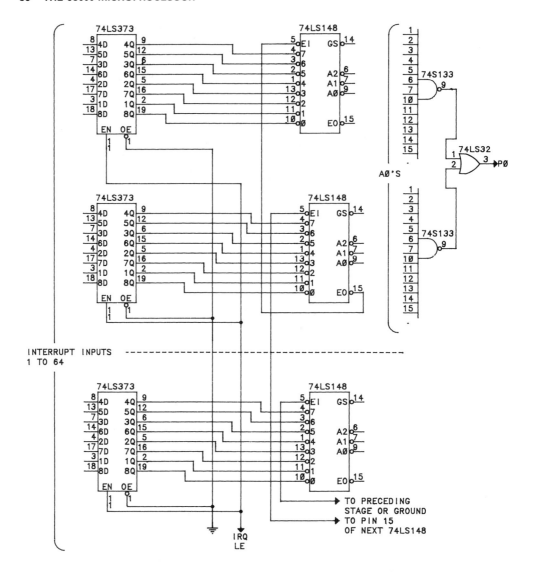

Fig. 6-7. Vectored, priority interrupt handling.

The A0 line from each of the 24 stages forms the A0 of the vector number through a NAND gate. Lines A1 and A2 are formed in a similar manner, as shown in Fig. 6-7. Bits 3 and 7 of the encoded interrupt are formed by NANDing selected GS outputs of the encoders. Bits 6 and 7 of the vector number differ from the corresponding bits of the encoded interrupt because of the offset of 64.

After the vector number has had sufficient time to propagate, latch no. 2, shown in Fig. 6-8, captures this number and allows the release of latch no. 1.

A final encoder encodes the priority level and transfers it to the MC68000 $\overline{\text{IPL}}$ lines. Figure 6-8 also shows how the $\overline{\text{DTACK}}$ and IACK signals are asserted.

EXCEPTION HANDLING 87

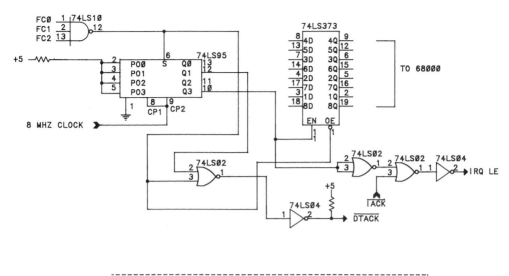

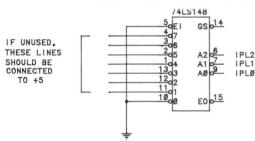

Fig. 6-8. Block diagram of user interrupt circuit with latches.

A user interrupting device is not limited to accessing only user interrupt vectors. For an interrupting device that does not have a vector register, the autovector concept can be used. External hardware, as shown in Fig. 6-9, can be used to recognize the IACK line and to assert the $\overline{VPA}$ (Valid Peripheral Address) to terminate the IACK cycle.

When the $\overline{VPA}$ is asserted, the MC68000 autovectors; that is, the processor branches to one of seven vector numbers used for this purpose (Nos. 25 through 31 in Table 6-2). Since each autovector number corresponds to one of the seven interrupt levels that the MC68000 accepts, a priority interrupt-system is set, as shown in Fig. 6-10.

The circuit in Fig. 6-11 allows peripheral devices of the MC68000 family to be connected.

The MC68000 peripheral devices have an interrupt request output (IRQ) and an IACK input. The circuit in Fig. 6-11 generates both of these signals. First, the 74LS138 decoder is asserted by the FC lines (all high, IACK) and the $\overline{AS}$ (asserted at the beginning of an IACK bus cycle). The 74LS148 encoder generates the priority interrupt level. The IACK level is generated by the binary value of

88 THE 68000 MICROPROCESSOR

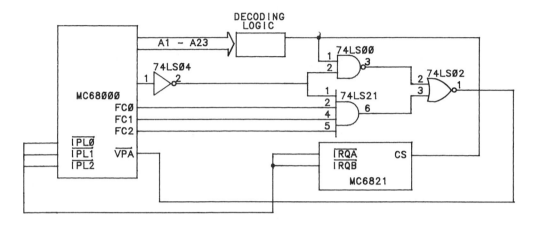

Fig. 6-9. Autovectoring.

A1, A2, and A3 on the control inputs of the decoder. Enable input E1 of the 74LS138 is asserted by lines A4 through A24 being high. This feature separates the IACK space of the MC68000 from the CPU space of the MC68020 and thus provides compatibility among the MC68000 family peripheral devices and future processors.

Several interrupting devices can share the same priority level in an MC68000 system, as the circuit in Fig. 6-12 demonstrates. This circuit functions in conjunction with the one in Fig. 6-11. The lower priority device (No. 2) receives an IACK from the MC68000 only if device No. 1 has not sent an interrupt request. That is, in this configuration, devices closer to the beginning of the chain have the higher priority.

Whenever a level-four interrupt is signaled, the FC lines are asserted and negate the preset inputs of both flip-flops. AS is also asserted at this stage. Thus, the circuit in Fig. 6-11 asserts IACK4. This causes the NOR gate (in Fig. 6-12) to clock in the current state of the IRQ output of each device to drive its respective

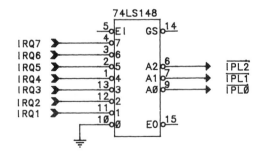

Fig. 6-10. Priority autovectoring.

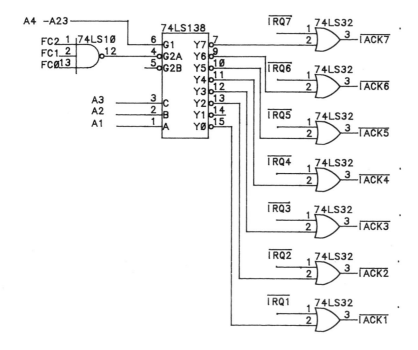

Fig. 6-11. IACK generation circuit.

IACK input. Clocking is inhibited for an interrupting device if the IRQ line of a higher-priority device in the chain is active.

Finally, an MC68000 system may have a combination of vectored and autovectored devices, as the circuit in Fig. 6-13 shows. Since this circuit is quite similar to the circuit in Fig. 6-11, no further discussion is needed.

A level-seven interrupt is nonmaskable; that is, a value of seven in the interrupt flags of the status register does not disable the interrupt. As with a maskable interrupt, a level-seven interrupt should remain on the $\overline{\text{IPL}}$ lines until an IACK bus cycle is initiated to guarantee the system's recognition of the interrupt.

A nonmaskable interrupt is edge-triggered by a transition from a lower-priority request to the level-seven request in contrast to the maskable interrupt levels one through six, which are level sensitive. Thus, if a level-seven interrupt is requested, it will be recognized only once, since only one low-priority-to-level-seven transition has occurred.

If more than one level-seven interrupt is to be recognized, one of two actions must take place. In both instances, $\overline{\text{IPL}}$ lines must hold a level between zero and six, and this level will be changed by a level-seven interrupt. Then, either one of two things happens, as follows:

1. The level remains on the pins until the initiation of the IACK bus cycle, in which event the interrupt request level later returns to a lower interrupt

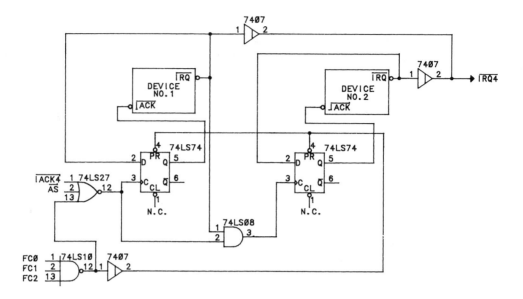

Fig. 6-12. "Daisy-Chain" interrupts.

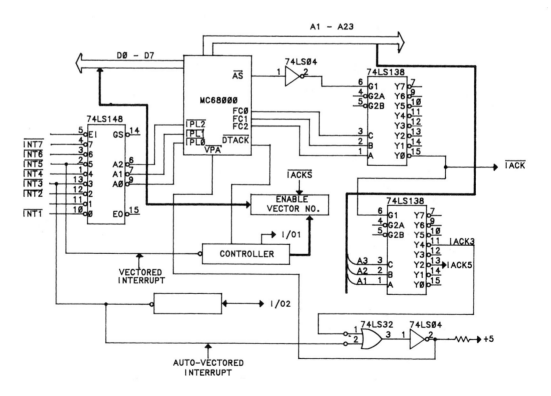

Fig. 6-13. Combination vector-autovector circuit.

request and finally back to level seven, thus causing a second transition on the $\overline{\text{IPL}}$ lines; or

2. The level-seven interrupt remains on the lines and, if the interrupt service routine for the level-seven interrupt lowers the interrupt mask level, a second level-seven interrupt will be recognized even though no transition has occurred on the $\overline{\text{IPL}}$ lines, and the interrupt mask in the status register will be set back to seven.

A $\overline{\text{BERR}}$ (Bus Error) signal also will terminate a bus cycle. This signal can be asserted because

1. The MC68000 tries to address nonresident memory, and the watchdog timer produces a timeout signal to set the $\overline{\text{BERR}}$ line.
2. A parity error causes a bus error and a rerun cycle.
3. An error caused by the memory management units asserts the bus error line.

Finally, a spurious interrupt causes a bus error. Although the $\overline{\text{IPL}}$ lines are synchronized to enhance noise immunity, noise that penetrates the external interrupt circuitry can initiate an erroneous IACK bus cycle. Since no device is requesting the service of an interrupt, neither $\overline{\text{DTACK}}$ nor $\overline{\text{VPA}}$ is asserted. Therefore, the system watchdog timer generates a bus error signal, and the MC68000 branches to the spurious interrupt vector.

Chapter 7
Peripheral Devices

INTRODUCTION

This chapter describes the connection of both serial and parallel input–output (I/O) devices to our hypothetical MC68000 system. The requirements for an adequate I/O configuration are as follows:

1. A serial connection to a telephone for communication with other systems
2. A serial connection to a terminal
3. A parallel connection to a printer based on the assumption that most available printers have the Centronix type parallel configuration
4. An audio cassette interface for secondary storage.

Motorola produces several devices that will accommodate such an I/O interface. The most likely candidates for our system are the MC6850 Asynchronous Communications Interface Adapter (ACIA) and the MC68230 Parallel Interface/Timer (PI/T) device. The latter can be used for the printer and the cassette interface.

MEMORY MAPPING OF I/O SPACE

Since the MC68000 uses memory-mapped I/O, an area must be reserved in our memory map to access the I/O registers of the peripheral devices. The area from $010000 to $01FFFF serves this purpose. The device's addresses are not fully decoded within this page, and thus each device can be accessed at different locations within the memory map.

Figure 7-1 shows the general block diagram of our I/O configuration.

MC6850 ACIA

The MC6850 ACIA—in use for quite some time—was one of the first devices adopted by the MC6800 eight-bit microprocessor systems for serial communication. The device has also been used as a cassette interface, although the PI/T is a better choice for our hypothetical computer.

Figure 7-2 sets forth the block diagram of the MC6850.

PERIPHERAL DEVICES 93

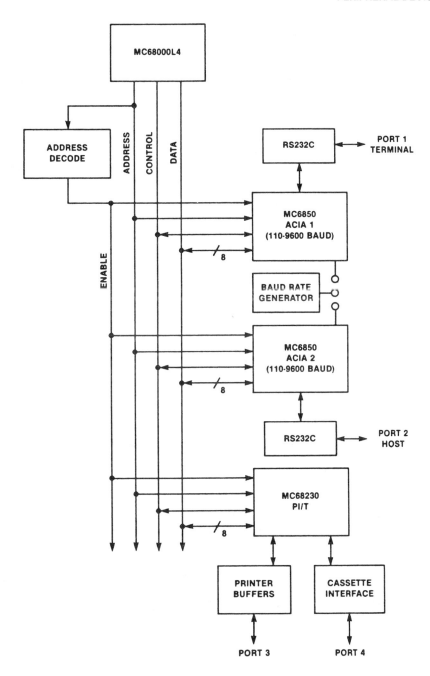

Fig. 7-1. I/O configuration of our system.

94 THE 68000 MICROPROCESSOR

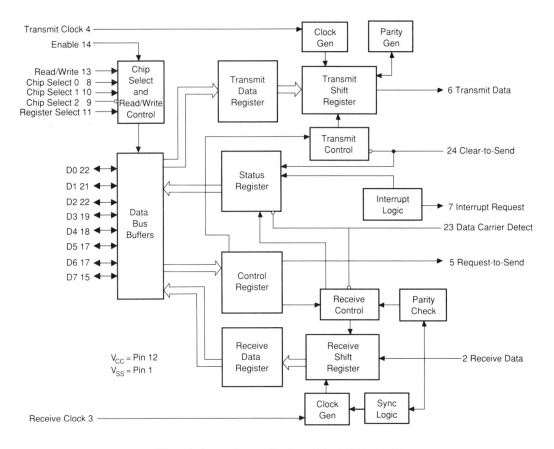

Fig. 7-2. Internal organization of the MC6850 ACIA.

The MC6850 is a "double device"; that is, there are two ACIA on the same chip. The following description applies to both sections of the device, since they function in the same manner. Only the addresses of the internal registers differ.

The MC6850 functions as an asynchronous receiver–transmitter (although, in our circuit, it is used in the synchronous mode). The device receives data from the system bus in parallel order and transmits the data to a serial device. The MC6850 also receives serial data from the external device and transfers the data to the system bus in parallel order. Four registers inside the ACIA store the outgoing data in parallel fashion and transmit the data serially and store the incoming data serially and transfer the data in parallel. The outgoing bit stream includes start, stop, and parity bits. Before an incoming bit stream is transferred to the parallel bus, the stream is stripped of these bits. Thus, two of the registers are "read only" and two are "write only." Only one register-select input is required to address all four registers since the R/W line provides the other select line.

The control registers in the ACIA determine the direction of the data flow. These registers can be programmed to assert the ACIA as an input or output device. Furthermore, a status register can be programmed to indicate whether the receiver–data register is full or the transmit register empty (RDA signal and TDRA signal). The status register also provides handshake between system and peripheral device by handling such signals as Request-to-Send ($\overline{\text{RTS}}$), Clear-to-Send ($\overline{\text{CTS}}$), and Data Carrier Detect ($\overline{\text{DCD}}$).

The status register maintains the current condition of internal ACIA activities. An eight-bit register, it is called a *read-only register* since the processor cannot store data in it.

The contents of the ACIA can be read by selecting the device through the CS0, CS1, and $\overline{\text{CS2}}$ lines, with the Register Select (RS) line held low (0) and the Read/Write line high (1).

A description of the eight status bit follows.

Bit 0: Receiver-Data Register Full (RDRF)

"1" = (a) Receiver-data register full.
     (b) The Interrupt Request bit ($\overline{\text{IRQ}}$), if enabled, is also set to 1 and remains set until the processor reads the data.

"0" = (a) The processor has read the contents of the receiver–data register. The data are retained there.
     (b) If there is loss of carrier, the $\overline{\text{Data Carrier Detect}}$ line is set high, and the RDRF bit is clamped at 0, indicating that the contents of the receiver–data register are not current.
     (c) A master reset condition also forces the RDRF bit to 0.

Bit 1: Transmit-Data Register Empty (TDRE)

"1" = (a) The contents of the transmit-data register have been transferred, and the register is ready to accept more data.
     (b) If enabled, the $\overline{\text{IRQ}}$ bit is also set to 1 and remains set until a write operation to the transmit–data register is completed.

"0" = (a) Transmit–data register is full.
     (b) When a 1 is present in the $\overline{\text{Clear to Send}}$ line ($\overline{\text{CTS}}$), causing Bit 3 of the status register to be set to 1, and thus indicating that it is not clear to send, Bit 0 of the TDRE is clamped to 0.

Bit 2: Data Carrier Detect ($\overline{\text{DCD}}$)

"1" = (a) No carrier from the modem.
     (b) If enabled, the $\overline{\text{IRQ}}$ bit is also set and remains set until the MC68000 reads the status and receiver–data registers or until a master reset occurs.
     (c) The RDRF bit is clamped at 0, inhibiting further interrupts from a receiver–data register full condition.

"0" = The carrier from the modem is present.

Bit 3: Clear-To-Send (CTS)
   "1" = The modem is not ready for data.
   "0" = The modem is ready to accept data.

Bit 4: Framing Error (FE)
   "1" = The absence of the first stop bit indicates that a received character is improperly framed by the start and stop bits. A state of 1 may also indicate a synchronization error, a faulty transmission, or a break condition. The error flag is set or reset during the receiver–data transfer time and is therefore present throughout the time the associated character is available.
   "0" = The received character is properly framed.

Bit 5: Receiver Overrun (OVRN)
   "1" = One or more characters in the data stream has been lost; that is, one or more characters has been received from the receiver–data register (RDR), but not read, before receipt of additional characters. An overrun condition begins midpoint in the last bit of the second character to be received in succession without the RDR having been read. An overrun does not occur in the status register until the valid character prior to an overrun is read. Character synchronization is maintained during the overrun condition. The overrun error flag is reset after the reading of data from the RDR. Overrun also is reset by a master reset.
   "0" = Absence of receiver overruns.

Bit 6: Parity Error (PE)
   "1" = The number of 1s in the character does not agree with the preselected odd or even parity. The parity-error indication is present as long as the data character is in the RDR. If no parity is selected, then both the transmitter parity generator output and the receiver parity check results are inhibited.
   "0" = No parity error.

Bit 7: Interrupt Request (IRQ)
   "1" = An interrupt that has caused the IRQ output line to go low is present. The interrupt is cleared by a read operation of the RDR, a write operation of the TDR, or a read of the SR, followed by a read of the RDR if this read is caused by DCD. A master reset always clears this bit.
   "0" = Absence of interrupts.

Two bytes are needed for the registers. One register can be loaded and another read at each byte address. Since the ACIA has an eight-bit wide bus, the device can be connected to either the low-order or high-order eight bits of the MC68000 data bus.

Although the name of the MC6850 includes the term *asynchronous,* the device is actually a synchronous bus interface that requires that a read or write to any of its registers be synchronized with the E clock (400 kHz).

MEMORY MAPPING OF ACIA

Table 7-1 provides the addresses of both ACIA. Their decoding is redundant with page $010000; i.e., both devices can be accessed every time address line A6 is "1" within this page.

GENERATING INTERRUPT REQUEST SIGNALS

We need to design a circuit that accepts the interrupt requests from both the ACIA and the PI/T and that generates the corresponding interrupt priority level on the $\overline{\text{IPL}}$ lines of the MC68000.

The circuit in Fig. 7-3 may well be called an *interrupt synchronizer.* First of all, an "abort" function would be useful in our system. This function generates a level-seven interrupt and returns control to the system's firmware; it differs from a reset, however, in that it does not reinitialize the system. Therefore, an abort function may be useful, e.g., in stopping a printer if the paper jams and thus in regaining control of processing without destroying previous system conditions or contents.

An abort function can be created with some software and the debounced switch arrangement in Fig. 7-3. Notice how the output of the abort switch is connected to input No. 7 (level-seven) of the 74LS148 priority encoder.

The circuit in Fig. 7-3 is easily deciphered. The octal D-type flip-flop device (74LS273) stores the five interrupt requests and also acts as the output of the interrupt priority levels.

Table 7-1. Address Space of ACIA.

ADDRESS (IN HEX)	REGISTER
010040	ACIA 1 Control Register (write only) Status Register (read only)
010041	ACIA 2 Control Register (write only) Status Register (read only)
010042	ACIA 1 Transmit–Data Register (write only) Receiver–Data Register (read only)
010043	ACIA 2 Transmit–Data Register (write only) Receiver–Data Register (read only)

98 THE 68000 MICROPROCESSOR

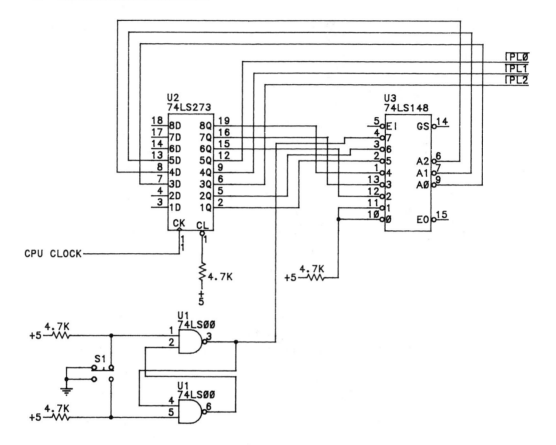

Fig. 7-3. Interrupt synchronizer.

The highest maskable priority is given to the modem ACIA (ACI1IRQ) so that, if our system is connected to a modem, incoming data will be protected from interruption by other maskable devices.

The next priority level is assigned to the terminal (ACI2IRQ). The other interrupt requests are clearly marked in Fig. 7-3. The lowest priority is given to the timer circuit of the PI/T (the audio–cassette interface is not used as frequently as a terminal).

Interrupt levels zero and one are not used and are negated via a pull-up resistor to the positive power supply (the 74LS148 requires active–low inputs). Inputs D2, D3, and D4 of the 74LS273 are connected to the outputs of the encoder. The outputs of the flip-flops are connected to the $\overline{IPL}$ lines of the MC68000. This scheme allows some timing delay so that the interrupt requests can be latched at the proper clock cycle.

With the interrupt-request circuitry designed, the interrupt-acknowledge signals must be generated. The system requires four major signals: one to the parallel port, one to the timer (cassette interface), one to the $\overline{VPA}$ input on the MC68000 (to complete the synchronous bus operation), and one to the bus-timeout-error watchdog timer.

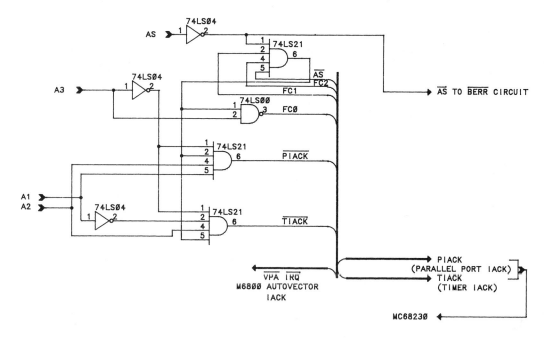

Fig. 7-4. Interrupt control signals.

Simple gating, as shown in Fig. 7-4, can provide all of the needed signals.

During an interrupt-acknowledge bus cycle, the FC lines and the $\overline{AS}$ are asserted. We can use the presence, or rather the absence, of $\overline{AS}$ to assert the Bus Error line ($\overline{BERR}$) of the timeout circuit.

An asserted $\overline{AS}$ is ANDed with the FC lines to provide the other interrupt-acknowledge signals. For example, the high outputs of the AND gate and address line A3 (one of the lines carrying a copy of the interrupt priority level) are inputs to the NAND gate; the $\overline{VPA}$ signal is output from this gate.

The circuit for the serial ports is shown in Fig. 7-5.

The 1488 and 1489 are line receivers and transmitters that provide the RS-232 protocol for the terminal and the modem. The MC14411 device provides selectable baud rates (maximum 9600 Baud) for the receipt and transmittal speeds of both ACIA.

It is important to set the control register of a 6850 correctly by loading the proper bit pattern into it. Table 7-2 indicates the setting of the bit pattern.

The terminal and modem sides of a serial interface use the same types of signals, but the modem side uses fewer. The Request-to-Send ($\overline{RTS}$) allows the processor to control a peripheral by entering the appropriate bit pattern into the control register of the ACIA. The other signals are Transmit Data (TX DATA), Receive Data (RX DATA), Data Terminal Ready (DTR), Clear-to-Send ($\overline{CTS}$), and Data Set Ready (DSR). These signals are needed to satisfy the RS-232 protocol between a 68000-based system and a terminal or modem.

The function of bits 0 and 1 requires further explanation. These two bits are associated with the baud rate at which ACIA receive and transmit data. As shown

100 THE 68000 MICROPROCESSOR

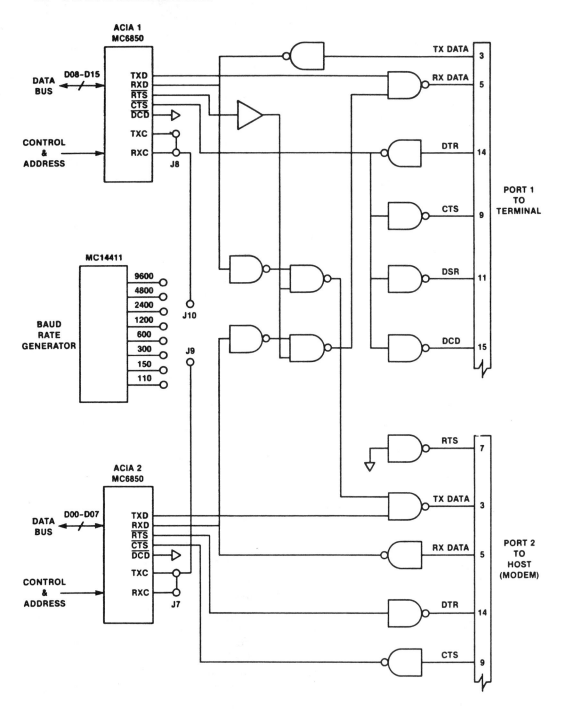

Fig. 7-5. Serial ports.

Table 7-2. ACIA Control Register Bit Setting Patterns.

BIT 7 RECEIVE INTERRUPT ENABLE	BITS 6, 5 TRANSMIT CONTROL	BITS 4, 3, 2 WORD SELECT	BITS 1, 0 COUNTER DIV.SEL
0–Disabled 1–Enabled	00–$\overline{\text{RTS}}$ low (transmit interrupt disabled) 01–$\overline{\text{RTS}}$ low (transmit interrupt enabled)	000– 7 bits, even parity, 2 stop bits 001–7, odd, 2 010–7, even, 1 011–7, odd, 1	00– ./.1 01– ./.16 10– ./.64 11–Master Reset
	10–$\overline{\text{RTS}}$ high (transmit interrupt disabled 11–$\overline{\text{RTS}}$ low (transmit interrupt disabled) Transmits a break level on transmit data output	100–8, none, 2 101–8, none, 1 110–8, even, 1 111–8, odd, 1	

in the circuit schematic in Fig. 7-5, this baud rate may be selected by various jumper connections. However, the clock divide ratio, as selected by bits 0 and 1 of the control register, affects the serial baud rate. The integrated circuit (MC14411) used for baud rate generation produces clocks that are 16 times higher in frequency than the desired serial baud rate. Thus, bits 0 and 1 set the internal counter of the ACIA to produce the proper division ratio. Use of a clock that is 16 times faster than the serial bit rate allows the ACIA to synchronize the clock with the incoming serial data. If the clock of the ACIA were equal to the serial bit rate, the ACIA could not synchronize the clock and the data. The maximum rate at which the 68000 can enter data is a function of the serial baud rate and the number of bits transmitted for each byte (including start, stop, and parity bits). This rate can be derived with the following expression:

$$\text{Update rate(bytes/second)} = \frac{\text{Baud rate(bits/second)}}{\text{No. of bits/byte}}$$

For example, if the requirement calls for 9600 baud and eight data bits with one stop bit and one start bit, the maximum update rate is 960 bytes/second (approximately one byte per msec).

The transmit-data register of the ACIA is double-buffered; that is, the register can allow a second byte to be transmitted during transmission of a first byte. The processor polls bit 1 of the ACIA status register (TDRE) to determine when data are being transferred from the transmit-data register so that new data may be entered while the previous data are being transmitted serially. An interrupt also can be generated if the transmitting interrupt bit is enabled.

102 THE 68000 MICROPROCESSOR

It is important to know, too, the function of the various bits in the ACIA status register, as previously explained.

Programming of a 6850 ACIA is fairly simple. A sample program is shown in Fig. 7-6. The program interfaces a 68000-based system with a host terminal via a 6850 ACIA. A similar program can be used for our hypothetical system.

According to the program, a character is received via the terminal and displayed on its screen. The processor determines whether transmission and reception of a character can occur by polling the status register until a character is received. The character is read by the processor and written into the ACIA's data register; from here it is transmitted to the display as soon as the transmit-data register is empty. The flowchart in Fig. 7-7 displays the activity of the program.

The EQUATE directives at the beginning of the program initialize the control, status, receiver, and transmit registers of one ACIA. If activation of both ACIA is required, the directives must be repeated (with different addresses, of course) for the second ACIA. The reset address is also assigned at this point in the program.

Several "directives" appear in the program. These are commands that a 68000 assembler uses but are not part of the processor's standard instruction set. Discussion of assemblers has been omitted from this text purposely, since discussion of any one assembler would not necessarily describe another because of their many special features.

```
            ACIASR  EQU     $0010040
            ACIACR  EQU     $0010040
            ACIADR  EQU     $0010042
            ACIATR  EQU     $0010042
            SYSTACK EQU     $0000786
            RESET   EQU     $0000008

                    DC.L    SYSTACK
                    DC.L    RESET
                    MOVE.B  #$03,ACIACR     ; Reset ACIA
                    MOVE.B  #$51,ACIACR     ; Initialize ACIA
    ERROR:          MOVE.B  ACIASR,D0       ; Get status
                    AND.B   #$7C,D0         ;  Mask IRQ,TDRA,RDA
                    BNE     ERROR           ; Any errors?

    READS1          BTST    #01,ACIASR
                    BNE     READS1
                    MOVE.B  ACIADR,D0       ; Read character

    READS2          BTST    #02,ACIASR      ; Is TDRA set?
                    BNE     READS2          ; Loop if not
                    MOVE.B  D0,ACIATR       ; Transmit character
                    BRA     ERROR           ; Start over
                    END
```

Fig. 7-6. Program to activate ACIA.

PERIPHERAL DEVICES 103

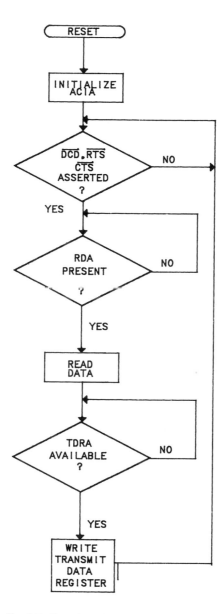

Fig. 7-7. Flowchart for program in Fig. 7-6.

The directive—DEFINE CONSTANT (DC)—allocates a 32-bit memory space that will hold the contents of the system stack pointer when the ACIA is activated. Another 32-bit space will hold the reset address.

The first instruction—MOVE.B #$03,ACIACR—produces a master reset of the ACIA by moving the following pattern into address 010040:

Bit : 7 6 5 4 3 2 1 0
0 0 0 0 0 0 1 1

The second instruction—MOVE.B #$51, ACIACR—moves the following bit pattern into the same address:

Bit : 7 6 5 4 3 2 1 0
0 1 0 1 0 0 0 1

That is, the interrupt bit is disabled, $\overline{RTS}$ is set high (transmit interrupt disabled), the data stream is set as eight bits—no parity—two stop bits, and the counter is set to divide by 16. The ACIA is thus initialized.

The next three instructions, or

```
ERROR: MOVE.B ACIASR, D0
       AND.B #$7C,D0
       BNE ERROR—
```

mask the $\overline{IRQ}$, TDRA, and RDA functions. If masking is unsuccessful, the program loops back to ERROR until masking is complete.

The next three instructions, or

```
READS1: BTST #01, ACIASR
        BNE READS1
        MOVE.B ACIADR,D0—
```

attempt to read a character. The first of these instruction tests the RDRF flag of the status register. Until this flag is set, the program reads characters and moves them into D0.

The next four instructions, or

```
READS2 : BTST #02, ACIASR
         BNE READS2
         MOVE.B D0, ACIATR
         BRA ERROR—
```

transmit a character. The TDRA flag is tested, and the character is transferred from D0, where it was originally placed during the reading operation, to the ACIA transmit register.

PARALLEL INTERFACE/TIMER

We have now come to the point of designing the printer and cassette interface. We have chosen to use the MC68230 PI/T for these circuits.

The block diagram of the MC68230 PI/T is shown in Fig. 7-8. This device provides two double-buffered, parallel-interface ports, eight general-purpose I/O pins, and one 24-bit programmable timer. The ports and the timer compose two independent sections within the PI/T. The port section consists of two eight-bit ports (Port A and Port B), four handshake lines (H1, H2, H3, and H4), and a third eight-bit

PERIPHERAL DEVICES 105

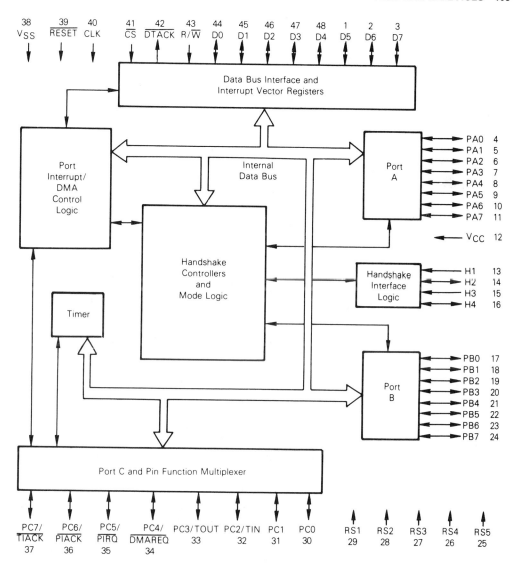

Fig. 7-8. Internal organization of the MC68230 PI/T.

port (Port C). Port C performs dual functions; six of its eight pins participate in a function associated with the timer, interrupts, or direct-memory-access requests. Ports A and B can function individually or be combined as one 16-bit parallel port. The parallel ports operate in both unidirectional and bidirectional modes. In the unidirectional mode, data-direction registers within the device determine whether the port pins are inputs or outputs. In the bidirectional mode, the registers are ignored, and the direction is determined dynamically by the state of the four handshake pins. These programmable pins provide an interface sufficiently flexible for connection to a wide variety of low-, medium-, or high-speed peripherals.

The second independent section within the PI/T, the timer, consists of a 24-bit, synchronous, presettable down-counter and a five-bit prescaler. Use of the prescaler is optional. The down-counter is clocked either by the output of the prescaler or by an external timer-input pin (one of the Port C dual-function pins). The prescaler, in turn, is clocked either by the system clock (CLK pin) or by the external timer-input pin. The MC68230 can generate periodic interrupts, a square wave, or a single interrupt after a programmed period of time. The timer can also measure elapsed time.

The PI/T has 23 registers that can be addressed from the system bus. The data bus interface is eight bits wide and connected to the low-order eight bits of the system data bus. Due to this arrangement, byte operations are valid only on odd addresses and on accesses to upper bytes; even addresses are invalid and result in a bus trap error. The PI/T occupies a 64-byte address space (32 words), although only 23 odd addresses are used for its programming. $\overline{\text{DTACK}}$ will be returned if, at any time, the other nine odd locations are accessed. These locations read as zeros, and writes to them are ignored.

DESIGNING THE PRINTER INTERFACE

The Centronix parallel printer interface is standard in the industry, and our circuit is designed to correspond to this interface.

Two real-time handshake signals are required: the $\overline{\text{DATA STROBE}}$ and $\overline{\text{ACKNLG}}$. Short data setup (50 nsec) and hold times are required with respect to the $\overline{\text{DATA STROBE}}$ signal.

Three additional printer-status signals—BUSY, PE (Printer Error), and SLCT (select)—are provided to maintain printer status. The diagram in Fig. 7-9 shows the timing requirements of the Centronix interface.

Whenever the PE signal is asserted, the printer is halted for a malfunction or other temporary interruption, such as an out-of-paper condition. Whenever SLCT is asserted, the printer is operational.

When the printer is first ready to receive data, its PE output signal furnishes a logic low, and its SLCT lines furnish a logic high. The first two signals may be connected to PC0 and PC1 of the PI/T, respectively, after inversion of the signals.

Once the printer accepts a data character, the printer returns an asserted $\overline{\text{ACKNLG}}$ pulse. After this pulse is inverted, it may be applied to the H1 line of the PI/T. The signal indicates that the printer is ready to accept a new character. If the printer is busy—either printing or performing another function, such as form feed—it outputs a BUSY signal to the PI/T. After inversion, this signal may be applied to the PA7 line of the PI/T; in this case, however, the $\overline{\text{ACKNLG}}$ signal is not asserted until the printer is again available. The interface is shown in Fig. 7-10.

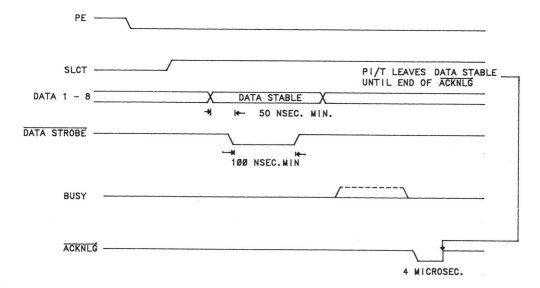

Fig. 7-9. Timing requirements of the Centronix printer interface.

Since the so-called expanded character set is not used, seven lines are adequate to transfer seven-bit ASCII-encoded characters from $20 to $7F, $0D (carriage return) and $0A (line feed). Characters that require an eight-bit ASCII code will be ignored and will be indicated by a $2E (period). Since data will be transferred from the system to the printer, the PI/T will be programmed in the unidirectional output mode, with double-buffered output transfers chosen for Port A. The term "double buffering" means that the PI/T is equipped internally with latches to hold not only the character to be transmitted but also a second character. Thus, on assertion of the corresponding transfer signals, a character becomes immediately available for transmission.

In our application, Port A is used for the transfer. Since Port B and handshake signals H3 and H4 are used, these lines may be attached to a second printer, if desired.

The seventh bit from Port A can be used as the BUSY input from the printer. When double-buffered output transfers are chosen, input pins, such as PA7, are unbuffered, and the processor can read the instantaneous level of the pin.

The H2 handshake pin is also buffered. It is used as an output DATA STROBE line to the printer and produces a four-clock cycle pulse (its duration depends on the clock speed of the processor) whenever new data are available at the pins of Port A. An ACKNLG signal from the printer is received at the H1 handshake line through a 74LS14 hex Schmitt-trigger inverted circuit. The H1 line is edge-sensitive; that is, a leading-edge pulse on H1 indicates that the printer is ready to accept new data.

108 THE 68000 MICROPROCESSOR

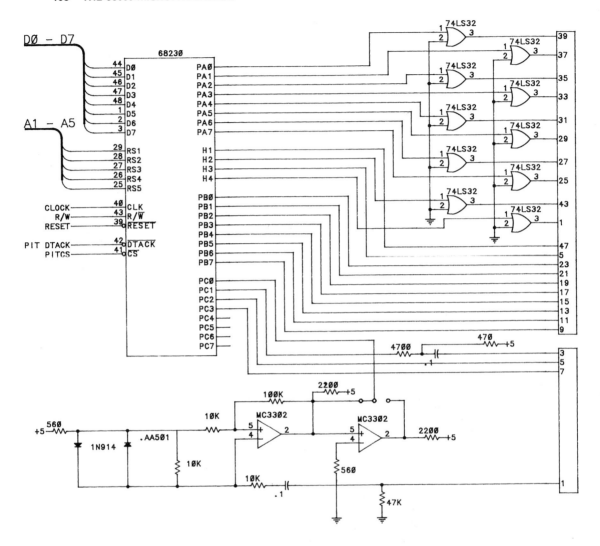

Fig. 7-10. Printer interface.

PROGRAMMING THE INTERFACE

The PI/T is located within the I/O address so that the device can be accessed whenever address line A6 equals zero. The general addressing area of the PI/T is $010000. As shown in Table 7-3, the various registers used in the printer interface are located within addresses $010001 to $01001B, inclusive. Table 7-4 shows the complete addressing range of the PI/T.

A typical program for a printer interface is shown in Fig. 7-11. The first part of the program assigns the general address of the PI/T. The other registers

Table 7-3. PI/T Registers.

REGISTER ADDRESS	7	6	5	REGISTER BIT 4	3	2	1	0	REGISTER NAME	PROGRAMMED VALUE
$10001	Port Mode Control		H34 Enable	H12 Enable	H4 Sense	H3 Sense	H2 Sense	H1 Sense	Port General Control Register	0000 0000
$10003	*	SVCRQ Select		Interrupt PFS		Port Interrupt Priority Control			Port Service Request Register	0000 0000
$10005	Bit 7	Bit 6	Bit 5	Bit 4	Bit 3	Bit 2	Bit 1	Bit 0	Port A Data Direction Register	1111 1111
$10007	Bit 7	Bit 6	Bit 5	Bit 4	Bit 3	Bit 2	Bit 1	Bit 0	Port B Data Direction Register	0000 0000
$1000D	Port A Submode		H2 Control			H2 Int Enable	H1 SVCRQ Enable	H1 Stat Ctrl	Port A Control Register	0110 0000
$1000F	Port B Submode		H4 Control			H4 Int Enable	H3 SVCRQ Enable	H3 Stat Ctrl	Port B Control Register	1010 0000
$10011	Bit 7	Bit 6	Bit 5	Bit 4	Bit 3	Bit 2	Bit 1	Bit 0	Port A Data Register	-- --
$10013	Bit 7	Bit 6	Bit 5	Bit 4	Bit 3	Bit 2	Bit 1	Bit 0	Port B Data Register	-- --
$1001B	H4 Level	H3 Level	H2 Level	H1 Level	H4S	H3S	H2S	H1S	Port Status Register	-- --

NOTE: A 0 (zero with a slash) in the programmed value indicates that the bit is programmed with different values depending on operation.

are accessed by use of the appropriate offset value from the general address. The second part of the program (LPOPEN) is the initialization routine for the interface. This routine sets up the PI/T for the unidirectional eight-bit mode; it also sets Port A as an output port and handshake Pin H2 as a pulsed output.

The first instruction in this routine is of particular interest. This instruction belongs to the Set Condition Code group. In this case, the instruction tests for the presence of the value FF in an address FINFLAG. If the value is present, the printer has finished printing and is idle. The FINFLAG label is part of the closing routine but not shown in the program.

The next five instructions move the proper bit patterns into the corresponding control registers of the PI/T (consult Table 7-3). For example, the instruction—MOVE.B #$7F, PADDR—moves the pattern 01111111 into the Port A data-direction register, making the seven bits of the register outputs and leaving bit 7 for use as a BUSY signal.

The third part of the program (LPWRITE) enables interrupts after checking the printer status. The PI/T generates an interrupt as soon as interrupts are enabled.

Table 7-4. PI/T addressing range.

ADDRESS($)	PI/T REGISTER
010001	Port General Control Register (PGCR)
010003	Port Service Request Register (PSRR)
010005	Port A Data Direction Register (PADDR)
010007	Port B Data Direction Register (PBDDR)
010009	Port C Data Direction Register (PCDDR)
01000B	Port Interrupt Vector Register (PIVR)
01000D	Port A Control Register (PACR)
01000F	Port B Control Register (PBCR)
010011	Port A Data Register (PADR)
010013	Port B Data Register (PBDR)
010015	Port A Alternate Register (PAAR)
010017	Port B Alternate Register (PBAR)
010019	Port C Data Register (PCDR)
01001B	Port Status Register (PSR)
010021	Timer Control Register (TCR)
010023	Timer Interrupt Vector Register (TIVR)
010027	Counter Preload Register High (CPRH)
010029	Counter Preload Register Middle (CPRM)
01002B	Counter Preload Register Low (CPRL)
01002F	Count Register High (CNTRH)
010031	Count Register Middle (CNTRM)
010033	Count Register Low (CNTRL)
010035	Timer Status Register (TSR)

NOTE: The PI/T address decode is redundant within page $010000. The PI/T can be accessed any time address line A6 = 0 within the page.

The fourth routine in the program (LPINTR) performs the printing task. It transfers characters from the buffer to the PI/T. After each character is received by the printer, an $\overline{ACKNLG}$ signal is sent back to the PI/T. This action moves another character to the output lines and also initiates movement of a new character to the double-buffered input.

DESIGN OF CASSETTE INTERFACE

The timer portion of the PI/T is used for the cassette interface circuitry. Information is sent to the tape as a serial stream of bits. Motorola uses the S-record, a description of which may be found in the Appendix. A logic one is represented by one period of a 2000-Hz, 50-percent duty-cycle square wave, and a logic zero is represented by one period of a 1000-Hz, 50-percent duty-cycle square wave. The serial data rate, then, is between 1000 and 2000 baud, depending on the bit stream being transmitted.

```
;                   CENTRONIX INTERFACE
;
PIT     EQU     $XXXX           ; Base address for PI/T
PGCR    EQU     PIT + 1         ; Port general control register
PSRR    EQU     PIT + 3         ; Port service request register
PADDR   EQU     PIT + 5         ; Port A data direction register
PIVR    EQU     PIT + $B        ; Port interrupt vector register
PACR    EQU     PIT + $D        ; Port A control register
PADR    EQU     PIT + $11       ; Port A data register
PCDR    EQU     PIT + $19       ; Port C data register
PSR     EQU     PIT + $1B       ; Port status register

;               LOPEN: Called once by a printer
;                      server routine.  It sets
;                      up the PI/T for unidi-
;                      rectional 8-bit mode,
;                      Port A output, H2 pulsed
;                      output handshake protocol
;
LOPEN   ST      FINFLAG         ; FF= Finished, idle
        MOVE.B  #$7F,PADDR      ; Pattern for data direction
                                ; register, 7 bits out, high bit in
        MOVE.B  #$78,PACR       ; Pattern for Port A control reg.
                                ; submode 01, pulsed
        MOVE.B  #$10,PGCR       ; Pattern for gen. control.reg.
                                ; Enable Port A, Mode 0
        MOVE.B  #$40,PIVR       ; Interrupt vector
        MOVE.B  #$18,PSRR       ; Enable interrupt pins
;
;
;               LPWRITE : User executes TRAP instruction.
;                         Trap handler sets up parameters:
;                         D0 = byte count, A0= buffer address
;                         If printer is online, routine
;                         enables just interrupts. D0=Return
;                         Status
LPWRITE CLR.B   FINFLAG         ; Starting
        MOVE.L  D0,BYTECNT      ; Save user parameters
        MOVE.L  A0,BUFFADDR
        BTST    #0,PCDR         ; In check?
        BEQ.S   NOGO
        BTST    #1,PCDR         ; On line?
        BEQ.S   LPWGO
;
NOGO    ST      D0              ; Set to all 1's
        RTS
;
LPWGO   BSET    1,PACR          ; Enable H1S interrupt
LPW1    TST.B   FINFLAG         ; Wait for FINFLAG EQU $FF
        BEQ.S   LPW1            ; OS buffering here
        CLR.B   D0              ; Normal status
        RTS                     ; Return
;
```

Fig. 7-11. Program for printer interface.

```
;
;                    LPINTR: Interrupt service routinje; it gets
;                            characters from buffer and sends them
;                            to PI/T for output to printer.
;                            Upon completion, interrupts are disabled.
;
;
LPINTR    MOVE.B    (A0)+,PADR      ; Move to PI/T
          SUBQ.L    #1,BYTECNT      ; Decrement character counter
          BEQ.L     EMPTY           ; Stop if out of characters
          BTST      #0,PSR          ; Is there room for another char?
          BNE.S     PRINTSOME       ; Yes, do it again
          BRA.S     NOTREADY        ; Not Ready
;
EMPTY     BCLR      #1,PACR         ; Disable H1S interrupts
          ST        FINFLAG         ; Set finished status
;
NOTREADY  MOVE.L    A0,BUFFADDR     ; Save buffer address
          MOVE.L    (SP)+,A0        ; Restore A0
          RTE
;
BUFFADDR  DC.L      0
BYTECNT   DC.L      0
FINFLAG   DC.L      0

          END
```

Fig. 7-11. Program for printer interface.

As with any data transfer using ASCII encoding, the effective baud rate, measured by the time required to transfer a block of data, is lower than the data rate on the transmission line. The same situation was discussed in connection with the ACIA. ASCII encoding generates a two-digit byte for every hexadecimal digit of data (for example, four becomes $34). This lower rate reduces the transfer rate by one-half. In addition, S-records require overhead bytes, such as type of S-record, address of data, number of bytes in the record, and checksums to be sent along with the data. These requirements result in an additional baud rate reduction of approximately one-third. The effective baud rate of the tape interface is between 300 and 500 baud, as opposed to the serial transmission rate of 1000 to 2000 baud.

The circuit for the cassette interface is shown in Fig. 7-12. Data are transmitted via the PC1 line of the PI/T. This line drives a voltage divider formed by R1 and R2 and is then AC-coupled to Pin 3 to the DATA OUT terminal. The voltage level from the PI/T is reduced by approximately 10-to-1 to avoid overdriving the tape-recorded input.

The DATA OUT line is normally connected to the auxiliary input of a tape recorder. The microphone input of a recorder, however, will work equally well. The various controls (tone and volume) are usually adjusted to compensate for the record-level variations between different recorders.

Data are transferred back to the processor via a DATA IN line. The Comparator U4B is used to square up the slowly changing transitions coming from the tape and to produce rapid transitions. Diodes CR1 and CR2 limit the input voltage

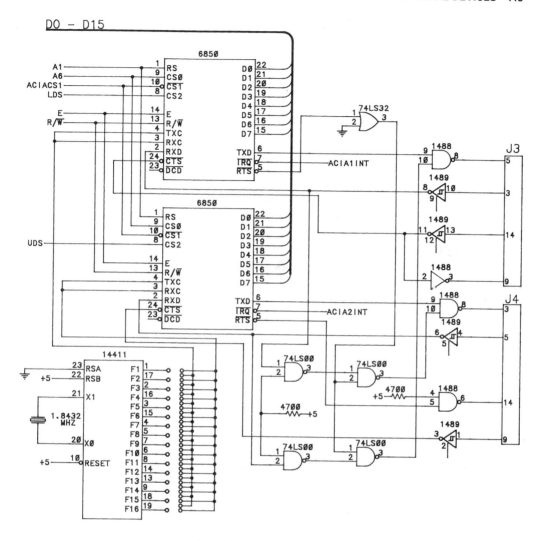

Fig. 7-12. Cassette interface.

swing of the comparator. Approximately 450 mV of hysteresis are used on the comparator.

A second comparator, U4A, is used to invert the output of U4B. This feature may or may not be required, depending on the type of recorder used. Some recorders play back a signal that is inverted from the original input signal; others return a noninverted signal. Comparator U4B simply inverts the playback signal. If the recorder does not produce a second inversion, one must be produced using the comparator U4A in order to provide the proper signal to the tape driver/receiver firmware. Such a program undoubtedly expects a noninverted signal.

Chapter 8
Another 68000-Based System

The hypothetical system described in the previous chapters is somewhat too complex to build on a prototyping board. It is, however, desirable for the reader to build a small system and to use it to gain programming experience.

The system described in this chapter was designed and built by Edward M. Carter of the United States Air Force Academy and A. B. Bonds of Vanderbilt University (members of their respective Computer Science Departments). Its builders named the system *VU68K*.

HARDWARE DESCRIPTION

The VU68K system is small and has a limited amount of memory and a limited number of input-output ports. The memory map, however, allows for expansion of both the memory capacity and the I/O capabilities.

Figure 8-1 shows the complete schematic of the VU68K. It is a good pedagogical tool, and the fact that only 15 integrated circuits are used attests to the system's simplicity. In fact, the system has many similarities to the hypothetical design described earlier. Several points on the VU68K, however, require further clarification.

Only the memories in the VU68K operate in the asynchronous mode. Since these devices do not have an acknowledge signal, the signal is synthesized with the 74161 counter instead. When $\overline{AS}$ goes low, an initial count of 1100 is loaded into the 74161. After four clock cycles, the high-order output bit of the counter, connected to the $\overline{DTACK}$ line, goes low, asserting $\overline{DTACK}$ and thereby signaling the availability of data. With a clock speed of 5 MHz, a transfer takes place in 800 nsec.

The baud-rate generator is the same circuit used in the hypothetical design. This circuit provides the receiving and transmitting speed for the two ACIA devices used in the design. ACIA No. 1 connects the VU68K to a terminal via IC15 and IC14 line transceivers. This ACIA resides at address $A00000 to $A00002. ACIA No. 2 may be used for connection with a modem. This ACIA resides at $C00000 to $C00002. When either ACIA is selected, address line A23, which is connected to the $\overline{VPA}$ line, must be high to assert $\overline{VPA}$ via inverter IC3. After a transfer, the processor resumes its synchronous operation. This scheme, however, limits addresses using A23 to synchronous devices only.

ANOTHER 68000-BASED SYSTEM 115

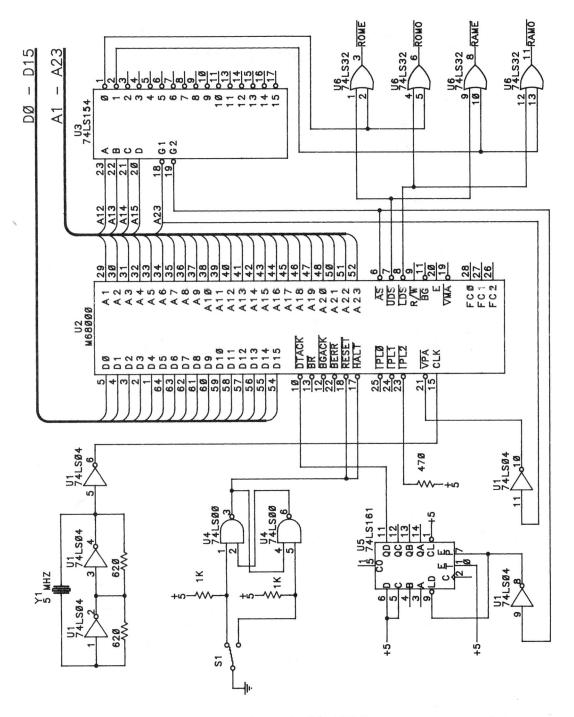

Fig.8-1 Schematic of the VU68K.
(part 1 of 3)

116 THE 68000 MICROPROCESSOR

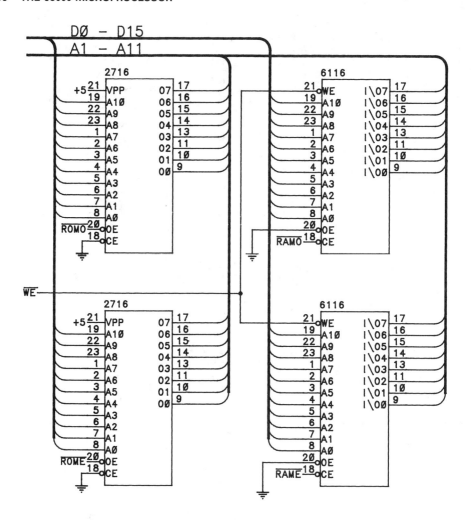

Fig.8-1 Schematic of the VU68K.
(part 2 of 3)

The VU68K uses the autovectored mode for interrupts and acknowledges only two levels of interrupt: Level 1 for keyboard serial-port interrupts and Level 2 for communication serial-port interrupts. The interrupts are signaled on the $\overline{IPL}$ lines. $\overline{IPL2}$ is always maintained high. This interrupt scheme allows the simultaneous use of the keyboard and the serial communication ports.

Address decoding is straightforward. The memory of the VU68K is divided into 2K-word by 16-bit blocks, with total expansion capability of 32K words. The reason for this arrangement is that the VU68K uses only 11 of the 68000's address bits for word selection and another four address bits for memory-block selection. The 11 bits select one of the 2K words, whereas the other four bits select one of the 16 2K-word blocks. Since each block contains 2K words, the total memory capacity is 2K by 16 or 32K words.

Fig. 8-1 Schematic of the VU68K.
(part 3 of 3)

The word-selection bits, A1 through A11, go directly to each of the ROM and RAM devices. The block-selection bits, A12 through A15, are connected to a 4-to-16 decoder. The decoder and some OR gates (IC6) assert a selected 2K-word block. The $\overline{\text{UDS}}$ and $\overline{\text{LDS}}$ lines are used, as previously described, to select byte or word accessing. Thus, four signals—$\overline{\text{ROME}}$, $\overline{\text{ROMO}}$, $\overline{\text{RAME}}$, and $\overline{\text{RAMO}}$—are used in conjunction with $\overline{\text{UDS}}$ and $\overline{\text{LDS}}$ to select the two ROM and the two RAM devices.

The memory map of the system is set forth in Table 8-1. Extension of the memory size and the number of peripheral devices is not complicated. Extended memory can reside in the lower 64K bytes of the memory map. The high-order bits of a new address in that area cause one of the pins of the address decoder to go low. The output from this pin can then be used by additional logic to select a new device. For example, assume that another 2K-word block of memory is to be added to the system. Two additional 6116 devices can reside at $002000 to $002FFF. The new RAM-select line will be Pin 3 of the IC5 decoder; two additional OR gates must be added to combine this select line with the $\overline{\text{LDS}}$ and $\overline{\text{UDS}}$ signals.

A new peripheral device, such as a 6850, can be added in an address that sets A23 high, i.e., between $800000 and $FFFFFF. For example, a new ACIA can be added in the addresses $900000 to $900002. This address area does not conflict with the other two ACIA devices. The high select-line will be A20, and the low select-line will be A21. To enhance the interrupt structure so that not all of the interrupts are handled in the autovectored mode, we must ensure that the synchronous mode-select line is still driven high when the terminal and serial ports are addressed. Discrete gates easily provide this facility.

THE OPERATING SYSTEM MONITOR

We now proceed to develop an operating system program, more commonly known as the *monitor*. This program oversees the entire operation of the VU68K by providing several services, such as commands to fill and examine memory, character input and output routines, trap handlers, and error-handling routines. We call this monitor *VUBUG*.

The VUBUG provides two support services. The first is buffered I/O for both the terminal and the serial communication port. All incoming and outgoing information is temporarily stored in an area in memory called "buffer." The interrupt-handling routines for these two I/O devices are at Levels 1 and 2, respectively. As an interrupt is generated during the transfer of a character, the port is read,

Table 8-1. Memory Map of the VU68K.

ADDRESS	DEVICE
$000000 to $000FFF	ROM
$001000 to $001FFF	RAM
$A00000 to $A00002	ACIA No. 1
$C00000 to $C00002	ACIA No. 2

Table 8-2. User-Interrupt Vectors.

VECTOR ADDRESS	INTERRUPT
$1000	User-Trap Vector B
$1004	User-Trap Vector C
$1008	User-Trap Vector D
$100C	User-Trap Vector E
$1010	User-Trap Vector F
$1014	User-Interrupt Vector 1
$1018	User-Interrupt Vector 2
$101C	User-Interrupt Vector 3
$1020	User-Interrupt Vector 4
$1024	User-Interrupt Vector 5
$1028	AutoVector Level 3
$102C	AutoVector Level 4
$1030	AutoVector Level 5
$1034	AutoVector Level 6
$1038	AutoVector Level 7

and the character is placed in a circular buffer that can store 16 bytes. Data are retrieved from the memory buffer area by a trap routine, which will be discussed later. Interrupts from the terminal's keyboard also cause the character typed to be echoed immediately. Writing to both the terminal and serial communication port is accomplished by a technique called *bus-wait* so that further interrupts are disabled until the I/O transfer is complete. Due to the location of these ports at different interrupt levels, separate interrupt routines and buffers are used, and both ports are accessible simultaneously.

The second support service of the VUBUG is interrupt handling by loading into memory five autovector, five user-interrupt vector, and five user-trap vector locations. See Table 8-2.

Each vector address in Table 8-2 may be used to hold a branch instruction to the corresponding user exception-handling routine. Each vector occupies a four-byte address, thus allowing a branch with a 16-bit displacement. Each exception-handling routine must terminate with an RTE instruction to ensure return to the correct location in the main program.

When the system is reset, the reset vector initializes the system stack, terminal and serial communication ports, and circular buffers. On completion of these tasks, the system enters the "command" mode; the user can then enter a desired command to have the monitor perform a task.

MONITOR COMMANDS

While a program is being executed, control of the system can be regained at any time by typing a ctrl-c (CONTROL-C), or output to the terminal's screen can be terminated by typing ctrl-s. Transmission to the screen can be resumed by typing ctrl-q. After ctrl-s and before ctrl-q, the processor is in a wait-state but will accept and place in buffer memory characters from either the terminal or modem port until the assigned buffer memory area is full. Thereafter, any new characters will be lost. Zero padding of all values is required.

We will now briefly describe the function of each command of the VUBUG. The number of "x's" denotes the number of characters to be entered; e.g., "xx" denotes two characters and "xxxx" denotes four characters. The notation "⟨cr⟩" denotes the "carriage return" or "enter" key on the terminal keyboard.

The "b" Command: Set/Remove Breakpoints

The "b" command implements the breakpoint function. A breakpoint is set by assigning an address to a command, as follows:

b+xxxx	Insert a breakpoint at address xxxx
b−xxxx	Remove a breakpoint at address xxxx
b⟨cr⟩	Show all breakpoints
b#	Remove all breakpoints

A breakpoint allows execution of a program segment up to the address of the breakpoint. The program is halted at that address, and VUBUG enters the command mode. At the next "g" (go) command, the original instruction is reinserted and executed. After execution, the breakpoint instruction is reinserted. Breakpoint and single-step modes cannot be active concurrently, but tracing is permitted with breakpoints.

The "c" Command: Copy Memory Blocks

The "c" command allows data blocks to be copied from one memory area to another. Its format is "c xxxx=yyyy,zzzz−i.e., copy from address yyyy through address zzzz to consecutively increasing addresses starting at xxxx.

The "d" Command: Display Data to Terminal

The "d" command displays data at some address block in memory on the screen. This command uses a memory examination pointer to "remember" the last block of data displayed. The starting address of data to be displayed is truncated to the nearest 16-byte boundary, and the terminating address is rounded to the next highest 16-byte boundary. The formats of this command are as follows:

d⟨cr⟩	Display the next 80 bytes from the last displayed address
d xxxx,⟨cr⟩	Display 80 bytes starting at address xxxx
d xxxx,yyyy	Display all data between locations xxxx and yyyy, inclusive

The "e" Command: Enter Terminal Emulator Mode

The "e" command allows the VU68K to communicate as a terminal with a host system attached to the serial communication port. The host system must operate in full duplex mode, and the terminal configuration must be set correctly, using either the "m" command or a user program. The VU68K remains in terminal emulator mode until the user types either ctrl-x or ctrl-l. The former terminates the emulator mode and places the VUBUG in command mode, whereas the latter also invokes the "l" command to allow transfer of data from the host via the serial communication port.

The "g" Command: Execute a User Program

The "g" command initiates execution of a user program from the address following the command or the last known address following a load, breakpoint, or single-step command. When a program is halted, a copy is made of all registers, including PC, SR, and address and data registers. The "g" command reinstates the values saved from the last program halt. These values may be modified by the "r" command. The formats of the "g" command are as follows:

g‹cr›	Execute user program starting at the address in the PC following a load, breakpoint, single-step, or "r" command
‹cr›	Same as g‹cr›
g xxxx	Execute a program starting at address xxxx

The "l" Command: Load Program from Host (S-format)

The "l" command allows the loading of a program from a host external system via the serial communication port. The program object code must be in the Motorola S-Format. Following the "l" command, the value saved in the user PC is the value of the start of the loaded program. The formats of the "l" command are as follows:

l‹cr›	Start program load
l xxxx	Start program load and offset each block by xxxx bytes

The "m" Command: Examine/Modify Memory

The "m" command examines and modifies the contents of a memory location. To facilitate its use, a pointer holds the memory location accessed last. The pointer is manipulated by several subcommands and maintains its value between invocations of the "m" command, the formats of which are as follows:

m‹cr›	Start memory mode
m xxxx	Start memory mode and set pointer at address xxxx
.xxxx	Set pointer to xxxx
=xx	Store value xx at address in pointer
,xx	Increment pointer and store xx
+	Increment pointer and display value at address in pointer
−	Decrement pointer and display value at address in pointer

The "p" Command: Load/Execute a Prototype Command

The "p" command allows execution of a prototype command in system mode. The only restriction placed on a prototype command is that is must be completed with an RTS instruction to relinquish control to the command processor. The formats of this command are as follows:

px yyyy	Associate with px the program starting at address yyyy, where x
px yyyy	is 1, 2, or 3
px‹cr›	Execute command px, where x is 1, 2, or 3

The "r" Command: Examine/Modify Registers

The "r" command is used to examine and modify the contents of any of the registers, including the user status register and user program counter. As with the "m" command, the "r" command maintains a pointer to the register accessed last, and all modifications are relative to this pointer. To exit the "r" command, an invalid subcommand is entered. The formats of the "r" command are as follows:

r‹cr›	Start register mode
r xx	Start register mode at register xx, where xx is:
	SR/sr Status Register
	PC/pc Program Counter
	D0/d0–D7/d7 Data registers
	A0/a0–A7/a7 Address registers
.xx	Set register pointer to register xx
=xxxxxxxx	Store value in register at pointer value for SR xxxx
‹cr›	Display values of all registers

The "s" Command: Single-Step Mode

The "s" command allows execution of a program, instruction-by-instruction. Invocation of the "s" command removes all breakpoints and turns the trace command off. The single-step command uses the T bit of the status register and, as with the trace command, is limited to single-step trap and interrupt-handling routines.

    The single-step function can be reinstated by setting the trace bit in the service routine. The displayed value of the program counter is the location of the next instruction to be executed. The single-step function does not start until the next "g" command for the user program is invoked. Consecutive single-stepping is accomplished by typing a carriage return.

    The formats of the "s" command are as follows:

s+	Start single-step function
s−	Stop single-step function

The "t" Command: Trace Program Execution

The "t" command traces a program instruction-by-instruction. The program counter value is printed *before* the execution of each instruction. Tracing and breakpoints are allowed to be active at the same time. The tracing of trap instructions renders the trace function inactive during the execution of the trap-handling routine; the function is reinstated, however, after the RTE instruction of the routine.

Traps may be traced by setting the trace bit in the status register upon entering the trap-handling routine. Tracing actually starts on issuance of the "g" command for a user program.

The formats of the "t" command are as follows:

t+	Start trace
t−	Stop trace

TRAPS

The VUBUG program provides eleven traps with which to service user-program requests. These traps are invoked by execution of the corresponding trap instruction shown in Table 8-3.

The value that the "get" trap returns in D0 is zero-padded so that the data read are of the correct size and do not contain erroneous bits. Data passed to the write functions need not be padded. The parameter to Trap No. 8 is the address of the string to be written. The string must be terminated by a zero. VUBUG uses address register A0 and data register D0 as working registers. Consequently, a user should not depend on values in these registers remaining the same before and after the execution of a trap.

In Table 8-3, a byte refers to two input characters that are converted to hexadecimal and packed into a single byte of memory, whereas a character is a single-

Table 8-3. VUBUG Traps.

TRAP	FUNCTION	PARAMETER	RETURN
0	Exit	None	None
1	Get byte	None	D0
2	Get word	None	D0
3	Get longword	None	D0
4	Write byte	D0	None
5	Write word	D0	None
6	Write longword	D0	None
7	Get character	None	D0
8	Write string	A0	None
9	Write character	D0	None
A	Write cr-lf	None	None

input character. In addition to the traps listed in Table 8-3, a user is provided with Traps B through F, with vectors at the locations shown in Table 8-2.

EXCEPTION PROCESSING

The VUBUG also makes provision for handling errors. The error-handling routine intercepts an interrupt caused by an error and displays a message on the terminal screen. In addition, register values are copied into the register save area, where they are accessible via the "r" command. Trapped errors include address/bus errors, illegal instruction errors, privilege violations, and a class of generic errors that share a single error-handling routine. The errors in this last category include zero-divide, CHK, TRAPV, and spurious interrupts.

THE MONITOR

We will now proceed with a detailed description of the monitor. This program, written by Edward M. Carter, is the property of the Computer Science Departments of the United States Air Force Academy and Vanderbilt University. VUBUG may be used in single systems for educational purposes but is not to be sold for commercial purposes.

The first part of the monitor assigns values to be used to structure a queue, as follows:

```
             ;Queue structure
                ORG     $0
     HEAD:      DC.W    #1,#0000
     TAIL:      DC.W    #1,#0000
     COUNT:     DC.W    #1,#0000
     QUEUE:     DB      #10,#00
```

The next part of the program defines constants that structure the breakpoint area:

```
             ;Breakpoint structure
                ORG $0
     INSTR:     DC.W    #1,#000
     ILOC:      DC.W    #1,#0000
```

The vector table must be located in the lower memory area. (A restriction at this point is that there should be no "ORG" directives to the addresses contained in the constants shown, because such directives will destroy the vector for interrupts and breakpoints.)

```
     ORG $0              ;Reset Vector
     DC.L  #1,STACK      ;System Stack
     DC.L  #1,START      ;Initial PC
     DC.L  #1,ABHLR      ;Bus Error
     DC.L  #1,ABHLR      ;Address Error
     DC.L  #1,BHLR       ;Illegal Instruction
     DC.L  #1,GHLR       ;Zero Divide
     DC.L  #1,GHLR       ;CHK
```

ANOTHER 68000-BASED SYSTEM

```
        DC.L #1,GHLR            ;TRAPV
        DC.L #1,PHLR            ;Privileged Instruction
        DC.L #1,THLR            ;Trace Routine
        DC.L #1,BHLR            ;Emulator Trap 1010
        DC.L #1,BHLR            ;Emulator Trap 1111
        ORG $3C
        DC.L #1,GHLR            ;Uninitialized Interrupt
        ORG $60
        DC.L #1,GHLR            ;Spurious Interrupt
```

As mentioned earlier, several errors share the same handling routine. For example, zero divide, CHK, and TRAPV all share the "GHLR" routine.

Examination of the vector table in Chap. 6 reveals that the ORG addresses the VUBUG uses in the assignment of vectors are the same as the vector addresses shown in the table. For example, ORG $3C is shown in the table as the vector address for the uninitialized interrupt-handling routine.

The autovector area is assigned next, as follows:

```
        DC.L #1,ININT           ;Terminal Vector
        DC.L #1,LPINT           ;Download-Line Vector
```

These locations are vector addresses $64 and $68, respectively, and correspond to autovector No. 1 and autovector No. 2. The locations are used for the terminal-handling routine and the serial communication-port routine.

The remaining autovectors, at $6C through $7C, are left for the user, as follows:

```
        DC.L #1,$1028           ;User Autovector No. 3
        DC.L #1,$102C           ;User Autovector No. 4
        DC.L #1,$1030           ;User Autovector No. 5
        DC.L #1,$1034           ;User Autovector No. 6
        DC.L #1,$1038           ;User Autovector No. 7
```

The traps in Table 8-3 are assigned next, as follows:

```
        DC.L #1,TEXIT           ;Trap 0, Exit
        DC.L #1,TGETB           ;Trap 1, Get Byte
        DC.L #1,TGETW           ;Trap 2, Get Word
        DC.L #1,TGETL           ;Trap 3, Get Longword
        DC.L #1,TWRTB           ;Trap 4, Write Byte
        DC.L #1,TWRTW           ;Trap 5, Write Word
        DC.L #1,TWRTL           ;Trap 6, Write Longword
        DC.L #1,TGETC           ;Trap 7, Get Character
        DC.L #1,TWRTS           ;Trap 8, Write String
        DC.L #1,TWRTC           ;Trap 9, Write Character
        DC.L #1,TCRLF           ;Trap 10, Write Carriage
                                ;Return, Line Feed
```

We can also define the user-trap vectors B through F in Table 8-2, as follows:

```
UTRPB:  DC.L #1,$1000           ;User Trap Vector B
UTRPC:  DC.L #1,$1004           ;User Trap Vector C
UTRPD:  DC.L #1,$1008           ;User Trap Vector D
UTRPE:  DC.L #1,$100C           ;User Trap Vector E
UTRPF:  DC.L #1,$1010           ;User Trap Vector F
```

These vectors are located within the trap vector area in Table 8-2 ($80 to $BC).

We must now assign a memory area for the system stack (80 words), an area for the storage table of breakpoint numbers, an area for the contents of all of the registers, and other areas clearly marked in the listing. The data area for these constants begins at $103C, a location past the vector area.

The asterisk used is an assembler directive and serves as the symbolic name of the assembler location counter. We may think of it as expressing the idea "*—the address of myself." For example, consider the instruction "10 JUMP ##*" situated at location 10. This instruction directs the processor, in effect, to "jump to myself" since the assembler location counter contains the value 10 in this example, and the instruction will be translated as a jump to location 10 *from* location 10. This scheme is used when the processor is to wait for an interrupt.

The assembler location counter should not be confused with the processor's program counter. The program counter always contains a value two bytes greater than that of the assembler location counter, and this is often the address of the next instruction to be executed. In the following case, the stack will be equated to hexadecimal address 113C [80 decimal is 50 hex; this is multiplied by 2 (word size), yielding hexadecimal 100].

```
            ORG $103C
SAREA:      DC.W #80,#0000      ;Clear an area of 80 words
                                ;to be used as system
                                ;stack
STACK:      EQU *
```

An area must be reserved for the breakpoint table (ten locations), as follows:

```
BKTAB:      DC.W #0A,#0000
```

Save areas must also be reserved for all of the registers. Each of these areas is 32 bits long, with the exception of that for the status register, which is 16 bits long. The save areas are as follows:

```
SR:         DC.W #1,#0000           ;Status Register Save Area
PC:         DC.L #1,#00000000       ;PC Save Area
D0:         DC.L #1,#00000000       ;D0 Save Area
D1:         DC.L #1,#00000000       ;D1 Save Area
D2:         DC.L #1,#00000000       ;D2 Save Area
D3:         DC.L #1,#00000000       ;D3 Save Area
D4:         DC.L #1,#00000000       ;D4 Save Area
D5:         DC.L #1,#00000000       ;D5 Save Area
D6:         DC.L #1,#00000000       ;D6 Save Area
D7:         DC.L #1,#00000000       ;D7 Save Area
A0:         DC.L #1,#00000000       ;A0 Save Area
A1:         DC.L #1,#00000000       ;A1 Save Area
A2:         DC.L #1,#00000000       ;A2 Save Area
A3:         DC.L #1,#00000000       ;A3 Save Area
A4:         DC.L #1,#00000000       ;A4 Save Area
A5:         DC.L #1,#00000000       ;A5 Save Area
A6:         DC.L #1,#00000000       ;A6 Save Area
A7:         DC.L #1,#00000000       ;A7 Save Area
```

Three word-length areas are reserved for the prototype table:

```
PTAB:       DC.W #3,#0000           ;Prototype Table
```

The register examination pointer and the memory examination pointer each require one word-length area:

```
REXAM:  DC.W #1,#0000    ;Register Examination Pointer
EXAM:   DC.W #1,#0000    ;Memory Examination Pointer
```

We now reserve five temporary work areas—each with the length of one word—that will be used by various subroutines:

```
        T1:     DC.W #1,#0000    ;Temporary Work Area
        T2:     DC.W #1,#0000
        T3:     DC.W #1,#0000
        T4:     DC.W #1,#0000
        T5:     DC.W #1,#0000
```

The following areas are reserved for the terminal buffer, user stack, breakpoint flag, ctrl-s, and ctrl-q:

```
        CTRLS:  DC.W #1,#0000    ;Ctrl-s, Ctrl-q Flag
        BKPTF:  EQU *-1          ;Breakpoint Flag
        LBUFF:  DC.W #0B,#0000   ;Load Buffer
        IBUFF:  DC.W #0B,#0000   ;Terminal Buffer
        USERS:  DC.W #80,#0000   ;User's Stack Area
        USTCK:  EQU *
```

Finally, we assign addresses for the terminal ACIA and the serial communication ACIA:

```
                ;Terminal
                ;
        TTYST:  EQU $A00000
        TTYD:   EQU $A00002
                ;Load Port
                ;
        LPST:   EQU $C00000
        LPD:    EQU $C00002
```

The main program starts at address $00C0. Three storage locations are defined first: for the sign-on message, for the carriage return and linefeed, and for the "bad command" message, which will be invoked whenever an incorrect command character is entered. All three character strings are terminated by a zero.

```
        ; Start of Monitor
        ;
                ORG $C0
        HOWDY:  DS "\cMC68000 Monitor VUBUG\0"
        RNNO:   DS "\r\n\n\0"
        BCOMM:  DS ": Bad Command\r\n\0"
```

Next we reserve space for seven user-interrupt vectors, which must remain at address $0100. The vectors include the bit pattern that must be inserted in the supervisor status register, with or without interrupts enabled. That is, the pattern 2000 (binary 0010000000000000) will set the S flag and keep the remaining flags at zero. The pattern 2700 will set the S flag and the interrupt mask pattern at the highest level (111), which will disable interrupts. Finally, storage is defined for the initial prompt (!).

```
        VECT1:  DC.L #1,$1014
```

128 THE 68000 MICROPROCESSOR

```
VECT2:  DC.L #1,$1018
VECT3:  DC.L #1,$101C
VECT4:  DC.L #1,$1020
VECT5:  DC.L #1,$1024
SSRI:   DC.W #1,#2000      ;Supervisor SR, interrupts
SSRN:   DC.W #1,#2700      ;Supervisor SR, no interrupts
PRMP:   DS "\r\n!\0"       ;Prompt (!)
```

The next sequence of events takes care of several "housekeeping chores"; for example, some typical tasks would be the following:

1. Initialize the input-output ports (ACIA)
2. Set up the various buffers and queues
3. Initialize various control variables
4. Clear the breakpoint table area
5. Clear the register save area
6. Set the user stack pointer
7. Clear the system stack
8. Enable interrupt mask
9. Display sign-on message
10. Enable interrupts for ports
11. Enter command mode

```
        START:  MOVE.B #03,TTYST       ;Set up terminal ACIA
                MOVE.B #09,TTYST
                MOVE.B #03,LPST        ;Set up serial communication
                                       ;for ACIA
                MOVE.B #09,LPST
                LEA IBUFF,A1           ;Set buffers
                MOVE #0,HEAD(A1)
                MOVE #FFFF,TAIL(A1)
                MOVE #0,COUNT(A1)
                LEA LBUFF,A1
                MOVE #0,HEAD(A1)       ;Set up queue for lp
                MOVE #FFFF,TAIL(A1)
                MOVE #0,COUNT(A1)
                MOVE #0,EXAM           ;Initialize control
                MOVE.B #0,CTRLS        ;Variables
                MOVE.B #0,BKPTF
                MOVEQ #4,D0            ;Clear breakpoint table
                LEA BKTAB,A1
        SLP:    MOVE.L #0,(A1)+
                DBF D0,SLP
                MOVE #0,SR             ;Clear register save area
                MOVE #10,D0
                LEA PC,A0
        SLP1:   MOVE.L #0,(A0)+
                DBF D0,SLP1
```

ANOTHER 68000-BASED SYSTEM

```
            LEA USTCK,A0          ;Set user stack pointer
            MOVE.L A0,A7
            LEA SAREA,A0          ;Clear system stack
            MOVEQ #3F,D0
    SLP2:   MOVE.L #0,(A0)+
            DBF D0,SLP2
    DONE:   MOVE SSRI,SR          ;Enable interrupt mask
            LEA HOWDY,A0          ;Display sign-on
            BSR WRITS
            MOVE.B #89,TTYST      ;Enable terminal ACIA
                                  ;interrupts
            MOVE.B #89,LPST       ;Enable serial communication
                                  ;ACIA
            BRA COMM              ;Enter command mode
```

The next several routines are concerned with output. The first routine outputs one byte held in D0 to the terminal ACIA; it begins by checking whether a ctrl-s has been typed (as we have mentioned, a ctrl-s terminates output to the terminal):

```
    WRIT:   BTST #0,CTRLS         ;Check for ctrl-s
            BEQ CWRIT             ;No, write byte
            STOP #2000            ;Yes, wait for next character
            BRA WRIT              ;When ready, try to echo
    CWRIT:  MOVE.B D0,TTYD        ;Write character to port
    WRITA:  MOVE.B TTYST,D0       ;Sample control register
            BTST #1,D0
            BEQ WRITA
            RTS
```

The next routine is associated with the serial communication port; the routine outputs a byte held in D0 to that port:

```
    WRITU:  MOVE.B D0,LPD         ;Write it
    WRITP:  MOVE.B LPST,D0        ;Wait for completion
            BTST #1,D0
            BEQ WRITP
            RTS
```

The following routine outputs a string, which must be terminated with a zero:

```
    WRITS:  MOVE.B (A0)+,D0       ;A0 is address of string
            BEQ DWRTS
            BSR WRIT
            BRA WRITS
    DWRTS:  RTS
```

The next routine outputs a word, byte, or longword:

```
    WRITB:  MOVE #1,T1            ;T1 is the number of bytes
            BRA WR
    WRITW:  MOVE #3,T1
            BRA WR
    WRITL:  MOVE #7,T1
    WR:     MOVEM.L #6002,-(A7)   ;Save registers
            MOVE T1,D2            ;Set count
```

```
              MOVE.B #00,t5+1           ;Write a zero at end
              LEA t5+1,A6               ;Use temporary register as
                                        ;a stack
```

The next set of instructions converts each hexadecimal digit to an ASCII byte. A character has already been read and is held in D0. The character is transferred to D1, and the routine determines whether the character is within the valid (0–9, A–F) hexadecimal limits.

```
    ALP:      MOVE D0,D1                ;Make each hex digit a
              ANDI.B #0F,D1             ;valid ASCII byte
              CMPI.B #0A,D1             ;Check if ABCDEF
              BLT OR3
              ORI.B #40,D1
              SUB.B #09,D1
              BRA M1
    OR3:      ORI.B #30,D1              ;Set high-order bits
    M1:       MOVE.B D1,-(A6)           ;Put on stack
              LSR.L #4,D0               ;Get next hex digit
              DBF D2,ALP
              MOVEA A6,A0               ;Write the stack
              BSR WRITS
              MOVEM.L (A7)+,#4006       ;Restore registers
              RTS
```

The next program segment constitutes the "command processor." The various characters entered via the keyboard will be checked for validity, and then control will be branched to a location defined by the command processor.

```
    CTAB:     DC.W #1,#4D00             ;m--memory update
              DC.W #1,mem
              DC.W #1,#4C00             ;l--load from host
              DC.W #1,load
              DC.W #1,0C00              ;ctrl-l, another load from
                                        ;host
              DC.W #1,lnoof
              DC.W #1,#4400             ;d--dump contents of
                                        ;memory
              DC.W #1,dump
              DC.W #1,#5300             ;s--single step
              DC.W #1,singl
              DC.W #1,#5400             ;t--trace
              DC.W #1,trace
              DC.W #1,#4700             ;g--execute program
              DC.W #1,go
              DC.W #1,#0D00             ;<cr>--short "g"
              DC.W #1,ggo               ;command
              DC.W #1,#4500             ;e--enter terminal
              DC.W #1,emul              ;emulator mode
              DC.W #1,#4200             ;b--set/remove
              DC.W #1,bkpt              ;breakpoints
              DC.W #1,#4300             ;c--copy memory blocks
              DC.W #1,copy
```

ANOTHER 68000-BASED SYSTEM

```
            DC.W #1,#5200           ;r--display/modify registers
            DC.W#1,regs
            DC.W #1,#5000           ;p--prototype command
            DC.W #1,proto
```

The next set of instructions constructs a routine in which the structure of each entry is command (com) and address of servicing routine (code):

```
    COM:    EQU $0
    CODE:   EQU $2
    COMM:   LEA PRMP,A0             ;Display prompt
            BSR WRITS
            BSR GETCH               ;Get command from buffer
            ANDI.B #DF,D0           ;Make upper-case
            LEA CTAB-4,A2           ;Set up search of command
                                    ;processor
            MOVEQ #0C,D2            ;Count is one less
    CLP:    ADDQ #4,A2
            CMP.B COM(A2),D0
            DBEQ D2,CLP
            BNE BAD                 ;Search fails
            MOVEA CODE(A2),A2       ;Get address for success
            JSR(A2)                 ;Go to it
            BRA COMM                ;Loop back for next command
    BAD:    LEA BCOMM,A0            ;Display "bad" message
            BSR WRITS
            BRA COMM
```

The next sequence of instruction is concerned with the input of a character from the keyboard. The routine stores an input character in a buffer whose address is contained in A1.

```
    ININT:  MOVE SSRN,SR            ;Disable interrupts
            MOVEM.L #C060,-(A7)     ;Save registers
            MOVE.B TTYD,D1          ;Get character
            BTST#3,BKPTF            ;In emulator mode?
            BEQ INCMP               ;No, so continue
            CMPI.B #0C,D1           ;Ctrl-1?
            BEQ INLD                ;Yes, so load
            CMP.B #18,D1            ;No, ctrl-x?
            BNE INWRU               ;No, so write it
    INLD:   BCLR #3,BKPTF           ;Exit emulator mode
            LEA EMUDN,A1            ;Set up return
            MOVE.L A1,#12(A7)       ;Put return deep in stack
            CMPI.B #0C,D1           ;Ctrl-1?
            BNE OUT                 ;No
            BRA INCMP               ;Check for ctrl-s or
                                    ;ctrl-q
    INWRU:  MOVE D1,D0              ;Write to host
            BSR WRITU
            BRA OUT
    INCMP:  CMPI.B #03,D1           ;Check for ctrl-c
```

132 THE 68000 MICROPROCESSOR

```
                BEQ RSTRT
                CMPI.B #13,D1           ;Check for ctrl-s
                BNE CTRLQ
                MOVE.B #1,CTRLS
                BRA OUT
        CTRLQ:  CMPI.B #11,D1           ;Check for ctrl-q
                BNE C1
                MOVE.B #0,CTRLS
                BRA OUT
        C1:     LEA IBUFF,A1            ;Get buffer address
                CMPI #10,COUNT(A1)      ;Overflow?
                BLT CONT                ;No
                BRA OUT                 ;Yes, so ignore
        CONT:   ADDQ #1,TAIL(A1)        ;Add character to buffer
                ADDQ #1,COUNT(A1)       ;Add one to count
                ANDI #0F,TAIL(A1)       ;Modulo-16
                MOVEA TAIL(A1),A2       ;Get offset of new entry
                LEA QUEUE(A1),A1        ;Get address of queue
                MOVE.B D1,#0(A1,A2)     ;Move byte into buffer
                MOVE.B D1,D0            ;Set up for echo
                BSR WRIT
        OUT:    MOVEM.L (A7)+,#0603     ;Restore registers
                RTE
```

A similar outine must be designed for the serial communications port:

```
        LPINT:  MOVE SSRN,SR            ;Disable interrupts
                MOVEM.L #C060,-(A7)     ;Save registers
                MOVE.B LPD,D1           ;Get character
                BTST #3,BKPTF           ;In emulator mode?
                BEQ LPLEA               ;No, so continue
                MOVE D1,D0              ;Echo for emulator mode
                BSR WRIT
                BRA LOUT
        LPLEA:  LEA LBUFF,A1            ;Queue a character
                CMPI #10,COUNT(A1)
                BLT LCONT
                BRA LOUT
        LCONT:  ADDQ #1,TAIL(A1)
                ADDQ #1,COUNT(A1)
                ANDI #0F,TAIL(A1)
                MOVEA TAIL(A1),A2
                LEA QUEUE(A1),A1
                MOVE.B D1,#0(A1,A2)
        LOUT:   MOVEM.L (A7)+,#0603
                RTE
```

The following routine gets a character from the queue of the serial communcation port (if a character is not available, the routine waits until a character is present):

```
        LGCH:   MOVEM.L #60,-(A7)       ;Save registers
        LAGN:   ORI #0700,SR            ;Disable interrupts
                LEA LBUFF,A1            ;Point at buffer
```

```
            MOVE  COUNT(A1),T1      ;See if there is a character
            BEQ   LWAIT             ;No, so wait
            MOVEA HEAD(A1),A2       ;Yes, find it and update
            ADDQ  #1,HEAD(A1)
            SUBQ  #1,COUNT(A1)
            ANDI  #0F,HEAD(A1)
            LEA   QUEUE(A1),A1      ;Return character
            MOVE.B #0(A1,A2),D0
            ANDI  #F8FF,SR          ;Enable interrupts
            MOVEM.L (A7)+,#0600     ;Restore registers
            RTS
    LWAIT:  STOP  #2000
            BRA   LAGN
```

The next routine produces a restart if ctrl-c has been typed; the important registers (user stack, status register, and PC) are restored, and the routine returns control to the command processor:

```
    RSTRT:  MOVEM.L (A7)+,#0603     ;Restore registers from
                                    ;interrupt
            MOVEM.L #FFFF,D0        ;Save registers
            MOVE  USP,A0            ;Save user stack pointer
            MOVE.L A0,A7
            MOVE  (A7)+,SR          ;Restore status
            MOVE.L (A7)+,PC         ;Restore program counter
            PEA   COMM              ;Fake a return to command
                                    ;loop
            MOVE  SSRI,-(A7)        ;Fake a new status register
            RTE
```

The next routine gets a character from the input queue; if a character is not available, the routine waits until one becomes available:

```
    GETCH:  MOVEM.L #60,-(A7)       ;Save registers
    TRYAG:  ORI   #0700,SR
            LEA   IBUFF,A1
            MOVE  COUNT(A1),T1
            BEQ   WAIT
            MOVEQ #0,D0
            MOVEA HEAD(A1),A2
            ADDQ  #1,HEAD(A1)
            SUBQ  #1,COUNT(A1)
            ANDI  #0F,HEAD(A1)
            LEA   QUEUE(A1),A1
            MOVE.B #0(A1,A2),D0
            ANDI  #F8FF,SR
            MOVEM.L (A7)+,#0600
            RTS
    WAIT:   STOP  #2000
            BRA   TRYAG
```

The next short routine outputs a carriage return and a linefeed; the routine is called in several places by the main program:

```
    CF:     DS    "\r\n\0"
```

```
              CRLF:   LEA CF,A0
                      BSR WRITS
                      RTS
```

The following routine fetches numbers of various sizes (byte, word, longword); one of the temporary storage areas (T1) is used as a counter of the number size:

```
              GETB:   MOVE #1,T1              ;T1 is byte count
                      BRA GB
              GETW:   MOVE #3,T1
                      BRA GB
              GETL:   MOVE #7,T1
              GB:     MOVEM.L #6000,-(A7)     ;Save registers
                      MOVE T1,D2
                      MOVEQ #0,D1
              BLP:    JSR (A0)                ;A0 holds address of port
                                              ;with number
                      CMPI.B #3A,D0           ;Check for abcdef
                      BLT N1
                      ADD.B #09,D0
              N1:     ANDI.B #0F,D0
                      ASL.L #4,D1             ;Place in next hex digit
                      OR.B D0,D1
                      DBF D2,BLP
                      MOVE.L D1,D0            ;Set up return in D0
                      MOVEM.L (A7)+,#6        ;Restore registers
                      RTS
```

The remainder of the monitor includes the routines that execute the various commands:

```
              ;Copy memory blocks
              ;
              CDMES:  DS "\n\rCopied\0"
              CTOM:   DS "\to\0"
              CFORM:  DS "for\0"
              CBYT:   DS "bytes\0"
              COPY:   BSR GETCH               ;Get past blank
                      LEA GETCH,A0            ;Set up for terminal input
                      BSR GETW                ;Get target address
                      MOVE D0,D2              ;Save it
                      MOVEA D0,A2
                      BSR GETCH               ;Get past =
                      BSR GETW                ;Get start address
                      MOVE D0,D3              ;Save it
                      MOVEA D0,A3             ;Again
                      BSR GETCH               ;Get past ","
                      BSR GETW                ;Get ending address
                      SUB D3,D0               ;Calculate byte count
                      MOVE D0,D4              ;Save it
                      ADDQ #1,D4
              COLP:   MOVE.B (A3)+,(A2)+      ;Start moving
                      DBF D0,COLP
```

```
                LEA  CDMES,A0       ;Say we're done
                BSR  WRITS
                MOVE D3,D0
                BSR  WRITW
                LEA  CTOM,A0
                BSR  WRITS
                MOVE D2,D0
                BSR  WRITW
                LEA  CFORM,A0
                BSR  WRITS
                MOVE D4,D0
                BSR  WRITW
                LEA  CBYT,A0
                BSR  WRITS
                RTS
```

The next routine examines and updates requested memory locations:

```
        ;Memory examine and update
        MTAB:   DC.W #1,#2E00       ;.
                DC.W #1,MDOT
                DC.W #1,#3D00       ;=
                DC.W #1,MEQU
                DC.W #1,#2C00       ;,
                DC.W #1,MCOM
                DC.W #1,#2B00       ;+
                DC.W #1,#MPLU
                DC.W #1,#2D00       ;-
                DC.W #1,MMIN
                DC.W #1,#0D00       ;<CR>
                DC.W #1,MLOC
        MMES:   DS "\n\n\rMemory Mode\0"
        MPRMP:  DS "\n\r:\0"
        MEQM:   DS "= = \0"
        MEM:    BSR  GETCH          ;Get delimiter
                CMPI.B #0D,D0       ;If <CR>, then enter M
                BEQ  MNOAD
                LEA  GETCH,A0       ;Else get the address
                BSR  GETW
                BRA  MPLP           ;Set the address
        MNOAD:  MOVEQ #0,D0         ;Start with no address
        MPLP:   MOVE D0,EXAM        ;Set the address
                LEA  MMES,A0        ;Load message
                BSR  WRITS
        MLP:    LEA  MPRMP,A0       ;Write memory prompt
                BSR  WRITS
                BSR  GETCH          ;Enter memory command loop
                MOVEQ #5,D2         ;Set for search
                LEA  MTAB-4,A0
        MMLP:   ADDQ #4,A0          ;Search loop like command
                CMP.B (A0),D0
                DBEQ D2,MMLP
```

136   THE 68000 MICROPROCESSOR

```
                BNE MEXIT               ;Exit if not found
                MOVEA #2(A0),A0         ;Get routine address
                JSR (A0)                ;Branch to it
                BRA MLP                 ;Stay in memory loop
    MEXIT:      RTS
    MDOT:       LEA GETCH,A0            ;Handle setting of address
                BSR GETW                ;Get address
                MOVE D0,EXAM            ;Set in pointer
                BSR MLOC                ;Print address and value
                RTS
    MEQU:       LEA GETCH,A0            ;Handle new value at
                                        ;pointer
                BSR GETB                ;Get new value
                MOVEA EXAM,A0           ;Set address
                MOVE.B D0,(A0)          ;Move new value
                BSR MLOC                ;Write new value
                RTS
    MCOM:       ADDQ #1,EXAM            ;Handle pointer increment
                                        ;by one
                BSR MEQU                ;Write new address and
                                        ;value
                RTS
    MPLU:       ADDQ #1,EXAM            ;Increment pointer
                BSR MLOC                ;Write value
                RTS
    MMIN:       SUBQ #1,EXAM            ;Decrement pointer
                BSR MLOC
                RTS
    MLOC:       BSR CRLF                ;Write address and value
                MOVE EXAM,D0            ;Write address
                BSR WRITW
                LEA MEQM,A0
                BSR WRITS
                MOVEA EXAM,A0
                MOVE.B (A0),D0          ;Write value
                BSR WRITB
                RTS
```

The next routine examines and modifies the registers:

```
            ;Regs -- Modify/examine
            ;
    RTAB:   DC.W #1,#2E00           ;.
            DC.W #1,RDOT
            DC.W #1,#3D00           ;=
            DC.W #1,REQU
            DC.W #1,#0D00           ;<CR>
            DC.W #1,RALL
    RTAB1:  DC.W #1,#CB00           ;Internal name/offset
            DS "SR"                 ;Print name
            DC.W #1,#9C02
```

```
                DS   "PC"
                DC.W #1,#D006
                DS   "D0"
                DC.W #1,#D10A
                DS   "D1"
                DC.W #1,#D20E
                DS   "D2"
                DC.W #1,D312
                DC   "D3"
                DC.W #1,#D416
                DS   "D4"
                DC.W #1,#D51A
                DS   "D5"
                DC.W #1,#D61E
                DS   "D6"
                DC.W #1,#D722
                DS   "D7"
                DC.W #1,#A026
                DS   "A0"
                DC.W #1,#A12A
                DS   "A1"
                DC.W #1,#A22E
                DS   "A2"
                DC.W #1,#A332
                DS   "A3"
                DC.W #1,#A436
                DS   "A4"
                DC.W #1,#A53A
                DS   "A5"
                DC.W #1,#A63E
                DS   "A6"
                DC.W #1,#A742
                DS   "A7"
RMES:           DS   "\n\n\rRegister Mode\0"
RPRMP:          DS   "\n\r:\0"
REQM:           DS   "= =\0"
REGS:           BSR  GETCH              ;Get delimiter
                CMPI.B #0D,D0           ;If <CR>, then start at SR
                BEQ  RNOAD
                LEA  GETCH,A0           ;Else set for terminal input
                BSR  GETB               ;Get register name
                BSR  RADDR              ;Set address
                BRA  RPLP               ;Set register pointer
RNOAD:          LEA  RTAB1,A3           ;Set default pointer value
                MOVE A3,REXAM
RPLP:           LEA  RMES,A0            ;Say hello
                BSR  WRITS
                BSR  RLOC               ;Write starting location
                                        ;value
```

138 THE 68000 MICROPROCESSOR

```
RLP:    LEA RPRMP,A0        ;Write register prompt
        BSR WRITS
        BSR GETCH           ;Get command
        MOVEQ #2,D2         ;Set for search
        LEA RTAB-4,A0
RMLP:   ADDQ #4,A0          ;Search
        CMP.B (A0),D0
        DBEQ D2,RMLP
        BNE REXIT           ;Exit if not found
        MOVEA #2(A0),A0     ;Found it, if so, go to it
        JSR (A0)
        BRA RLP             ;Go again
REXIT:  RTS
RDOT:   LEA GETCH,A0        ;Set register pointer
        BSR GETB
        BSR RADDR           ;Set input address
        BSR RLOC            ;Write register and value
        RTS
REQU:   LEA GETCH,A0        ;Set new value
        MOVEA REXAM,A3
        MOVEQ #0,D1         ;Clear D1
        MOVE.B #1(A3),D1    ;Get offset
        BEQ REQUS           ;Branch if SR is register
        BSR GETL            ;Get new value
        LEA SR,A4           ;Find save area offset
        ADDA D1,A4          ;Add offset
        MOVE.L D0,(A4)      ;Move in new value
        BRA REQUR           ;Print it
REQUS:  BSR GETW            ;Same as above but for SR
        MOVE D0,SR
REQUR:  BSR RLOC            ;Write new value
        RTS
RALL:   LEA RTAB1-4,A3      ;Write all registers
        MOVEQ #11,D2        ;Set count
RALP:   ADDQ #4,A3          ;Loop
        MOVE A3,REXAM
        BSR RLOC
        DBF D2,RALP
        RTS
RADDR:  MOVE #11,D4         ;Find offset in save area
        LEA RTAB1-4,A3
RADLP:  ADDQ #4,A3
        CMP.B (A3),D0
        DBEQ D4,RADLP
        BNE REXIT
        MOVE A3,REXAM       ;Set register pointer
        RTS
RLOC:   BSR CRLF            ;Print register name and
                            ;value
```

ANOTHER 68000-BASED SYSTEM

```
                MOVEA   REXAM,A4
                MOVE.B  #2(A4),D0       ;Write name
                BSR     WRIT
                MOVE.B  #3(A4),D0
                BSR     WRIT
                LEA     REQM,A0
                BSR     WRITS
                MOVEQ   #0,D0
                MOVE.B  #1(A4),D0       ;Write value
                BEQ     RPSR            ;Branch if SR
                LEA     SR,A0           ;Find offset
                ADDA    D0,A0           ;Add offset
                MOVE.L  (A0),D0         ;Move in new value
                BSR     WRITL
                BRA     RRTS
        RPSR:   MOVE    SR,D0           ;Write SR value
                BSR     WRITW
        RRTS:   RTS
```

The next set of instructions loads a program via the serial communication port (loading is carried out in S-Format, which is described fully in the Appendix A):

```
        ;Load data via the serial communication port
        ;
        LMES:   DS      "\n\rLoad...\0"
        SLMES:  DS      "\n\rUser PC = =\0"
        ELMES:  DS      "\n\rLoad Done...\0"
        LOAD:   BSR     GETCH
                CMPI.B  #0D,D0          ;If <CR>, then no offset
                BEQ     LNOOF
                LEA     GETCH,A0        ;Get offset
                BSR     GETW
                MOVE.L  D0,PC           ;Save load point for go
                                        ;command
                BRA     LD1
        LNOOF:  MOVE.L  #0,PC
        LD1:    LEA     LBUFF,A1        ;Point at LBUFF
                MOVE    #0,HEAD(A1)     ;Set queue for lp
                MOVE    #FFFF,TAIL(A1)
                MOVE    #0,COUNT(A1)
                LEA     LMES,A0         ;Print starting message
                BSR     WRITS
        LLP:    BSR     LGCH            ;Get S
                CMPI.B  #53,D0
                BNE     LLP             ;No -- start over
                BSR     LGCH            ;Get one or nine
                CMPI.B  #39,D0          ;Nine, then done
                BEQ     LDONE
                CMPI.B  #31,D0          ;One, then another record
                BNE     LLP
                LEA     LGCH,A0         ;Setup for GETB and GETW
```

```
                BSR  GETB              ;Get byte count
                MOVE D0,D1
                SUBQ #4,D1             ;Remove count for check
                BSR  GETW
                ADD.L PC,D0            ;Add offset
                MOVEA D0,A1            ;Save starting address
        LBLP:   BSR  GETB              ;Get actual data byte
                MOVE.B D0,(A1)+        ;Move to memory
                DBF  D1,LBLP           ;Loop for count
                BSR  GETW              ;Gobble up check and crlf
                BRA  LLP               ;Try another record
        LDONE:  BSR  LGCH              ;Gobble up byte count
                BSR  LGCH
                BSR  GETW              ;Get address from end
                                       ;macro
                ADD.L PC,D0            ;Add offset
                MOVE D0,D1             ;Save it
                MOVE.L D0,PC           ;Set starting address for
                                       ;go
                MOVE #0,SR             ;Set status register
                MOVE #10,D0
                LEA  D0,A1
        LREG:   MOVE.L #0,(A1)+
                DBF  D0,LREG
                LEA  USTCK,A0
                MOVE.L A0,A7           ;Set user stack
                LEA  SLMES,A0          ;Write message
                BSR  WRITS
                MOVE D1,D0
                BSR  WRITW             ;Write starting address
                MOVE #03,D1            ;Gobble up last four bytes
        LL2:    BSR  LGCH
                DBF  D1,LL2
                LEA  ELMES,A0          ;Send last message
                BSR  WRITS
                RTS
```

The "e" command allows the system to enter a terminal emulator mode. Thus, any character other than ctrl-x may be sent to a host system. The character ctrl-x is the escape sequence for getting out of the terminal emulator mode. The Ctrl-l character serves the same purpose, but a load (1) command is placed in the command buffer.

The emulation routine is short. Storage is assigned for two messages. The emulator mode message is displayed first, and the system waits for an interrupt. If the interrupt is received, the interrupt-handling routine will save in the buffer any input character and display it on the screen. At the end of the interrupt-handling routine, the emulation routine will display the termination message and return to the main program.

ANOTHER 68000-BASED SYSTEM 141

```
        ;e -- Emulation routine
        ;
EMMES:  DS "\n\rExit terminal mode\0"
ENMES:  DS "\n\rTerminal mode:\n\r\0"
EMUL:   LEA ENMES,A0            ;Write starting message
        BSR WRITS
        BSET #3,BKPTF           ;Set emulator mode
EMU1:   STOP #2000              ;Wait for interrupt. If
                                ;interrupted, the interrupt
                                ;routine will buffer and
                                ;echo input
        BRA EMUL
EMUDN:  LEA EMMES,A0            ;Entered from interrupt
                                ;handler
        BSR WRITS
        RTS
```

The next set of instructions allows the use of prototype commands, designed by a programmer; the command is executed while the VU68K is in system mode:

```
        ;Proto -- Prototype command in RAM
        ;
PMESS:  DS "\n\rPrototype\0"
PM1:    DS "running:\n\r\0"
PM2:    DS "installed\r\0"
PROTO:  BSR GETCH               ;Get prototype number
        MOVE.L D0,D1            ;Save number
        ANDI #0F,D1             ;Strip leading hex digit
        SUBQ #1,D1              ;Normalize to zero
        LSL #1,D1               ;Multiply by two
        LEA PTAB,A1             ;Set starting address
        ADDA D1,A1              ;Add offset
        BSR GETCH               ;Get delimiter
        CMPI.B #0D,D0           ;If <CR>, then do command
        BEQ PRUN
        LEA GETCH,A0            ;Else install in table
        BSR GETW                ;Get address
        MOVE D0,(A1)            ;Move in address
        LEA PMESS,A0
        BSR WRITS
        LEA PM2,A0
        BSR WRITS
        BRA PRTS
PRUN:   MOVEA (A1),A1           ;Run prototype command
        LEA PMESS,A0
        BSR WRITS
        LEA PM1,A0
        BSR WRITS
        JSR (A1)                ;Go do it
PRTS:   RTS
```

142 THE 68000 MICROPROCESSOR

The following routine sets and removes breakpoints. This routine and the memory dump routine are perhaps the longest. The breakpoint routine expects a character in D0. If this character is a carriage return, then all of the existing breakpoints are listed. The routine next makes two comparisons in order to add (+) or remove (−) a breakpoint. A #sign following the "b" command will remove the breakpoints and display the message, "breakpoints removed." The routine discards any characters not associated with it and displays an error message.

```
        ;Bkpt -- Set/Remove breakpoints
        ;
BRMES:  DS  "\n\rBkpts removed\0"
BDMES:  DS  "\n\rBkpts at:\n\r\0"
BPMES:  DS  "\n\rBkpt added at \0"
BMMES:  DS  "\n\rBkpt deleted at \0"
BBMES:  DS  "\n\rBkpt error \0"
BKIN:   BKPT                    ;Instruction constant
BKPT:   BSR GETCH               ;Get delimiter
        CMPI.B #0D,D0           ;If <CR>, then print all
                                ;breakpoints
        BEQ BDIS
        CMPI.B #2B,D0           ;If +, add a breakpoint
        BEQ BPLS
        CMPI.B #2D,D0           ;If -, delete a breakpoint
        BEQ BMIN
        CMPI.B #23,D0           ;If #, delete all break-
                                ;points
        BNE BBAD                ;Else it's a bad message
BREM:   MOVEQ #4,D1             ;Remove all breakpoints
        LEA BKTAB-4,A1          ;Set for loop
BLP1:   ADDA #4,A1
        MOVEA ILOC(A1),A0       ;Get address from table
        CMPA #00,A0             ;If zero, then not an entry
        BEQ BNO
        MOVE INSTR(A1),(A0)     ;Else move instruction
                                ;back
        MOVE.L #0,INSTR(A1)     ;Clear table entry
BNO:    BDF D1,BLP1             ;Loop
        BCLR #0,BKPTF           ;Clear breakpoint if in
                                ;one
        BTST #2,BKPTF           ;In trace?
        BNE BRNO                ;Yes
        ANDI #7FFF,SR           ;Else clear trace bit
BRNO:   LEA BRMES,A0            ;Say done
        BSR WRITS
        BRA BRTS
BDIS:   LEA BDMES,A0            ;Display all breakpoints
        BSR WRITS
        LEA BKTAB-4,A1          ;Set loop
        MOVEQ #4,D1
```

ANOTHER 68000-BASED SYSTEM   143

```
BDLP:   ADDA #4,A1              ;Loop
        MOVE ILOC(A1),D0        ;Get breakpoint
        BEQ BELP                ;If zero, then not an entry
        BSR WRITW
        BSR CRLF
BELP:   DBF D1,BDLP             ;Loop
        BRA BRTS
BPLS:   LEA BKTAB-4,A1          ;Add a breakpoint
        MOVE #4,D1              ;Set for loop
        LEA GETCH,A0            ;Set up to get address
        BSR GETW
B12:    ADDA #4,A1              ;Loop
        CMP ILOC(A1),D0         ;Found entry already in
                                ;table?
        BNE BM0                 ;Yes
        MOVEA D0,A2             ;Reset it to make sure
        MOVE BKIN,(A2)          ;Set instruction
        BRA BFND                ;Exit for found
BM0:    MOVE ILOC(A1),D2        ;Move to set condition
                                ;codes
        DBEQ D1,B12             ;Exit if zero entry found
        BNE BBAD                ;If exit is on count and
                                ;not zero
        MOVE D0,ILOC(A1)        ;Move in address
        MOVEA D0,A2             ;Point at location
        MOVE (A2),INSTR(A1)     ;Get instruction into table
        MOVE BKIN,(A2)          ;Set breakpoint instruction
BFND:   LEA BPMES,A0            ;Load message
        BSR WRITS
        MOVE A2,D0
        BSR WRITW
        BCLR #1,BKPTF           ;Clear in-single flag
        BTST #2,BKPTF           ;In trace?
        BNE BRTS                ;Yes
        ANDI #7FFF,SR           ;Clear trace bit
        BRA BRTS
BMIN:   LEA BKTAB-4,A1          ;Delete a breakpoint entry
        MOVE #4,D1              ;Set up for search
        LEA GETCH,A0            ;Set up for terminal input
        BSR GETW
B13:    ADDA #4,A1              ;Loop
        CMP ILOC(A1),D0         ;Is this the one?
        DBEQ D1,B13             ;If yes, then exit,
                                ;else loop
        BNE BBAD                ;Exit on count?
        MOVEA D0,A2             ;No, so get address
        MOVE INSTR(A1),(A2)     ;Return instruction
        MOVE.L #0,INSTR(A1)     ;Clear table entry
        BTST #0,BKPTF           ;In breakpoint?
```

```
                    BEQ   BOK              ;No
                    CMP.L PC,D0            ;Yes, this breakpoint?
                    BNE   BOK              ;No
                    BCLR  #0,BKPTF         ;Yes, so clear handling it
                    BTST  #2,BKPTF         ;In trace?
                    BNE   BOK              ;Yes
                    ANDI  #7FFF,SR         ;Else clear trace flag
         BOK:       LEA   BMMES,A0         ;Load message
                    BSR   WRITS
                    MOVE  A2,D0            ;Print address
                    BSR   WRITW
                    BRA   BRTS
         BBAD:      LEA   BBMES,A0         ;Error handler
                    BSR   WRITS
         BRTS:      RTS
```

A memory dump can be displayed in the following three ways:

1. By invoking the "d" command and a carriage return, the 64 bytes following the location last examined will be displayed.

2. By invoking the "d" command, an address, and a carriage return, the 64 bytes next following the address requested will be displayed.

3. By invoking the "d" command, a starting address, and an ending address, the bytes between the two addresses will be displayed.

The screen displays rows of 16 bytes, numbered at the top row from 0 to F. The starting address of each row is displayed in a left-hand column. If a byte is equivalent to an ASCII character, this character is displayed on the right-hand side of the screen. Any non-ASCII bytes are displayed as dots.

The first lines of the routine define the storage for the memory dump message, the 0 to F numbers of the top row, and a carriage return and linefeed.

```
         ; Dump -- Dump memory
         ;
         DMES:      DS    "\n\n\rMemory Dump\n\r\0"
         DHED:      DS    "\n\r 0 1 2 3"
                    DS    " 4 5 6 7 8 9 A"
                    DS    " B C D E F"
         DCR:       DS    "\n\r\0"
```

The DUMP portion of the routine expects the command character; if the character is a carriage return, then the routine performs a dump from the starting pointer. If the character is not a carriage return, the routine jumps to DEXAM. If the character is a ‹cr›, the routine saves the ending address and adds 64 to the starting address for the length of the dump. The actual dump is carried out by the DGO) portion of the routine.

```
         DUMP:      LEA   GETCH,A0         ;Set for terminal input
                    BSR   GETCH            ;Get delimiter
                    CMPI.B #0D,D0          ;If <cr>, then dump from
                                           ;pointer
                    BNE   DEXAM            ;Else get address
                    MOVEA EXAM,A1          ;Get exam
                    MOVEA A1,A2            ;Save it for ending address
```

ANOTHER 68000-BASED SYSTEM

```
        ADDA #40,A2              ;Add 64 for length of dump
        BRA DGO                  ;Go do it
```

The DEXAM portion of the routine takes care of the remaining two ways by which to display a memory dump—"d" ‹address› and "d" ‹starting address›,‹ending address›. DEXAM does this by examining the delimiter at the end of the first address.

```
DEXAM:  BSR GETW                 ;Get starting address
        MOVEA D0,A1
        BSR GETCH                ;Get delimiter
        CMPI.B #2C,D0            ;If ",", then get ending
                                 ;address
        BNE DCOM
        BSR GETW                 ;Get address
        MOVEA D0,A2              ;Save it
        BRA DGO                  ;Do a dump
```

The DCOM part of the routine provides 64 bytes of dump in those cases in which only one address has been entered:

```
DCOM:   MOVEA A1,A2              ;Default to 64 byte dump
        ADDA #40,A2
```

DGO begins by displaying the memory dump message and the 0 to F in the top row. It continues by setting the boundary of the dump to 16 bytes and rounding the ending address to that boundary. Finally, DGO moves the byte count (0 to 15) to D1.

```
DGO:    LEA DMES,A0              ;Display message
        BSR WRITS
        LEA DHED,A0              ;Print top row hex nos.
        BSR WRITS
        MOVE A1,D0               ;Set starting address at
                                 ;16 bytes
        ANDI.B #F0,D0
        MOVEA D0,A1
        MOVE A2,D0               ;Round ending address to
                                 ;boundary
        ORI.B #0F,D0
        MOVEA D0,A2
        MOVE #0F,D1              ;Move byte count to D1
```

The next segment in the routine is D11, which writes out the starting address and saves it in A3.

```
D11:    MOVE A1,D0               ;Write starting address
        BSR WRITW
        MOVEA A1,A3              ;Save starting address
```

Segment DFLP does the actual writing of the bytes on the screen. This part first outputs a space between the starting address of each row and the byte following the address value and then continues by getting the next byte and leaving a space between bytes. When the 16-byte count is reached, DFLP resets the counter, gets another row starting address, and outputs a space.

```
DFLP:   MOVE #20,D0              ;Write a space
```

```
              BSR  WRIT
              MOVE.B (A1)+,D0       ;Get next byte
              BSR  WRITB            ;Write it
              DBF  D1,DFLP          ;Loop
              MOVE #0F,D1           ;Reset byte count
              MOVEA A3,A1           ;Refetch starting address
              MOVE #20,D0           ;Write a space
              BSR  WRIT
```

The next three segments—DSLP, DOK, and DWRT—write the ASCII character or the dot on the right-hand side of the screen. The last segment, DWRT, checks for the end of a line in order to generate a carriage return/linefeed to the next line. The segment also resets the byte count; if the 16 bytes have not been displayed, it loops back for more bytes.

```
     DSLP:    MOVE.B (A1)+,D0       ;Write the byte ASCII
                                    ;equivalent
              CMPI.B #20,D0         ;If not printable, then
                                    ;dot
              BGE  DOK
              MOVE.B #2E,D0         ;Move in the dot
              BRA  DWRT
     DOK:     CMPI.B #7F,D0         ;Printable again?
              BLT  DWRT             ;Yes
              MOVE.B #2E,D0         ;No, move in a dot
     DWRT:    BSR  WRITS            ;Write it
              DBF  D1,DSLP          ;Line done?
              LEA  DCR,A0           ;Yes, so crlf
              BSR  WRITS
              MOVE #10,D1           ;Reset byte count
              CMPA A1,A2            ;Done?
              DBLT D1,D11           ;No, so loop
              MOVE A1,EXAM          ;Yes, so update exam
              RTS
```

The trace mode segment starts by displaying the Trace On or Trace Off message as soon as the appropriate character is entered (T+ or T−). The TRACE segment determines whether the system is in breakpoint mode. If so, then the trace mode is not cancelled since both modes are allowed to be present simultaneously. If the system is not at a breakpoint, the trace is cleared, and the next segment (TCLR) carries out the clearing of the trace mode.

```
     TMES:    DS   "\n\rTrace \0"
     TONM:    DS   "on\0"
     TOFFM:   DS   "off\0"
     TRACE:   BSR  GETCH            ;Get command
              MOVE D0,D1            ;Save it
              LEA  TMES,A0          ;Write message
              BSR  WRITS
              CMPI.B #2B,D1         ;Is it a +?
              BEQ  TON              ;Yes
              BTST #0,BKPTF         ;In breakpoint?
              BNE  TCLR             ;Yes, so don't clear trace
```

ANOTHER 68000-BASED SYSTEM 147

```
        ANDI #7FFF,SR         ;Clear trace
TCLR:   BCLR #2,BKPTF         ;Turn off in-trace flag
        LEA TOFFM,A0          ;Load off message
        BRA TDONE             ;Exit
TON:    ORI #8000,SR          ;Set trace bit
        BCLR #1,BKPTF         ;Clear single step
        BSET #2,BKPTF         ;Set in-trace flag
        LEA TONM,A0           ;Write message
TDONE:  BSR WRITS
        RTS
```

The single-step segment accomplishes basically the same task as the trace mode. The single-step mode, however, removes all breakpoints and turns the trace off. The segment begins by reserving storage for the header.

```
        SMES:   DS "\n\rSingle step\0"
        SONM:   DS "on\0"
        SOFFM:  DS "off\0"
```

The SINGL segment, which is similar to the TRACE segment, accepts and saves the command character, displays the header, and checks whether the next character is a "+". If it is, the single-step mode begins. The segment ends by checking whether the program also has breakpoints. If a breakpoint is present, the trace mode (also associated with single-stepping) is not turned off. If there are no breakpoints, the segment clears the trace bit.

```
SINGL:  BSR GETCH             ;Get command
        MOVE D0,D1            ;Save it
        LEA SMES,A0           ;Write message
        BSR WRITS
        CMPI.B #2B,D1         ;Is it a "+"?
        BEQ SON               ;Yes
        BTST #0, BKPTF        ;In breakpoint?
        BNE SCLR              ;Yes, so don't clear trace
        ANDI #7FFF,SR         ;Clear trace bit
```

The segment SCLR clears the single-trace flag, displays a "single-trace off" message, and ends the single-step mode:

```
SCLR:   BCLR #1,BKPTF         ;Turn off in-single flag
        LEA SOFFM,A0          ;Write off message
        BSR WRITS
        BRA SDONE             ;Exit
```

The SON segment sets the stage for the single-step mode. The segment clears the breakpoint flag and sets the single-step flag. SON clears the trace-mode flag and displays the "single step on" message. Finally, the segment removes all breakpoints and sets the trace bit in the status register.

```
SON:    BCLR #0,BKPTF         ;Clear in-breakpoint flag
        BSET #1,BKPTF         ;Set in-single flag
        BCLR #2,BKPTF         ;Clear in-trace flag
        LEA SONM,A0           ;Write message
        BSR WRITS
        BSR BREM              ;Remove all breakpoints
                              ;for single stepping
        ORI #8000,SR          ;Set trace bit
```

The SDONE segment exits to the main program:

                        SDONE: RTS

The "go" mode of the monitor executes a program either from the starting address of the last load or from an address that a value following the "g" command specifies.

The routine starts with the GMES segment, reserving space for the message "Program:". The segment then accepts a character and checks whether it is a carriage return. If it is, execution starts at the address given in the command of the last known address from load, breakpoint, or single step. If the character is not a carriage return, then execution begins from the address specified in the command.

```
        GMES:   DS "\cProgram:\n\n\r\0"
        GO:     BSR GETCH              ;Get separator
                CMPI.B #0D,D0          ;If <CR>, then start from
                                       ;default
                BEQ GG0
        GGET:   LEA GETCH,A0           ;Else get starting address
                                       ;as given in command
                BSR GETW
                MOVE.L D0,PC           ;Set for return
```

The GG0 segment displays the message "Program:"; however, it does so only if the program is not in single-step mode.

```
        GG0:    BTST #1,BKPTF          ;Single step?
                BNE GNOM               ;Yes, so no message
                LEA GMES,A0            ;Write message
                BSR WRITS
```

The last segments—GNOM and GBMOV—perform some stacking operations. They also set the return address for the program counter and the return pattern for the status register and enable the interrupts.

```
        GNOM:   ADDQ #4,A7             ;Pop the stack
                MOVEM.L D0,#7FFF       ;Get saved values
                MOVE.L A7,T1           ;Save system-stack pointer
                MOVEA.L A7,A7          ;Get saved user-stack
                                       ;pointer
                MOVE A7,USP            ;Reset user stack
                MOVEA.L T1,A7          ;Reset system stack
        GBMOV:  MOVE.L PC,-(A7)        ;Set up return PC
                ANDI #F8FF,SR          ;Enable interrupts
                MOVE SR,-(A7)          ;Set up return SR
                RTE
```

The last part of the VUBUG lists the various interrupt, trap, and other handling routines.

```
                ;Generic trap handler
                ;
        GHMES:  DS "\n\rTrap at \0"
        GHLR:   MOVEM.L #FFFF,D0       ;Save all registers
                MOVE USP,A6            ;Get and save user-stack
                                       ;pointer
```

ANOTHER 68000-BASED SYSTEM   149

```
                MOVE.L A6,A7
                MOVE (A7)+,SR           ;Save current SR
                MOVE.L (A7)+,PC         ;Save current return value
                PEA COMM                ;Set for return to command
                MOVE SSRI,-(A7)         ;Enable interrupts on return
GHPR:           LEA GHMES,A0            ;Write message
GHPR1:          BSR WRITS
                MOVE.L PC,D0
                BSR WRITL
                RTE
;
;Breakpoint handler
;
BHMES:          DS "\n\rBreakpoint at \0"
BININ:          DS "\n\rBad Instruction at \0"
BHLR:           MOVE SSRN,SR            ;Disable interrupts
                MOVEM.L #FFFF,D0        ;Save registers
                MOVE USP,A6             ;Get and save user-stack
                                        ;pointer
                MOVE.L A6,A7
                MOVE (A7)+,SR           ;Save Status Register
                MOVE.L (A7)+,PC         ;Save Program Counter
                PEA COMM                ;Set for return to command
                MOVE SSRI,-(A7)         ;Enable interrupts on return
                MOVEA.L PC,A0           ;Get PC on interrupt
                CMPI #FFFF,(A0)         ;Was interrupt caused by
                                        ;breakpoint input?
                BEQ BSND                ;Yes
                LEA BININ,A0            ;No, invalid instruction
                BRA GHPR1               ;Go write message
BSND:           LEA BHMES,A0            ;Write breakpoint message
                BSR WRITS
                MOVE.L PC,D0
                BSR WRITW
                BSR CRLF
                LEA BKTAB-4,A1          ;Find the breakpoint entry
                MOVE #4,D1              ;Maximum of five
                MOVE.L PC,D0            ;This is where it happened
BHL:            ADDA #4,A1
                CMP ILOC(A1),D0         ;Is this the entry?
                DBEQ D1,BHL             ;Loop if not
                BNE BHRTE               ;Not found, so quit
                MOVEA D0,A2             ;Point at it
                MOVE INSTR(A1),(A2)     ;Move instruction back in
                ORI #8000,SR            ;Set trace mode on
                BSET #0,BKPTF           ;Set in-breakpoint flag
BHRTE:          RTE
;
;Trace handler
;
```

```
         TLOCM:  DS "\n\rPC == \0"
         THLR:   MOVE SSRN,SR           ;Disable interrupts
                 MOVE.L A0,A0           ;Save used registers
                 MOVE.L D0,D0
                 BTST #0,BKPTF          ;Handling a breakpoint?
                 BEQ TREAL              ;No, so it's a real trace
                 MOVEA.L PC,A0          ;Yes, find where it occurred
                 MOVE BKIN,(A0)         ;Reset breakpoint instruction
                 BCLR #0,BKPTF          ;Clear in-progress break-
                                        ;point
                 BTST #2,BKPTF          ;In trace mode
                 BNE TREAL              ;Yes, go trace it
         THMA0:  ANDI #7FFF,(A7)        ;No, so clear the trace
                                        ;bit
                 BRA TRTE
         TREAL:  MOVE.L #2(A7),PC       ;Not (just) a breakpoint
                                        ;but trace or single step
                 BTST #1,BKPTF          ;Trace?
                 BEQ TRPR               ;Yes
                 MOVEM.L #FFFF,D0       ;No, single step
                 MOVE USP,A6            ;Save registers and stack
                                        ;pointer
                 MOVE.L A6,A7
                 MOVE (A7)+,SR          ;Save Status Register
                 MOVE.L (A7)+,PC        ;Save PC
                 PEA COMM               ;Fake return to command
                 MOVE SSRI,-(A7)        ;Enable interrupts on return
         TRPR:   LEA TLOCM,A0           ;Write message
                 BSR WRITS
                 MOVE.L PC,D0
                 BSR WRITL
         TRTE:   MOVEA.L A0,A0          ;Restore used registers
                 MOVE.L D0,D0
         TR:     RTE
         ;
         ;Privilege violation handler
         ;
         PRMES:  DS "\n\rPrivilege Error at \0"
         PHLR:   MOVEM.L #FFFF,D0
                 MOVE USP,A6
                 MOVE.L A6,A7
                 MOVE (A7)+,SR
                 MOVE.L (A7)+,PC
                 PEA COMM
                 MOVE SSRI,-(A7)
         PRPR:   LEA PRMES,A0
                 BRA GHPR1
         ;
         ;Address error/bus error trap
         ;
```

```
ABMES:  DS "\n\rAddress Error at \0"
ABHLR:  MOVEM.L #FFFF,D0
        MOVE.L A6,A7            ;Same as above but...
        MOVE #8(A7),SR          ;Status Register is deeper
                                ;in stack
        MOVE.L #A(A7),PC        ;So is PC
        PEA COMM
        MOVE SSRI,-(A7)
ABPR:   LEA ABMES,A0
        BRA GHPR1
;
;Macro instruction handlers
;
;
;Exit
;
TEXIT:  MOVEM.L #FFFF,D0        ;Save register values
        MOVE USP,A6             ;Save user-stack pointer
        MOVE.L A6,A7
        MOVE (A7)+,SR           ;Save Status Register
        MOVE.L (A7)+,PC         ;Save PC
        LEA STACK, A7           ;Reset system mode stack
        PEA COMM                ;Fake return to command
        MOVE SSRI,-(A7)         ;Do same for status
        RTE
;
;Getb
;
TGETB:  LEA GETCH,A0
        BSR GETB
        RTE
;
;Getw
;
TGETW:  LEA GETCH,A0
        BSR GETW
        RTE
;
;Getl
;
TGETL:  LEA GETCH,A0
        BSR GETL
        RTE
;
;Wrtb
;
TWRTB:  BSR WRITB
        RTE
;
;Wrtw
```

```
                ;
        TWRTW:  BSR WRITW
                RTE
        ;
        ;Wrtl
        ;
        TWRTL:  BSR WRITL
                RTE
        ;
        ;Getc
        ;
        TGETC:  BSR GETCH
                RTE
        ;
        ;Wrts
        ;
        TWRTS:  BSR WRITS
                RTE
        ;
        ;Wrtc
        ;
        TWRTC:  BSR WRIT
                RTE
        ;
        ;Crlf
        ;
        TCRLF:  BSR CRLF
                RTE
        ;
                END START
```

The monitor set forth in this chapter has been assembled and tested. A listing of the object code is provided in the Appendix for those readers who wish to program EPROM devices without having to assemble the code.

Appendix A
S-RECORD OUTPUT FORMAT

The S-record format for output modules was devised for the purpose of encoding programs or data files in a printable format for transportation between computer systems. The transportation process can thus be visually monitored and the S-records more easily edited.

S-RECORD CONTENT

When viewed by the user, S-records are essentially character strings made of several fields that identify the record type, record length, memory address, code/data, and checksum. Each byte of binary data is encoded as a 2-character hexadecimal number: the first character representing the high-order 4 bits of the byte, and the second, the low-order 4 bits.

The 5 fields that comprise an S-record are shown below:

type	record	length	code/data	checksum

where the fields are composed as follows:

FIELD	PRINTABLE CHARACTERS	CONTENTS
Type	2	S-record type: S0, S1, etc.
Record length	2	The count of character pairs in the record, excluding type and record length.
Address	4, 6, or 8	The 2-, 3-, or 4-byte address at which the data field is to be loaded into memory.
Code/data	0–2n	From 0 to n bytes of executable code, memory-loadable data, or descriptive information. For compatibility with teletypewriters, some programs may limit the number of bytes to as few as 28 (56 printable characters in the S-record).
Checksum	2	The least significant byte of the one's complement of the sum of the values represented by the pairs of characters making up the record length, address, and code/data fields.

Each record may be terminated with a CR/LF/NULL. Additionally, an S-record may have an initial field to accommodate other data, such as line numbers generated by some time-sharing systems.

Accuracy of transmission is ensured by the record length (byte count) and checksum fields.

S-RECORD TYPES

Eight types of S-records have been defined to accommodate the several needs of the encoding, transportation, and decoding functions. The various Motorola upload, download, and other record transportation control programs, as well as cross assemblers, linkers, and other file-creating or debugging programs, utilize only those S-records that serve the purpose of the program. For specific information on which S-records are supported by a particular program, the user's manual for that program must be consulted. TUTOR—the firmware supplied with the educational computer—supports S0, S1, S2, S8, and S9 records. The S2 and S8 records are not often used, however, because all of the on-board RAM and ROM can be addressed with a 2-byte address.

An S-record-format module may contain S-records of the following types:

S0 The header record for each block of S-records. The code/data field may contain any descriptive information identifying the following block of S-records. Under VERSAdos, the resident linker's IDENT command can be used to designate module name, version number, revision number, and description information that will make up the header record. The address field is normally made up of zeros.

S1 A record containing code/data and the 2-byte address at which the code/data is to reside.

S2 A record containing code/data and the 3-byte address at which the code/data is to reside.

S3 A record containing code/data and the 4-byte address at which the code/data is to reside.

S5 A record containing the number S1, S2, and S3 records transmitted in a particular block. This count appears in the address field; there is no code/data field.

S7 A termination record for a block of S3 records. The address field may optionally contain the 4-byte address of the instruction to which control is to be passed. There is no code/data field.

S8 A termination record for a block of S2 records. The address field may optionally contain the 3-byte address of the instruction to which control is to be passed. There is no code/data field.

S9 A termination record for a block of S1 records. The address field may optionally contain the 2-byte address of the instruction to which control is to be passed. Under VERSAdos, the resident linker's ENTRY command can be used to specify this address. If not specified, the first entry point

APPENDIX A

specification encountered in the object module input will be used. There is no code/data field.

Only one termination record is used for each block of S-records. As a rule, S7 and S8 records are used only when control is to be passed to a 3- or 4-byte address. Normally, only one header record is used, although it is possible for multiple header records to occur.

CREATION OF S-RECORDS

S-record-format programs may be produced by several dump utilities, debuggers, VERSAdos' resident linkage editor, or several cross assemblers or cross linkers. On EXORmacs, the Build Load Module (MBLM) utility allows an executable load module to be built from S-records and has a counterpart utility in BUILDS, which allows an S-record file to be created from a load module.

Several programs are available for downloading a file in S-record format from a host system to an 8-bit or 16-bit microprocessor-based system. Programs are also available for uploading an S-record file to or from an EXORmacs system.

EXAMPLE

Shown below is a typical S-record-format module, as printed or displayed:

```
S00600004844521B
S1130000285F245F2212226A000424290008237C2A
S11300100002000800082629001853812341001813
S113002041E900084E42234300182342000824A952
S107003000144ED492
S9030000FC
```

The module consists of one S0 record, four S1 records, and an S9 record.
The S0 record is comprised of the following character pairs:

S0 S-record type S0, indicating that it is a header record
06 Hexadecimal 06 (decimal 6), indicating that six character pairs (or ASCII bytes) follow
00
00 Four-character 2-byte address field, zeros in this example
48
44 ASCII H, D, and R - "HDR"
52
1B The checksum

The first S1 records is explained as follows:

S1 S-record type S1, indicating that it is a code/data record to be loaded/verified at a 2-byte address
13 Hexadecimal 13 (decimal 19), indicating that 19 character pairs, representing 19 bytes of binary data, follow

00 Four-character 2-byte address field; hexadecimal address 0000,
00 where the data that follows is to be loaded

The next 16 character pairs of the first S1 record are the ASCII bytes of the actual program code/data. In this assembly language example, the hexadecimal opcodes of the program are written in sequence in the code/data fields of the S1 records:

OPCODE	INSTRUCTION	
285F	MOVE.L	(A7)+,A4
245F	MOVE.L	(A7)+,A2
2212	MOVE.L	(A2),D1
226A0004	MOVE.L	4(A2),A1
24290008	MOVE.L	FUNCTION (A1), D2
237C	MOVE.L	#FORCEFUNC,FUNCTION(A1)
.	(The balance of this code is continued in the	
.	code/data fields of the remaining S1 records	
.	and stored in memory location 0010, etc.)	
2A	The checksum of the first S1 record.	

The second and third S1 records each also contain $13 (19) character pairs and are ended with checksums 13 and 52, respectively. The fourth S1 record contains 07 character pairs and has a checksum of 92.

The S9 record is explained as follows:

S9 S-record type S9, indicating a termination record
03 Hexadecimal 03, indicating that three character pairs (3 bytes) follow
00
00 The address field, zeros
FC The checksum of the S9 record

Each printable character in an S-record is encoded in hexadecimal (ASCII in this example) representation of the binary bits which are actually transmitted. For example, the first S1 record above is sent as shown by the table on the following page.

type		length		address						code/data						checksum	
S	1	1	3	0	0	0	0	3	0	2	8	5	F	...	6	2	A
5 3	3 1	3 1	3 3	3 0	3 0	3 0	3 0	3 3	3 0	3 2	3 8	3 5	3 4	...	3 6	3 2	4 1
0101 0011	0011 0001	0011 0001	0011 0011	0011 0000	0011 0000	0011 0000	0011 0000	0011 0011	0011 0000	0011 0010	0011 1000	0011 0101	0100 0110	...	0100 0110	0011 0010	0100 0001

Appendix B
INSTRUCTION SET DETAILS

B.1 INTRODUCTION

This appendix contains detailed information about each instruction in the MC68000 instruction set. They are arranged in alphabetical order with the mnemonic heading set in large bold type for easy reference.

B.2 ADDRESSING CATEGORIES

Effective address modes may be categorized by the ways in which they may be used. The following classifications will be used in the instruction definitions.

- Data   If an effective address mode may be used to refer to data operands, it is considered a data addressing effective address mode.
- Memory If an effective address mode may be used to refer to memory operands, it is considered a memory addressing effective address mode.
- Alterable If an effective address mode may be used to refer to alterable (writable) operands, it is considered an alterable addressing effective address mode.
- Control   If an effective address mode may be used to refer to memory operands without an associated size, it is considered a control addressing effective address mode.

Table B-1 shows the various categories to which each of the effective address modes belong.

Table B-1. Effective Addressing Mode Categories

Addressing Mode	Mode	Register	Addressing Categories				Assembler Syntax
			Data	Memory	Control	Alterable	
Data Register Direct	000	reg. no.	X	—	—	X	Dn
Address Register Direct	001	reg. no.	—	—	—	X	An
Address Register Indirect	010	reg. no.	X	X	X	X	(An)
Address Register Indirect with Postincrement	011	reg. no.	X	X	—	X	(An) +
Address Register Indirect with Predecrement	100	reg. no.	X	X	—	X	– (An)
Address Register Indirect with Displacement	101	reg. no	X	X	X	X	d(An)
Address Register Indirect with Index	110	reg. no.	X	X	X	X	d(An, ix)
Absolute Short	111	000	X	X	X	X	xxx.W
Absolute Long	111	001	X	X	X	X	xxx.L
Program Counter with Displacement	111	010	X	X	X	—	d(PC)
Program Counter with Index	111	011	X	X	X	—	d(PC, ix)
Immediate	111	100	X	X	—	—	#xxx

These categories may be combined so that additional, more restrictive, classifications may be defined. For example, the instruction descriptions use such classifications as alterable memory or data alterable. The former refers to those addressing modes which are both alterable and memory addresses, and the latter refers to addressing modes which are both data and alterable.

B.3 INSTRUCTION DESCRIPTION

The formats of each instruction are given in the following pages. Figure B-1 illustrates what information is given.

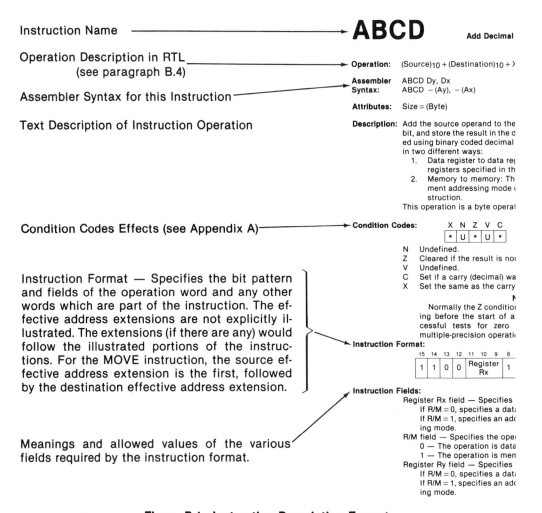

Figure B-1. Instruction Description Format

B.4 REGISTER TRANSFER LANGUAGE DEFINITIONS

The following register transfer language definitions are used for the operation description in the details of the instruction set.

OPERANDS:

An	— address register	**SSP**	— supervisor stack pointer
Dn	— data register	**USP**	— user stack pointer
Rn	— any data or address register	**SP**	— active stack pointer (equivalent to A7)
PC	— program counter	**X**	— extend operand (from condition codes)
SR	— status register		
CCR	— condition codes (low order byte of status register)	**Z**	— zero condition code
		V	— overflow condition code
Immediate Data	— immediate data from the instruction		
d	— address displacement	**Destination**	— destination effective address
Source	— source effective address	**Vector**	— location of exception vector

SUBFIELDS AND QUALIFIERS:

<bit> OF <operand>	selects a single bit of the operand
<operand>[<bit number>:<bit number>]	selects a subfield of an operand
(<operand>)	the contents of the referenced location
<operand>$_{10}$	the operand is binary coded decimal; operations are to be performed in decimal.
(<address register>)	the register indirect operator which indicates that the operand register points to the memory location of the instruction operand. The optional mode qualifiers are $-$, $+$, (d) and (d, ix); these are explained in Section 2.
$-$(<address register>)	
(<address register>)$+$	

OPERATIONS: Operations are grouped into binary, unary, and other.

Binary — These operations are written <operand> <op> <operand> where <op> is one of the following:

$\rightarrow$	the left operand is moved to the location specified by the right operand
$\leftrightarrow$	the contents of the two operands are exchanged
$+$	the operands are added
$-$	the right operand is subtracted from the left operand
$*$	the operands are multiplied
$/$	the first operand is divided by the second operand
$\wedge$	the operands are logically ANDed
$\vee$	the operands are logically ORed
$\oplus$	the operands are logically exclusively ORed
$<$	relational test, true if left operand is less than right operand
$>$	relational test, true if left operand is not equal to right operand
shifted by rotated by	the left operand is shifted or rotated by the number of positions specified by the right operand

Unary:

$\sim$ <operand>	the operand is logically complemented
<operand> sign-extended	the operand is sign extended, all bits of the upper half are made equal to high order bit of the lower half
<operand> tested	the operand is compared to 0, the results are used to set the condition codes

Other:

TRAP	equivalent to PC$\rightarrow$(SSP)$-$; SR$\rightarrow$(SSP)$-$; (vector)$\rightarrow$PC
STOP	enter the stopped state, waiting for interrupts

If <condition> **then** <operations> **else** <operations> The condition is tested. If true, the operations after the "then" are performed. If the condition is false and the optional "else" clause is present, the operations after the "else" are performed. If the condition is false and the optional "else" clause is absent, the instruction performs no operation.

ABCD   Add Decimal with Extend   ABCD

Operation: $(Source)_{10} + (Destination)_{10} + X \rightarrow$ Destination

Assembler Syntax: ABCD Dy, Dx
                ABCD $-(Ay), -(Ax)$

Attributes: Size = (Byte)

Description: Add the source operand to the destination operand along with the extend bit, and store the result in the destination location. The addition is performed using binary coded decimal arithmetic. The operands may be addressed in two different ways:
1. Data register to data register: The operands are contained in the data registers specified in the instruction.
2. Memory to memory: The operands are addressed with the predecrement addressing mode using the address registers specified in the instruction.

This operation is a byte operation only.

Condition Codes:

X	N	Z	V	C
*	U	*	U	*

     N   Undefined.
     Z   Cleared if the result is non-zero. Unchanged otherwise.
     V   Undefined.
     C   Set if a carry (decimal) was generated. Cleared otherwise.
     X   Set the same as the carry bit.

NOTE

Normally the Z condition code bit is set via programming before the start of an operation. This allows successful tests for zero results upon completion of multiple-precision operations.

Instruction Format:

15	14	13	12	11	10	9	8	7	6	5	4	3	2	1	0
1	1	0	0	\multicolumn{3}{c}{Register Rx}		1	0	0	0	R/M	\multicolumn{3}{c}{Register Ry}		

Instruction Fields:

     Register Rx field — Specifies the destination register:
         If R/M = 0, specifies a data register.
         If R/M = 1, specifies an address register for the predecrement addressing mode.
     R/M field — Specifies the operand addressing mode:
         0 — The operation is data register to data register.
         1 — The operation is memory to memory.
     Register Ry field — Specifies the source register:
         If R/M = 0, specifies a data register.
         If R/M = 1, specifies an address register for the predecrement addressing mode.

ADD

Add Binary

ADD

Operation: (Source) + (Destination) → Destination

Assembler ADD <ea>, Dn
Syntax: ADD Dn, <ea>

Attributes: Size = (Byte, Word, Long)

Description: Add the source operand to the destination operand, and store the result in the destination location. The size of the operation may be specified to be byte, word, or long. The mode of the instruction indicates which operand is the source and which is the destination as well as the operand size.

Condition Codes:

X	N	Z	V	C
*	*	*	*	*

N Set if the result is negative. Cleared otherwise.
Z Set if the result is zero. Cleared otherwise.
V Set if an overflow is generated. Cleared otherwise.
C Set if a carry is generated. Cleared otherwise.
X Set the same as the carry bit.

Instruction Format:

15	14	13	12	11 10 9	8 7 6	5 4 3	2 1 0
1	1	0	1	Register	Op-Mode	Effective Address Mode	Register

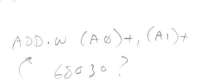

Instruction Fields:

Register field — Specifies any of the eight data registers.
Op-Mode field —

Byte	Word	Long	Operation
000	001	010	(<Dn>) + (<ea>) → <Dn>
100	101	110	(<ea>) + (<Dn>) → <ea>

Effective Address field — Determines addressing mode:
  a. If the location specified is a source operand, then all addressing modes are allowed as shown:

Addressing Mode	Mode	Register	Addressing Mode	Mode	Register
Dn	000	register number	d(An, Xi)	110	register number
An*	001	register number	Abs.W	111	000
(An)	010	register number	Abs.L	111	001
(An)+	011	register number	d(PC)	111	010
-(An)	100	register number	d(PC, Xi)	111	011
d(An)	101	register number	Imm	111	100

*Word and Long only.

— Continued —

ADD Add Binary ADD

Effective Address field (Continued)

b. If the location specified is a destination operand, then only alterable memory addressing modes are allowed as shown:

Addressing Mode	Mode	Register	Addressing Mode	Mode	Register
Dn	—	—	d(An, Xi)	110	register number
An	—	—	Abs.W	111	000
(An)	010	register number	Abs.L	111	001
(An) +	011	register number	d(PC)	—	—
− (An)	100	register number	d(PC, Xi)	—	—
d(An)	101	register number	Imm	—	—

Notes:
1. If the destination is a data register, then it cannot be specified by using the destination <ea> mode, but must use the destination Dn mode instead.
2. ADDA is used when the destination is an address register. ADDI and ADDQ are used when the source is immediate data. Most assemblers automatically make this distinction.

ADDA   Add Address   ADDA

Operation: (Source) + (Destination) → Destination

Assembler Syntax: ADD <ea>, An

Attributes: Size = (Word, Long)

Description: Add the source operand to the destination address register, and store the result in the address register. The size of the operation may be specified to be word or long. The entire destination address register is used regardless of the operation size.

Condition Codes: Not affected.

Instruction Format:

15	14	13	12	11 10 9	8 7 6	5 4 3	2 1 0
1	1	0	1	Register	Op-Mode	Effective Address Mode	Register

Instruction Fields:

    Register field — Specifies any of the eight address registers. This is always the destination.

    Op-Mode field — Specifies the size of the operation:

        011 — word operation. The source operand is sign-extended to a long operand and the operation is performed on the address register using all 32 bits.

        111 — long operation.

    Effective Address field — Specifies the source operand. All addressing modes are allowed as shown:

Addressing Mode	Mode	Register	Addressing Mode	Mode	Register
Dn	000	register number	d(An, Xi)	110	register number
An	001	register number	Abs.W	111	000
(An)	010	register number	Abs.L	111	001
(An)+	011	register number	d(PC)	111	010
−(An)	100	register number	d(PC, Xi)	111	011
d(An)	101	register number	Imm	111	100

ADDI — Add Immediate — ADDI

Operation: Immediate Data + (Destination) → Destination

Assembler Syntax: ADDI #<data>,<ea>

Attributes: Size = (Byte, Word, Long)

Description: Add the immediate data to the destination operand, and store the result in the destination location. The size of the operation may be specified to be byte, word, or long. The size of the immediate data matches the operation size.

Condition Codes:

```
X N Z V C
* * * * *
```

- N Set if the result is negative. Cleared otherwise.
- Z Set if the result is zero. Cleared otherwise.
- V Set if an overflow is generated. Cleared otherwise.
- C Set if a carry is generated. Cleared otherwise.
- X Set the same as the carry bit.

Instruction Format:

15	14	13	12	11	10	9	8	7	6	5	4	3	2	1	0
0	0	0	0	0	1	1	0	Size		Effective Address Mode | Register					
Word Data (16 bits)								Byte Data (8 bits)							
Long Data (32 bits, including previous word)															

Instruction Fields:

Size field — Specifies the size of the operation:
- 00 — byte operation.
- 01 — word operation.
- 10 — long operation.

Effective Address field — Specifies the destination operand. Only data alterable addressing modes are allowed as shown:

Addressing Mode	Mode	Register	Addressing Mode	Mode	Register
Dn	000	register number	d(An, Xi)	110	register number
An	—	—	Abs.W	111	000
(An)	010	register number	Abs.L	111	001
(An)+	011	register number	d(PC)	—	—
-(An)	100	register number	d(PC, Xi)	—	—
d(An)	101	register number	Imm	—	—

Immediate field — (Data immediately following the instruction):
If size = 00, then the data is the low order byte of the immediate word.
If size = 01, then the data is the entire immediate word.
If size = 10, then the data is the next two immediate words.

ADDQ

Add Quick

ADDQ

Operation: Immediate Data + (Destination) → Destination

Assembler Syntax: ADDQ #<data>, <ea>

Attributes: Size = (Byte, Word, Long)

Description: Add the immediate data to the operand at the destination location. The data range is from 1 to 8. The size of the operation may be specified to be byte, word, or long. Word and long operations are also allowed on the address registers and the condition codes are not affected. The entire destination address register is used regardless of the operation size.

Condition Codes:

X	N	Z	V	C
*	*	*	*	*

N Set if the result is negative. Cleared otherwise.
Z Set if the result is zero. Cleared otherwise.
V Set if an overflow is generated. Cleared otherwise.
C Set if a carry is generated. Cleared otherwise.
X Set the same as the carry bit.

The condition codes are not affected if an addition to an address register is made.

Instruction Format:

15	14	13	12	11	10	9	8	7	6	5	4	3	2	1	0
0	1	0	1	Data			0	Size		Effective Address					
										Mode			Register		

Instruction Fields:

Data field — Three bits of immediate data, 0, 1-7 representing a range of 8, 1 to 7 respectively.

Size field — Specifies the size of the operation:
  00 — byte operation.
  01 — word operation.
  10 — long operation.

Effective Address field — Specifies the destination location. Only alterable addressing modes are allowed as shown:

Addressing Mode	Mode	Register	Addressing Mode	Mode	Register
Dn	000	register number	d(An, Xi)	110	register number
An*	001	register number	Abs.W	111	000
(An)	010	register number	Abs.L	111	001
(An)+	011	register number	d(PC)	—	—
−(An)	100	register number	d(PC, Xi)	—	—
d(An)	101	register number	Imm	—	—

*Word and Long only.

ADDX Add Extended ADDX

Operation: (Source) + (Destination) + X → Destination

Assembler Syntax:
ADDX Dy, Dx
ADDX −(Ay), −(Ax)

Attributes: Size = (Byte, Word, Long)

Description: Add the source operand to the destination operand along with the extend bit and store the result in the destination location. The operands may be addressed in two different ways:
1. Data register to data register: the operands are contained in data registers specified in the instruction.
2. Memory to memory: the operands are addressed with the predecrement addressing mode using the address registers specified in the instruction.

The size of the operation may be specified to be byte, word, or long.

Condition Codes:

X	N	Z	V	C
*	*	*	*	*

N Set if the result is negative. Cleared otherwise.
Z Cleared if the result is non-zero. Unchanged otherwise.
V Set if an overflow is generated. Cleared otherwise.
C Set if a carry is generated. Cleared otherwise.
X Set the same as the carry bit.

NOTE
Normally the Z condition code bit is set via programming before the start of an operation. This allows successful tests for zero results upon completion of multiple-precision operations.

Instruction Format:

15	14	13	12	11	10	9	8	7	6	5	4	3	2	1	0
1	1	0	1	Register Rx			1	Size		0	0	R/M	Register Ry		

Instruction Fields:

Register Rx field — Specifies the destination register:
If R/M = 0, specifies a data register.
If R/M = 1, specifies an address register for the predecrement addressing mode.

Size field — Specifies the size of the operation:
00 — byte operation.
01 — word operation.
10 — long operation.

— Continued —

ADDX

Add Extended

ADDX

Instruction Fields: (Continued)

    R/M field — Specifies the operand addressing mode:
        0 — The operation is data register to data register.
        1 — The operation is memory to memory.
    Register Ry field — Specifies the source register:
        If R/M = 0, specifies a data register.
        If R/M = 1, specifies an address register for the predecrement addressing mode.

AND

AND Logical

AND

Operation: (Source)∧(Destination) → Destination

Assembler AND <ea>, Dn
Syntax: AND Dn, <ea>

Attributes: Size = (Byte, Word, Long)

Description: AND the source operand to the destination operand and store the result in the destination location. The size of the operation may be specified to be byte, word, or long. The contents of an address register may not be used as an operand.

Condition Codes:

X	N	Z	V	C
—	*	*	0	0

N Set if the most significant bit of the result is set. Cleared otherwise.
Z Set if the result is zero. Cleared otherwise.
V Always cleared.
C Always cleared.
X Not affected.

Instruction Format:

15	14	13	12	11	10	9	8	7	6	5	4	3	2	1	0
1	1	0	0	\multicolumn{3}{Register}			\multicolumn{3}{Op-Mode}			\multicolumn{3}{Effective Address Mode}			Register		

15	14	13	12	11	10	9	8	7	6	5	4	3	2	1	0
1	1	0	0	Register			Op-Mode			Effective Address				
										Mode			Register		

Instruction Fields:

Register field — Specifies any of the eight data registers.
Op-Mode field —

Byte	Word	Long	Operation
000	001	010	(<Dn>) ∧ (<ea>) → <Dn>
100	101	110	(<ea>) ∧ (<Dn>) → <ea>

Effective Address field — Determines addressing mode:
  If the location specified is a source operand then only data addressing modes are allowed as shown:

Addressing Mode	Mode	Register	Addressing Mode	Mode	Register
Dn	000	register number	d(An, Xi)	110	register number
An	—	—	Abs.W	111	000
(An)	010	register number	Abs.L	111	001
(An)+	011	register number	d(PC)	111	010
−(An)	100	register number	d(PC, Xi)	111	011
d(An)	101	register number	Imm	111	100

— Continued —

AND

AND Logical

AND

Effective Address field (Continued)

If the location specified is a destination operand then only alterable memory addressing modes are allowed as shown:

Addressing Mode	Mode	Register	Addressing Mode	Mode	Register
Dn	—	—	d(An, Xi)	110	register number
An	—	—	Abs.W	111	000
(An)	010	register number	Abs.L	111	001
(An)+	011	register number	d(PC)	—	—
−(An)	100	register number	d(PC, Xi)	—	—
d(An)	101	register number	Imm	—	—

Notes:
1. If the destination is a data register, then it cannot be specified by using the destination <ea> mode, but must use the destination Dn mode instead.
2. ANDI is used when the source is immediate data. Most assemblers automatically make this distinction.

ANDI ANDI

AND Immediate

Operation: Immediate Data ∧ (Destination) → Destination

Assembler Syntax: ANDI #<data>, <ea>

Attributes: Size = (Byte, Word, Long)

Description: AND the immediate data to the destination operand and store the result in the destination location. The size of the operation may be specified to be byte, word, or long. The size of the immediate data matches the operation size.

Condition Codes:

X	N	Z	V	C
—	*	*	0	0

N Set if the most significant bit of the result is set. Cleared otherwise.
Z Set if the result is zero. Cleared otherwise.
V Always cleared.
C Always cleared.
X Not affected.

Instruction Format:

15	14	13	12	11	10	9	8	7	6	5	4	3	2	1	0
0	0	0	0	0	0	1	0	\multicolumn{2}{c}{Size}	\multicolumn{2}{c}{Effective Address Mode}	\multicolumn{2}{c}{Register}		
\multicolumn{8}{l}{Word Data (16 bits)}	\multicolumn{8}{l}{Byte Data (8 bits)}							
\multicolumn{16}{l}{Long Data (32 bits, including previous word)}															

Instruction Fields:

Size field — Specifies the size of the operation:
  00 — byte operation.
  01 — word operation.
  10 — long operation.

Effective Address field — Specifies the destination operand. Only data alterable addressing modes are allowed as shown:

Addressing Mode	Mode	Register	Addressing Mode	Mode	Register
Dn	000	register number	d(An, Xi)	110	register number
An	—	—	Abs.W	111	000
(An)	010	register number	Abs.L	111	001
(An)+	011	register number	d(PC)	—	—
−(An)	100	register number	d(PC, Xi)	—	—
d(An)	101	register number	Imm	—	—

Immediate field — (Data immediately following the instruction):
  If size = 00, then the data is the low order byte of the immediate word.
  If size = 01, then the data is the entire immediate word.
  If size = 10, then the data is the next two immediate words.

ANDI to CCR

AND Immediate to Condition Codes

Operation: (Source)∧CCR → CCR

Assembler Syntax: ANDI #xxx, CCR

Attributes: Size = (Byte)

Description: AND the immediate operand with the condition codes and store the result in the low-order byte of the status register.

Condition Codes:

X	N	Z	V	C
*	*	*	*	*

- N — Cleared if bit 3 of immediate operand is zero. Unchanged otherwise.
- Z — Cleared if bit 2 of immediate operand is zero. Unchanged otherwise.
- V — Cleared if bit 1 of immediate operand is zero. Unchanged otherwise.
- C — Cleared if bit 0 of immediate operand is zero. Unchanged otherwise.
- X — Cleared if bit 4 of immediate operand is zero. Unchanged otherwise.

Instruction Format:

15	14	13	12	11	10	9	8	7	6	5	4	3	2	1	0
0	0	0	0	0	0	1	0	0	0	1	1	1	1	0	0
0	0	0	0	0	0	0	0	\multicolumn{8}{c}{Byte Data (8 bits)}

ANDI to SR

AND Immediate to the Status Register (Privileged Instruction)

Operation: If supervisor state
then (Source)∧SR → SR
else TRAP

Assembler Syntax: ANDI #xxx, SR

Attributes: Size = (Word)

Description: AND the immediate operand with the contents of the status register and store the result in the status register. All bits of the status register are affected.

Condition Codes:

X	N	Z	V	C
*	*	*	*	*

N Cleared if bit 3 of immediate operand is zero. Unchanged otherwise.
Z Cleared if bit 2 of immediate operand is zero. Unchanged otherwise.
V Cleared if bit 1 of immediate operand is zero. Unchanged otherwise.
C Cleared if bit 0 of immediate operand is zero. Unchanged otherwise.
X Cleared if bit 4 of immediate operand is zero. Unchanged otherwise.

Instruction Format:

15	14	13	12	11	10	9	8	7	6	5	4	3	2	1	0
0	0	0	0	0	0	1	0	0	1	1	1	1	1	0	0
Word Data (16 bits)															

ASL, ASR   Arithmetic Shift   ASL, ASR

Operation: (Destination) Shifted by <count> → Destination

Assembler Syntax:
ASd Dx, Dy
ASd #<data>, Dy
ASd <ea>

Attributes: Size = (Byte, Word, Long)

Description: Arithmetically shift the bits of the operand in the direction specified. The carry bit receives the last bit shifted out of the operand. The shift count for the shifting of a register may be specified in two different ways:
1. Immediate: the shift count is specified in the instruction (shift range, 1-8).
2. Register: the shift count is contained in a data register specified in the instruction.

The size of the operation may be specified to be byte, word, or long. The content of memory may be shifted one bit only and the operand size is restricted to a word.

For ASL, the operand is shifted left; the number of positions shifted is the shift count. Bits shifted out of the high order bit go to both the carry and the extend bits; zeroes are shifted into the low order bit. The overflow bit indicates if any sign changes occur during the shift.

ASL:
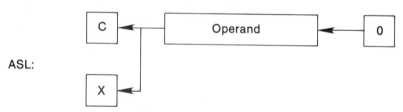

For ASR, the operand is shifted right; the number of positions shifted is the shift count. Bits shifted out of the low order bit go to both the carry and the extend bits; the sign bit is replicated into the high order bit.

ASR:
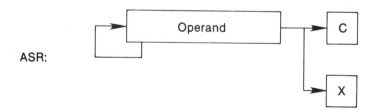

— Continued —

ASL, ASR   Arithmetic Shift   ASL, ASR

Condition Codes:

X	N	Z	V	C
*	*	*	*	*

- N Set if the most significant bit of the result is set. Cleared otherwise.
- Z Set if the result is zero. Cleared otherwise.
- V Set if the most significant bit is changed at any time during the shift operation. Cleared otherwise.
- C Set according to the last bit shifted out of the operand. Cleared for a shift count of zero.
- X Set according to the last bit shifted out of the operand. Unaffected for a shift count of zero.

Instruction Format (Register Shifts):

15	14	13	12	11	10	9	8	7	6	5	4	3	2	1	0
1	1	1	0	Count/Register			dr	Size		i/r	0	0	Register		

Instruction Fields (Register Shifts):

Count/Register field — Specifies shift count or register where count is located:

  If i/r = 0, the shift count is specified in this field. The values 0, 1-7 represent a range of 8, 1 to 7 respectively.

  If i/r = 1, the shift count (modulo 64) is contained in the data register specified in this field.

dr field — Specifies the direction of the shift:

  0 — shift right.
  1 — shift left.

Size field — Specifies the size of the operation:

  00 — byte operation.
  01 — word operation.
  10 — long operation.

i/r field —

  If i/r = 0, specifies immediate shift count.
  if i/r = 1, specifies register shift count.

Register field — Specifies a data register whose content is to be shifted.

Instruction Format (Memory Shifts):

15	14	13	12	11	10	9	8	7	6	5	4	3	2	1	0
1	1	1	0	0	0	0	dr	1	1	Effective Address					
										Mode			Register		

— Continued —

ASL, ASR Arithmetic Shift ASL, ASR

Instruction Fields (Memory Shifts):

dr field — Specifies the direction of the shift:
 0 — shift right.
 1 — shift left.

Effective Address field — Specifies the operand to be shifted. Only memory alterable addressing modes are allowed as shown:

Addressing Mode	Mode	Register	Addressing Mode	Mode	Register
Dn	—	—	d(An, Xi)	110	register number
An	—	—	Abs.W	111	000
(An)	010	register number	Abs.L	111	001
(An)+	011	register number	d(PC)	—	—
−(An)	100	register number	d(PC, Xi)	—	—
d(An)	101	register number	Imm	—	—

Bcc   Branch Conditionally   Bcc

Operation: If (condition true) then PC + d → PC

Assembler Syntax: Bcc <label>

Attributes: Size = (Byte, Word)

Description: If the specified condition is met, program execution continues at location (PC) + displacement. Displacement is a twos complement integer which counts the relative distance in bytes. The value in PC is the current instruction location plus two. If the 8-bit displacement in the instruction word is zero, then the 16-bit displacement (word immediately following the instruction) is used. "cc" may specify the following conditions:

CC	carry clear	0100	$\overline{C}$	LS	low or same	0011	$C + Z$
CS	carry set	0101	C	LT	less than	1101	$N \cdot \overline{V} + \overline{N} \cdot V$
EQ	equal	0111	Z	MI	minus	1011	N
GE	greater or equal	1100	$N \cdot V + \overline{N} \cdot \overline{V}$	NE	not equal	0110	$\overline{Z}$
GT	greater than	1110	$N \cdot V \cdot \overline{Z} + \overline{N} \cdot \overline{V} \cdot \overline{Z}$	PL	plus	1010	$\overline{N}$
HI	high	0010	$\overline{C} \cdot \overline{Z}$	VC	overflow clear	1000	$\overline{V}$
LE	less or equal	1111	$Z + N \cdot \overline{V} + \overline{N} \cdot V$	VS	overflow set	1001	V

Condition Codes: Not affected.

Instruction Format:

15	14	13	12	11	10	9	8	7	6	5	4	3	2	1	0
0	1	1	0	\multicolumn{4}{}{Condition}				\multicolumn{8}{}{8-bit Displacement}							
\multicolumn{16}{}{16-bit Displacement if 8-bit Displacement = 0}															

Instruction Fields:

Condition field — One of fourteen conditions discussed in description.

8-bit Displacement field — Twos complement integer specifying the relative distance (in bytes) between the branch instruction and the next instruction to be executed if the condition is met.

16-bit Displacement field — Allows a larger displacement than 8 bits. Used only if the 8-bit displacement is equal to zero.

Note: A short branch to the immediately following instruction cannot be done because it would result in a zero offset which forces a word branch instruction definition.

BCHG

Test a Bit and Change

BCHG

Operation: ~(<bit number>) OF Destination → Z;
~(<bit number>) OF Destination → <bit number> OF Destination

Assembler Syntax: BCHG Dn, <ea>
BCHG #<data>, <ea>

Attributes: Size = (Byte, Long)

Description: A bit in the destination operand is tested and the state of the specified bit is reflected in the Z condition code. After the test, the state of the specified bit is changed in the destination. If a data register is the destination, then the bit numbering is modulo 32 allowing bit manipulation on all bits in a data register. If a memory location is the destination, a byte is read from that location, the bit operation performed using the bit number modulo 8, and the byte written back to the location with zero referring to the least-significant bit. The bit number for this operation may be specified in two different ways:
1. Immediate — the bit number is specified in a second word of the instruction.
2. Register — the bit number is contained in a data register specified in the instruction.

Condition Codes:

X	N	Z	V	C
—	—	*	—	—

N Not affected.
Z Set if the bit tested is zero. Cleared otherwise.
V Not affected.
C Not affected.
X Not affected.

Instruction Format (Bit Number Dynamic):

15	14	13	12	11	10	9	8	7	6	5	4	3	2	1	0
0	0	0	0	\multicolumn{3}{c}{Register}	1	0	1	\multicolumn{3}{c}{Effective Address Mode}	\multicolumn{3}{c}{Register}

Instruction Fields (Bit Number Dynamic):

Register field — Specifies the data register whose content is the bit number.

Effective Address field — Specifies the destination location. Only data alterable addressing modes are allowed as shown:

Addressing Mode	Mode	Register	Addressing Mode	Mode	Register
Dn*	000	register number	d(An, Xi)	110	register number
An	—	—	Abs.W	111	000
(An)	010	register number	Abs.L	111	001
(An)+	011	register number	d(PC)	—	—
−(An)	100	register number	d(PC, Xi)	—	—
d(An)	101	register number	Imm	—	—

*Long only; all others are byte only.

— Continued —

BCHG Test a Bit and Change BCHG

Instruction Format (Bit Number Static):

15	14	13	12	11	10	9	8	7	6	5	4	3	2	1	0
0	0	0	0	1	0	0	0	0	1	\multicolumn{6}{c}{Effective Address Mode | Register}
0	0	0	0	0	0	0	0	\multicolumn{8}{c}{bit number}

Instruction Fields (Bit Number Static):

Effective Address field — Specifies the destination location. Only data alterable addressing modes are allowed as shown:

Addressing Mode	Mode	Register	Addressing Mode	Mode	Register
Dn	000	register number	d(An, Xi)	110	register number
An	—	—	Abs.W	111	000
(An)	010	register number	Abs.L	111	001
(An)+	011	register number	d(PC)	—	—
−(An)	100	register number	d(PC, Xi)	—	—
d(An)	101	register number	Imm	—	—

*Long only; all others are byte only.

bit number field — Specifies the bit numbers.

BCLR

Test a Bit and Clear

BCLR

Operation: ~(<bit number>) OF Destination)→Z;
0→<bit number> OF Destination

Assembler BLCR Dn, <ea>
Syntax: BCLR #<data>, <ea>

Attributes: Size = (Byte, Long)

Description: A bit in the destination operand is tested and the state of the specified bit is reflected in the Z condition code. After the test, the specified bit is cleared in the destination. If a data register is the destination, then the bit numbering is modulo 32 allowing bit manipulation on all bits in a data register. If a memory location is the destination, a byte is read from that location, the bit operation performed using the bit number modulo 8, and the byte written back to the location with zero referring to the least-significant bit. The bit number for this operation may be specified in two different ways:
1. Immediate — the bit number is specified in a second word of the instruction.
2. Register — the bit number is contained in a data register specified in the instruction.

Condition Codes:

X	N	Z	V	C
—	—	*	—	—

N Not affected.
Z Set if the bit tested is zero. Cleared otherwise.
V Not affected.
C Not affected.
X Not affected.

Instruction Format (Bit Number Dynamic):

15	14	13	12	11	10	9	8	7	6	5	4	3	2	1	0
0	0	0	0	Register			1	1	0	Effective Address				
										Mode			Register		

Instruction Fields (Bit Number Dynamic):

Register field — Specifies the data register whose content is the bit number.

Effective Address field — Specifies the destination location. Only data alterable addressing modes are allowed as shown:

Addressing Mode	Mode	Register	Addressing Mode	Mode	Register
Dn*	000	register number	d(An, Xi)	110	register number
An	—	—	Abs.W	111	000
(An)	010	register number	Abs.L	111	001
(An)+	011	register number	d(PC)	—	—
−(An)	100	register number	d(PC, Xi)	—	—
d(An)	101	register number	Imm	—	—

*Long only; all others are byte only.

— Continued —

BCLR Test a Bit and Clear BCLR

Instruction Format (Bit Number Static):

15	14	13	12	11	10	9	8	7	6	5 4 3	2 1 0
0	0	0	0	1	0	0	0	1	0	Effective Address Mode	Register
0	0	0	0	0	0	0	0	\multicolumn{4}{c}{bit number}				

15	14	13	12	11	10	9	8	7	6	5	4	3	2	1	0
0	0	0	0	1	0	0	0	1	0	\multicolumn{3}{c	}{Effective Address Mode}	\multicolumn{3}{c	}{Register}
0	0	0	0	0	0	0	0	\multicolumn{8}{c	}{bit number}

Instruction Fields (Bit Number Static):

Effective Address field — Specifies the destination location. Only data alterable addressing modes are allowed as shown:

Addressing Mode	Mode	Register	Addressing Mode	Mode	Register
Dn*	000	register only	d(An, Xi)	110	register number
An	—	—	Abs.W	111	000
(An)	010	register number	Abs.L	111	001
(An)+	011	register number	d(PC)	—	—
−(An)	100	register number	d(PC, Xi)	—	—
d(An)	101	register number	Imm	—	—

*Long only; all others are byte only.

bit number field — Specifies the bit number.

BRA   Branch Always   BRA

Operation: PC + d → PC

Assembler Syntax: BRA <label>

Attributes: Size = (Byte, Word)

Description: Program execution continues at location (PC) + displacement. Displacement is a twos complement integer which counts the relative distance in bytes. The value in PC is the current instruction location plus two. If the 8-bit displacement in the instruction word is zero, then the 16-bit displacement (word immediately following the instruction) is used.

Condition Codes: Not affected.

Instruction Format:

15	14	13	12	11	10	9	8	7	6	5	4	3	2	1	0
0	1	1	0	0	0	0	0	8-bit Displacement							
16-bit Displacement if 8-bit Displacement = 0															

Instruction Fields:

     8-bit Displacement field — Twos complement integer specifying the relative distance (in bytes) between the branch instruction and the next instruction to be executed if the condition is met.

     16-bit Displacement field — Allows a larger displacement than 8 bits. Used only if the 8-bit displacement is equal to zero.

Note: A short branch to the immediately following instruction cannot be done because it would result in a zero offset which forces a word branch instruction definition.

BSET

Test a Bit and Set

BSET

Operation: ~(<bit number>) OF Destination → Z
1 → <bit number> OF Destination

Assembler Syntax: BSET Dn, <ea>
BSET #<data>, <ea>

Attributes: Size = (Byte, Long)

Description: A bit in the destination operand is tested and the state of the specified bit is reflected in the Z condition code. After the test, the specified bit is set in the destination. If a data register is the destination, then the bit numbering is modulo 32, allowing bit manipulation on all bits in a data register. If a memory location is the destination, a byte is read from that location, the bit operation performed using the bit number modulo 8, and the byte written back to the location with zero referring to the least-significant bit. The bit number for this operation may be specified in two different ways:
1. Immediate — the bit number is specified in a second word of the instruction.
2. Register — the bit number is contained in a data register specified in the instruction.

Condition Codes:

X	N	Z	V	C
—	—	*	—	—

N Not affected.
Z Set if the bit tested is zero. Cleared otherwise.
V Not affected.
C Not affected.
X Not affected.

Instruction Format (Bit Number Dynamic):

15	14	13	12	11	10	9	8	7	6	5	4	3	2	1	0
0	0	0	0	\multicolumn{3}{Register}			1	1	1	\multicolumn{3}{Effective Address}		
										Mode			Register		

Instruction Fields (Bit Number Dynamic):

Register field — Specifies the data register whose content is the bit number.

Effective Address field — Specifies the destination location. Only data alterable addressing modes are allowed as shown:

Addressing Mode	Mode	Register	Addressing Mode	Mode	Register
Dn*	000	register number	d(An, Xi)	110	register number
An	—	—	Abs.W	111	000
(An)	010	register number	Abs.L	111	001
(An)+	011	register number	d(PC)	—	—
-(An)	100	register number	d(PC, Xi)	—	—
d(An)	101	register number	Imm	—	—

*Long only; all others are byte only

— Continued —

BSET

Test a Bit and Set

BSET

Instruction Format (Bit Number Static):

15	14	13	12	11	10	9	8	7	6	5 4 3	2 1 0
0	0	0	0	1	0	0	0	1	1	Effective Address Mode	Register
0	0	0	0	0	0	0	0	\multicolumn{4}{c	}{bit number}	

Instruction Fields (Bit Number Static):

Effective Address field — Specifies the destination location. Only data alterable addressing modes are allowed as shown:

Addressing Mode	Mode	Register	Addressing Mode	Mode	Register
Dn*	000	register number	d(An, Xi)	110	register number
An	—	—	Abs.W	111	000
(An)	010	register number	Abs.L	111	001
(An)+	011	register number	d(PC)	—	—
−(An)	100	register number	d(PC, Xi)	—	—
d(An)	101	register number	Imm	—	—

*Long only; all others are byte only.

bit number field — Specifies the bit number.

185

BSR

Branch to Subroutine

BSR

Operation: PC → −(SP); PC + d → PC

Assembler Syntax: BSR <label>

Attributes: Size = (Byte, Word)

Description: The long word address of the instruction immediately following the BSR instruction is pushed onto the system stack. Program execution then continues at location (PC) + displacement. Displacement is a twos complement integer which counts the relative distances in bytes. The value in PC is the current instruction location plus two. If the 8-bit displacement in the instruction word is zero, then the 16-bit displacement (word immediately following the instruction) is used.

Condition Codes: Not affected.

Instruction Format:

15	14	13	12	11	10	9	8	7	6	5	4	3	2	1	0
0	1	1	0	0	0	0	1	\multicolumn{8}{c}{8-bit Displacement}
\multicolumn{16}{c}{16-bit Displacement if 8-bit Displacement = 0}

Instruction Fields:

8-bit Displacement field — Twos complement integer specifying the relative distance (in bytes) between the branch instruction and the next instruction to be executed if the condition is met.

16-bit Displacement field — Allows a larger displacement than 8 bits. Used only if the 8-bit displacement is equal to zero.

Note: A short subroutine branch to the immediately following instruction cannot be done because it would result in a zero offset which forces a word branch instruction definition.

BTST

BTST Test a Bit **BTST**

Operation: ~(<bit number>) OF Destination → Z

Assembler BTST Dn, <ea>
Syntax: BTST #<data>, <ea>

Attributes: Size = (Byte, Long)

Description: A bit in the destination operand is tested and the state of the specified bit is reflected in the Z condition code. If a data register is the destination, then the bit numbering is modulo 32, allowing bit manipulation on all bits in a data register. If a memory location is the destination, a byte is read from that location, and the bit operation performed using the bit number modulo 8 with zero referring to the least-signifcant bit. The bit number for this operation may be specified in two different ways:
1. Immediate — the bit number is specified in a second word of the instruction.
2. Register — the bit number is contained in a data register specified in the instruction.

Condition Codes:

X	N	Z	V	C
—	—	*	—	—

N Not affected.
Z Set if the bit tested is zero. Cleared otherwise.
V Not affected.
C Not affected.
X Not affected.

Instruction Format (Bit Number Dynamic):

15	14	13	12	11	10	9	8	7	6	5	4	3	2	1	0
0	0	0	0	Register			1	0	0	Effective Address				
										Mode			Register		

Instruction Fields (Bit Number Dynamic):

Register field — Specifies the data register whose content is the bit number.

Effective Address field — Specifies the destination location. Only data addressing modes are allowed as shown:

Addressing Mode	Mode	Register	Addressing Mode	Mode	Register
Dn*	000	register number	d(An, Xi)	110	register number
An	—	—	Abs.W	111	000
(An)	010	register number	Abs.L	111	001
(An)+	011	register number	d(PC)	111	010
-(An)	100	register number	d(PC, Xi)	111	011
d(An)	101	register number	Imm	111	100

*Long only; all others are byte only.

— Continued —

BTST　　　Test a Bit　　　BTST

Instruction Format (Bit Number Static):

15	14	13	12	11	10	9	8	7	6	5	4	3	2	1	0
0	0	0	0	1	0	0	0	0	0	\multicolumn{3}{c}{Effective Address Mode}			Register
0	0	0	0	0	0	0	0	\multicolumn{8}{c}{bit number}							

15-10	9-8	7-6	5-3	2-0
000010	00	00	Effective Address Mode	Register
00000000			bit number	

Instruction Fields (Bit Number Static):

Effective Address field — Specifies the destination location. Only data addressing modes are allowed as shown:

Addressing Mode	Mode	Register	Addressing Mode	Mode	Register
Dn*	000	register number	d(An, Xi)	110	register number
An	—	—	Abs.W	111	000
(An)	010	register number	Abs.L	111	001
(An)+	011	register number	d(PC)	111	010
−(An)	100	register number	d(PC, Xi)	111	011
d(An)	101	register number	Imm	—	—

*Long only; all others are byte only.

bit number field — Specifies the bit number.

CHK

Check Register Against Bounds

Operation: If Dn<0 or Dn>(<ea>) then TRAP

Assembler Syntax: CHK <ea>, Dn

Attributes: Size = (Word)

Description: The content of the low order word in the data register specified in the instruction is examined and compared to the upper bound. The upper bound is a twos complement integer. If the register value is less than zero or greater than the upper bound contained in the operand word, then the processor initiates exception processing. The vector number is generated to reference the CHK instruction exception vector.

Condition Codes:

X	N	Z	V	C
—	*	U	U	U

N Set if Dn<0; cleared if Dn>(<ea>). Undefined otherwise.
Z Undefined.
V Undefined.
C Undefined.
X Not affected.

Instruction Format:

15	14	13	12	11	10	9	8	7	6	5	4	3	2	1	0
0	1	0	0	Register			1	1	0	Effective Address					
										Mode			Register		

Instruction Fields:

Register field — Specifies the data register whose content is checked.
Effective Address field — Specifies the upper bound operand word. Only data addressing modes are allowed as shown:

Addressing Mode	Mode	Register	Addressing Mode	Mode	Register
Dn	000	register number	d(An, Xi)	110	register number
An	—	—	Abs.W	111	000
(An)	010	register number	Abs.L	111	001
(An)+	011	register number	d(PC)	111	010
−(An)	100	register number	d(PC, Xi)	111	011
d(An)	101	register number	Imm	111	100

CLR

Clear an Operand

CLR

Operation: 0 → Destination

**Assembler
Syntax:** CLR <ea>

Attributes: Size = (Byte, Word, Long)

Description: The destination is cleared to all zero bits. The size of the operation may be specified to be byte, word, or long.

Condition Codes:

X	N	Z	V	C
—	0	1	0	0

N Always cleared.
Z Always set.
V Always cleared.
C Always cleared.
X Not affected.

Instruction Format:

15	14	13	12	11	10	9	8	7	6	5	4	3	2	1	0
0	1	0	0	0	0	1	0	Size		Effective Address					
										Mode			Register		

Instruction Fields:

Size field — Specifies the size of the operation:
- 00 — byte operation.
- 01 — word operation.
- 10 — long operation.

Effective Address field — Specifies the destination location. Only data alterable addressing modes are allowed as shown:

Addressing Mode	Mode	Register	Addressing Mode	Mode	Register
Dn	000	register number	d(An, Xi)	110	register number
An	—	—	Abs.W	111	000
(An)	010	register number	Abs.L	111	001
(An)+	011	register number	d(PC)	—	—
−(An)	100	register number	d(PC, Xi)	—	—
d(An)	101	register number	Imm	—	—

Note: A memory destination is read before it is written to.

CMP   Compare   CMP

Operation: (Destination) − (Source)

Assembler Syntax: CMP <ea>, Dn

Attributes: Size = (Byte, Word, Long)

Description: Subtract the source operand from the destination operand and set the condition codes according to the result; the destination location is not changed. The size of the operation may be specified to be byte, word, or long.

Condition Codes:

X	N	Z	V	C
—	*	*	*	*

N Set if the result is negative. Cleared otherwise.
Z Set if the result is zero. Cleared otherwise.
V Set if an overflow is generated. Cleared otherwise.
C Set if a borrow is generated. Cleared otherwise.
X Not affected.

Instruction Format:

15	14	13	12	11	10	9	8	7	6	5	4	3	2	1	0
1	0	1	1	\multicolumn{3}{c}{Register}	\multicolumn{3}{c}{Op-Mode}	\multicolumn{3}{c}{Effective Address Mode}	\multicolumn{3}{c}{Register}

Instruction Fields:

Register field — Specifies the destination data register.
Op-Mode field —

Byte	Word	Long	Operation
000	001	010	(<Dn>) − (<ea>)

Effective Address field — Specifies the source operand. All addressing modes are allowed as shown:

Addressing Mode	Mode	Register	Addressing Mode	Mode	Register
Dn	000	register number	d(An, Xi)	110	register number
An*	001	register number	Abs.W	111	000
(An)	010	register number	Abs.L	111	001
(An)+	011	register number	d(PC)	111	010
−(An)	100	register number	d(PC, Xi)	111	011
d(An)	101	register number	Imm	111	100

*Word and Long only.

Note: CMPA is used when the destination is an address register. CMPI is used when the source is immediate data. CMPM is used for memory to memory compares. Most assemblers automatically make this distinction.

CMPA   Compare Address   CMPA

Operation: (Destination) − (Source)

Assembler Syntax: CMPA <ea>, An

Attributes: Size = (Word, Long)

Description: Subtract the source operand from the destination address register and set the condition codes according to the result; the address register is not changed. The size of the operation may be specified to be word or long. Word length source operands are sign extended to 32 bit quantities before the operation is done.

Condition Code:

X	N	Z	V	C
—	*	*	*	*

N   Set if the result is negative. Cleared otherwise.
Z   Set if the result is zero. Cleared otherwise.
V   Set if an overflow is generated. Cleared otherwise.
C   Set if a borrow is generated. Cleared otherwise.
X   Not affected.

Instruction Format:

15	14	13	12	11 10 9	8 7 6	5 4 3	2 1 0
1	0	1	1	Register	Op-Mode	Effective Address Mode	Register

Instruction Fields:

Register field — Specifies the destination address register.

Op-Mode field — Specifies the size of the operation:
    011 — word operation. The source operand is sign-extended to a long operand and the operation is performed on the address register using all 32 bits.
    111 — long operation.

Effective Address field — Specifies the source operand. All addressing modes are allowed as shown:

Addressing Mode	Mode	Register	Addressing Mode	Mode	Register
Dn	000	register number	d(An, Xi)	110	register number
An	001	register number	Abs.W	111	000
(An)	010	register number	Abs.L	111	001
(An)+	011	register number	d(PC)	111	010
−(An)	100	register number	d(PC, Xi)	111	011
d(An)	101	register number	Imm	111	100

CMPI   Compare Immediate   CMPI

Operation: (Destination) − Immediate Data

Assembler Syntax: CMPI #<data>, <ea>

Attributes: Size = (Byte, Word, Long)

Description: Subtract the immediate data from the destination operand and set the condition codes according to the result; the destination location is not changed. The size of the operation may be specified to be byte, word, or long. The size of the immediate data matches the operation size.

Condition Codes:

X	N	Z	V	C
—	*	*	*	*

- N Set if the result is negative. Cleared otherwise.
- Z Set if the result is zero. Cleared otherwise.
- V Set if an overflow is generated. Cleared otherwise.
- C Set if a borrow is generated. Cleared otherwise.
- X Not affected.

Instruction Format:

15	14	13	12	11	10	9	8	7	6	5	4	3	2	1	0
0	0	0	0	1	1	0	0	\multicolumn{2}{c}{Size}	\multicolumn{4}{c}{Effective Address Mode | Register}			
\multicolumn{8}{c}{Word Data (16 bits)}	\multicolumn{8}{c}{Byte Data (8 bits)}															
\multicolumn{16}{c}{Long Data (32 bits, including previous word)}																

Instruction Fields:

Size field — Specifies the size of the operation:
- 00 — byte operation.
- 01 — word operation.
- 10 — long operation.

Effective Address field — Specifies the destination operand. Only data alterable addressing modes are allowed as shown:

Addressing Mode	Mode	Register	Addressing Mode	Mode	Register
Dn	000	register number	d(An, Xi)	110	register number
An	—	—	Abs.W	111	000
(An)	010	register number	Abs.L	111	001
(An)+	011	register number	d(PC)	—	—
−(An)	100	register number	d(PC, Xi)	—	—
d(An)	101	register number	Imm	—	—

Immediate field — (Data immediately following the instruction):
  If size = 00, then the data is the low order byte of the immediate word.
  If size = 01, then the data is the entire immediate word.
  If size = 10, then the data is the next two immediate words.

CMPM   Compare Memory   CMPM

Operation: (Destination) − (Source)

Assembler Syntax: CMPM (Ay)+ , (Ax)+

Attributes: Size = (Byte, Word, Long)

Description: Subtract the source operand from the destination operand, and set the condition codes according to the results; the destination location is not changed. The operands are always addressed with the postincrement addressing mode using the address registers specified in the instruction. The size of the operation may be specified to be byte, word, or long.

Condition Codes:

X	N	Z	V	C
—	*	*	*	*

N Set if the result is negative. Cleared otherwise.
Z Set if the result is zero. Cleared otherwise.
V Set if an overflow is generated. Cleared otherwise.
C Set if a borrow is generated. Cleared otherwise.
X Not affected.

Instruction Format:

15	14	13	12	11	10	9	8	7	6	5	4	3	2	1	0
1	0	1	1	\multicolumn{3}{c}{Register Rx}	1	\multicolumn{2}{c}{Size}	0	0	1	\multicolumn{3}{c}{Register Ry}

Instruction Fields:

Register Rx field — (always the destination) Specifies an address register for the postincrement addressing mode.

Size field — Specifies the size of the operation:
  00 — byte operation.
  01 — word operation.
  10 — long operation.

Register Ry field — (always the source) Specifies an address register for the postincrement addressing mode.

DBcc   Test Condition, Decrement, and Branch   DBcc

Operation: If (condition false)
then Dn − 1 → Dn;
If Dn ≠ −1
then PC + d → PC
else PC + 2 → PC (Fall through to next instruction)

Assembler Syntax: DBcc Dn, <label>

Attributes: Size = (Word)

Description: This instruction is a looping primitive of three parameters: a condition, a data register, and a displacement. The instruction first tests the condition to determine if the termination condition for the loop has been met, and if so, no operation is performed. If the termination condition is not true, the low order 16 bits of the counter data register are decremented by one. If the result is −1, the counter is exhausted and execution continues with the next instruction. If the result is not equal to −1, execution continues at the location indicated by the current value of PC plus the sign-extended 16-bit displacement. The value in PC is the current instruction location plus two "cc" may specify the following conditions:

CC	carry clear	0100	$\overline{C}$		LS	low or same	0011	$C + Z$
CS	carry set	0101	C		LT	less than	1101	$N \cdot \overline{V} + \overline{N} \cdot V$
EQ	equal	0111	Z		MI	minus	1011	N
F	false	0001	0		NE	not equal	0110	$\overline{Z}$
GE	greater or equal	1100	$N \cdot V + \overline{N} \cdot \overline{V}$		PL	plus	1010	$\overline{N}$
GT	greater than	1110	$N \cdot V \cdot \overline{Z} + \overline{N} \cdot \overline{V} \cdot \overline{Z}$		T	true	0000	1
HI	high	0010	$\overline{C} \cdot \overline{Z}$		VC	overflow clear	1000	$\overline{V}$
LE	less or equal	1111	$Z + N \cdot \overline{V} + \overline{N} \cdot V$		VS	overflow set	1001	V

Condition Codes: Not affected.

Instruction Format:

15	14	13	12	11	10	9	8	7	6	5	4	3	2	1	0
0	1	0	1	Condition				1	1	0	0	1	Register		
Displacement															

Instruction Fields:
Condition field — One of the sixteen conditions discussed in description.
Register field — Specifies the data register which is the counter.
Displacement field — Specifies the distance of the branch (in bytes).

Notes: 1. The terminating condition is like that defined by the UNTIL loop constructs of high-level languages. For example: DBMI can be stated as "decrement and branch until minus."

— Continued —

DBcc   Test Condition, Decrement and Branch   DBcc

Notes: (Continued)
2. Most assemblers accept DBRA for DBF for use when no condition is required for termination of a loop.
3. There are two basic ways of entering a loop; at the beginning or by branching to the trailing DBcc instruction. If a loop structure terminated with DBcc is entered at the beginning, the control index count must be one less than the number of loop executions desired. This count is useful for indexed addressing modes and dynamically specified bit operations. However, when entering a loop by branching directly to the trailing DBcc instruction, the control index should equal the loop execution count. In this case, if a zero count occurs, the DBcc instruction will not branch causing complete bypass of the main loop.

DIVS   Signed Divide   DIVS

Operation: (Destination)/(Source) → Destination

Assembler Syntax: DIVS <ea>, Dn

Attributes: Size = (Word)

Description: Divide the destination operand by the source operand and store the result in the destination. The destination operand is a long operand (32 bits) and the source operand is a word operand (16 bits). The operation is performed using signed arithmetic. The result is a 32-bit result such that:
1. The quotient is in the lower word (least significant 16-bits).
2. The remainder is in the upper word (most significant 16-bits).

The sign of the remainder is always the same as the dividend unless the remainder is equal to zero. Two special conditions may arise:
1. Division by zero causes a trap.
2. Overflow may be detected and set before completion of the instruction. If overflow is detected, the condition is flagged but the operands are unaffected.

Condition Codes:

X	N	Z	V	C
—	*	*	*	0

N   Set if the quotient is negative. Cleared otherwise. Undefined if overflow.
Z   Set if the quotient is zero. Cleared otherwise. Undefined if overflow.
V   Set if division overflow is detected. Cleared otherwise.
C   Always cleared.
X   Not affected.

Instruction Format:

15	14	13	12	11 10 9	8	7	6	5 4 3	2 1 0
1	0	0	0	Register	1	1	1	Effective Address Mode	Register

Instruction Fields:

Register field — Specifies any of the eight data registers. This field always specifies the destination operand.

Effective Address field — Specifies the source operand. Only data addressing modes are allowed as shown:

Addressing Mode	Mode	Register	Addressing Mode	Mode	Register
Dn	000	register number	d(An, Xi)	110	register number
An	—	—	Abs.W	111	000
(An)	010	register number	Abs.L	111	001
(An)+	011	register number	d(PC)	111	010
−(An)	100	register number	d(PC, Xi)	111	011
d(An)	101	register number	Imm	111	100

Note: Overflow occurs if the quotient is larger than a 16-bit signed integer.

DIVU   Unsigned Divide   DIVU

Operation: (Destination)/(Source) → Destination

Assembler Syntax: DIVU <ea>, Dn

Attributes: Size = (Word)

Description: Divide the destination operand by the source operand and store the result in the destination. The destination operand is a long operand (32 bits) and the source operand is a word (16 bit) operand. The operation is performed using unsigned arithmetic. The result is a 32-bit result such that:
    1. The quotient is in the lower word (least significnat 16 bits).
    2. The remainder is in the upper word (most significant 16 bits).
Two special conditions may arise:
    1. Division by zero causes a trap.
    2. Overflow may be detected and set before completion of the instruction. If overflow is detected, the condition is flagged but the operands are unaffected.

Condition Codes:

X	N	Z	V	C
—	*	*	*	0

    N   Set if the most significant bit of the quotient is set. Cleared otherwise. Undefined if overflow.
    Z   Set if the quotient is zero. Cleared otherwise. Undefined if overflow.
    V   Set if division overflow is detected. Cleared otherwise.
    C   Always cleared.
    X   Not affected.

Instruction Format:

15	14	13	12	11	10	9	8	7	6	5	4	3	2	1	0
1	0	0	0	\multicolumn{3}{}{Register}			0	1	1	\multicolumn{6}{}{Effective Address}					

| 1 | 0 | 0 | 0 | Register | 0 | 1 | 1 | Effective Address Mode \| Register |

Instruction Fields:

    Register field — specifies any of the eight data registers. This field always specifies the destination operand.

    Effective Address field — Specifies the source operand. Only data addressing modes are allowed as shown:

Addressing Mode	Mode	Register	Addressing Mode	Mode	Register
Dn	000	register number	d(An, Xi)	110	register number
An	—	—	Abs.W	111	000
(An)	010	register number	Abs.L	111	001
(An)+	011	register number	d(PC)	111	010
−(An)	100	register number	d(PC, Xi)	111	011
d(An)	101	register number	Imm	111	100

Note: Overflow occurs if the quotient is larger than a 16-bit unsigned integer.

EOR

Exclusive OR Logical

EOR

Operation: (Source) ⊕ (Destination) → Destination

Assembler Syntax: EOR Dn, \<ea>

Attributes: Size = (Byte, Word, Long)

Description: Exclusive OR the source operand to the destination operand and store the result in the destination location. The size of the operation may be specified to be byte, word, or long. This operation is restricted to data registers as the source operand. The destination operand is specified in the effective address field.

Condition Codes:

X	N	Z	V	C
—	*	*	0	0

N Set if the most significant bit of the result is set. Cleared otherwise.
Z Set if the result is zero. Cleared otherwise.
V Always cleared.
C Always cleared.
X Not affected.

Instruction Format:

15	14	13	12	11	10	9	8	7	6	5	4	3	2	1	0
1	0	1	1	\multicolumn{3}{c}{Register}	\multicolumn{3}{c}{Op-Mode}	\multicolumn{3}{c}{Effective Address Mode}	\multicolumn{3}{c}{Register}

Instruction Fields:

Register field — Specifies any of the eight data registers.
Op-Mode field —

Byte	Word	Long	Operation
100	101	110	(\<ea>) ⊕ (\<Dx>) → \<ea>

Effective Address field — Specifies the destination operand. Only data alterable addressing modes are allowed as shown:

Addressing Mode	Mode	Register	Addressing Mode	Mode	Register
Dn	000	register number	d(An, Xi)	110	register number
An	—	—	Abs.W	111	000
(An)	010	register number	Abs.L	111	001
(An)+	011	register number	d(PC)	—	—
−(An)	100	register number	d(PC, Xi)	—	—
d(An)	101	register number	Imm	—	—

Note: Memory to data register operations are not allowed. EORI is used when the source is immediate data. Most assemblers automatically make this distinction.

EORI

Exclusive OR Immediate

EORI

Operation: Immediate Data ⊕ (Destination) → Destination

Assembler Syntax: EORI #<data>,<ea>

Attributes: Size = (Byte, Word, Long)

Description: Exclusive OR the immediate data to the destination operand and store the result in the destination location. The size of the operation may be specified to be byte, word, or long. The immediate data matches the operation size.

Condition Codes:

X	N	Z	V	C
—	*	*	0	0

N Set if the most significant bit of the result is set. Cleared otherwise.
Z Set if the result is zero. Cleared otherwise.
V Always cleared.
C Always cleared.
X Not affected.

Instruction Format:

15	14	13	12	11	10	9	8	7	6	5	4	3	2	1	0
0	0	0	0	1	0	1	0	Size		Effective Address					
										Mode			Register		
Word Data (16 bits)								Byte Data (8 bits)							
Long Data (32 bits, including previous word)															

Instruction Fields:

Size field — Specifies the size of the operation:
  00 — byte operation.
  01 — word operation.
  10 — long operation.

Effective Address field — Specifies the destination operand. Only data alterable addressing modes are allowed as shown:

Addressing Mode	Mode	Register	Addressing Mode	Mode	Register
Dn	000	register number	d(An, Xi)	110	register number
An	—	—	Abs.W	111	000
(An)	010	register number	Abs.L	111	001
(An)+	011	register number	d(PC)	—	—
−(An)	100	register number	d(PC, Xi)	—	—
d(An)	101	register number	Imm	—	—

Immediate field — (Data immediately following the instruction):
  If size = 00, then the data is the low order byte of the immediate word.
  If size = 01, then the data is the entire immediate word.
  If size = 10, then the data is the next two immediate words.

EORI to CCR

Exclusive OR Immediate to Condition Codes

EORI to CCR

Operation: (Source) ⊕ CCR → CCR

Assembler Syntax: EORI #xxx, CCR

Attributes: Size = (Byte)

Description: Exclusive OR the immediate operand with the condition codes and store the result in the low-order byte of the status register.

Condition Codes:

X	N	Z	V	C
*	*	*	*	*

- N Changed if bit 3 of immediate operand is one. Unchanged otherwise.
- Z Changed if bit 2 of immediate operand is one. Unchanged otherwise.
- V Changed if bit 1 of immediate operand is one. Unchanged otherwise.
- C Changed if bit 0 of immediate operand is one. Unchanged otherwise.
- X Changed if bit 4 of immediate operand is one. Unchanged otherwise.

Instruction Format:

15	14	13	12	11	10	9	8	7	6	5	4	3	2	1	0
0	0	0	0	1	0	1	0	0	0	1	1	1	1	0	0
0	0	0	0	0	0	0	0	Byte Data (8 bits)							

EORI to SR

Exclusive OR Immediate to the Status Register
(Privileged Instruction)

EORI to SR

Operation: If supervisor state
then (Source) $\oplus$ SR $\rightarrow$ SR
else TRAP

Assembler Syntax: EORI #xxx, SR

Attributes: Size = (Word)

Description: Exclusive OR the immediate operand with the contents of the status register and store the result in the status register. All bits of the status register are affected.

Condition Codes:

X	N	Z	V	C
*	*	*	*	*

N Changed if bit 3 of immediate operand is one. Unchanged otherwise.
Z Changed if bit 2 of immediate operand is one. Unchanged otherwise.
V Changed if bit 1 of immediate operand is one. Unchanged otherwise.
C Changed if bit 0 of immediate operand is one. Unchanged otherwise.
X Changed if bit 4 of immediate operand is one. Unchanged otherwise.

Instruction Format:

15	14	13	12	11	10	9	8	7	6	5	4	3	2	1	0
0	0	0	0	1	0	1	0	0	1	1	1	1	1	0	0
Word Data (16 bits)															

EXG

Exchange Registers

EXG

Operation: Rx ↔ Ry

Assembler Syntax: EXG Rx, Ry

Attributes: Size = (Long)

Description: Exchange the contents of two registers. This exchange is always a long (32 bit) operation. Exchange works in three modes:
1. Exchange data registers.
2. Exchange address registers.
3. Exchange a data register and an address register.

Condition Codes: Not affected.

Instruction Format:

15	14	13	12	11 10 9	8	7 6 5 4 3	2 1 0
1	1	0	0	Register Rx	1	Op-Mode	Register Ry

Instruction Fields:

Register Rx field — Specifies either a data register or an address register depending on the mode. If the exchange is between data and address registers, this field always specifies the data register.

Op-Mode field — Specifies whether exchanging:
  01000 — data registers.
  01001 — address registers.
  10001 — data register and address register.

Register Ry field — Specifies either a data register or an address register depending on the mode. If the exchange is between data and address registers, this field always specifies the address register.

EXT

Sign Extend

Operation: (Destination) Sign-extended → Destination

Assembler Syntax: EXT Dn

Attributes: Size = (Word, Long)

Description: Extend the sign bit of a data register from a byte to a word or from a word to a long operand depending on the size selected. If the operation is word sized, bit [7] of the designated data register is copied to bits [15:8] of that data register. If the operation is long sized, bit [15] of the designated data register is copied to bits [31:16] of that data register.

Condition Codes:

X	N	Z	V	C
—	*	*	0	0

- N Set if the result is negative. Cleared otherwise.
- Z Set if the result is zero. Cleared otherwise.
- V Always cleared.
- C Always cleared.
- X Not affected.

Instruction Format:

15	14	13	12	11	10	9	8	7	6	5	4	3	2	1	0
0	1	0	0	1	0	0	Op-Mode			0	0	0	Register		

Instruction Fields:

Op-Mode Field — Specifies the size of the sign-extension operation:
- 010 — Sign-extend low order byte of data register to word.
- 011 — Sign-extend low order word of data register to long.

Register field — Specifies the data register whose content is to be sign-extended.

ILLEGAL   Illegal Instruction   ILLEGAL

Operation: PC→ −(SSP); SR→ −(SSP)
(Illegal Instruction Vector)→ PC

Attributes: None

Description: This bit pattern causes an illegal instruction exception. All other illegal instruction bit patterns are reserved for future extension of the instruction set.

Condition Codes: Not affected.

Instruction Format:

15	14	13	12	11	10	9	8	7	6	5	4	3	2	1	0
0	1	0	0	1	0	1	0	1	1	1	1	1	1	0	0

JMP   Jump   JMP

Operation: Destination → PC

Assembler Syntax: JMP <ea>

Attributes: Unsized

Description: Program execution continues at the effective address specified by the instruction. The address is specified by the control addressing modes.

Condition Codes: Not affected.

Instruction Format:

15	14	13	12	11	10	9	8	7	6	5 4 3	2 1 0
0	1	0	0	1	1	1	0	1	1	Effective Address Mode	Register

Instruction Fields:

Effective Address field — Specifies the address of the next instruction. Only control addressing modes are allowed as shown:

Addressing Mode	Mode	Register	Addressing Mode	Mode	Register
Dn	—	—	d(An, Xi)	110	register number
An	—	—	Abs.W	111	000
(An)	010	register number	Abs.L	111	001
(An)+	—	—	d(PC)	111	010
−(An)	—	—	d(PC, Xi)	111	011
d(An)	101	register number	Imm	—	—

JSR   Jump to Subroutine   JSR

Operation: PC → −(SP); Destination → PC

Assembler Syntax: JSR <ea>

Attributes: Unsized

Description: The long word address of the instruction immediately following the JSR instruction is pushed onto the system stack. Program execution then continues at the address specifed in the instruction.

Condition Codes: Not affected.

Instruction Format:

15	14	13	12	11	10	9	8	7	6	5 4 3	2 1 0
0	1	0	0	1	1	1	0	1	0	Effective Address Mode	Register

Instruction Fields:

Effective Address field — Specifies the address of the next instruction. Only control addressing modes are allowed as shown:

Addressing Mode	Mode	Register	Addressing Mode	Mode	Register
Dn	—	—	d(An, Xi)	110	register number
An	—	—	Abs.W	111	000
(An)	010	register number	Abs.L	111	001
(An)+	—	—	d(PC)	111	010
−(An)	—	—	d(PC, Xi)	111	011
d(An)	101	register number	Imm	—	—

LEA LEA

Load Effective Address

Operation: Destination → An

Assembler Syntax: LEA <ea>, An

Attributes: Size = (Long)

Description: The effective address is loaded into the specified address register. All 32 bits of the address register are affected by this instruction.

Condition Codes: Not affected.

Instruction Format:

15	14	13	12	11	10	9	8	7	6	5	4	3	2	1	0
0	1	0	0	\multicolumn{3}{c}{Register}	1	1	1	\multicolumn{3}{c}{Effective Address Mode}	\multicolumn{3}{c}{Register}

Instruction Fields:

Register field — Specifies the address register which is to be loaded with the effective address.

Effective Address field — Specifies the address to be loaded into the address register. Only control addressing modes are allowed as shown:

Addressing Mode	Mode	Register	Addressing Mode	Mode	Register
Dn	—	—	d(An, Xi)	110	register number
An	—	—	Abs.W	111	000
(An)	010	register number	Abs.L	111	001
(An)+	—	—	d(PC)	111	010
−(An)	—	—	d(PC, Xi)	111	011
d(An)	101	register number	Imm	—	—

LINK   Link and Allocate   LINK

Operation: An → −(SP); SP → An; SP + d → SP

Assembler Syntax: LINK An, #<displacement>

Attributes: Unsized

Description: The current content of the specified address register is pushed onto the stack. After the push, the address register is loaded from the updated stack pointer. Finally, the 16-bit sign-extended displacement is added to the stack pointer. The content of the address register occupies two words on the stack. A negative displacement is specified to allocate stack area.

Condition Codes: Not affected.

Instruction Format:

15	14	13	12	11	10	9	8	7	6	5	4	3	2	1	0
0	1	0	0	1	1	1	0	0	1	0	1	0	\multicolumn{3}{c}{Register}
\multicolumn{16}{c}{Displacement}

Instruction Fields:

    Register field — Specifies the address register through which the link is to be constructed.

    Displacement field — Specifies the twos complement integer which is to be added to the stack pointer.

Note: LINK and UNLK can be used to maintain a linked list of local data and parameter areas on the stack for nested subroutine calls.

LSL, LSR   Logical Shift   LSL, LSR

Operation: (Destination) Shifted by <count> → Destination

Assembler LSd Dx, Dy
Syntax: LSd #<data>, Dy
               LSd <ea>

Attributes: Size = (Byte, Word, Long)

Description: Shift the bits of the operand in the direction specified. The carry bit receives the last bit shifted out of the operand. The shift count for the shifting of a register may be specified in two different ways:
1. Immediate — the shift count is specified in the instruction (shift range 1-8).
2. Register — the shift count is contained in a data register specified in the instruction.

The size of the operation may be specified to be byte, word, or long. The content of memory may be shifted one bit only and the operand size is restricted to a word.

For LSL, the operand is shifted left; the number of positions shifted is the shift count. Bits shifted out of the high order bit go to both the carry and the extend bits; zeroes are shifted into the low order bit.

LSL:
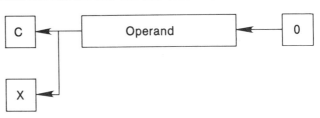

For LSR, the operand is shifted right; the number of positions shifted is the shift count. Bits shifted out of the low order bit go to both the carry and the extend bits; zeroes are shifted into the high order bit.

LSR:
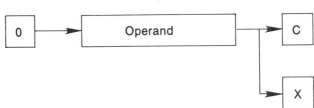

— Continued —

LSL, LSR   Logical Shift   LSL, LSR

Condition Codes:

X	N	Z	V	C
*	*	*	0	*

- N   Set if the result is negative. Cleared otherwise.
- Z   Set if the result is zero. Cleared otherwise.
- V   Always cleared.
- C   Set according to the last bit shifted out of the operand. Cleared for a shift count of zero.
- X   Set according to the last bit shifted out of the operand. Unaffected for a shift count of zero.

Instruction Format (Register Shifts):

15	14	13	12	11 10 9	8	7 6	5	4	3	2 1 0
1	1	1	0	Count/Register	dr	Size	i/r	0	1	Register

Instruction Fields (Register Shifts):

Count/Register field —
    If i/r = 0, the shift count is specified in this field. The values 0, 1-7 represent a range of 8, 1 to 7 respectively.
    If i/r = 1, the shift count (modulo 64) is contained in the data register specified in this field.

dr field — Specifies the direction of the shift:
    0 — shift right.
    1 — shift left.

Size field — Specifies the size of the operation:
    00 — byte operation.
    01 — word operation.
    10 — long operation.

i/r field —
    If i/r = 0, specifies immediate shift count.
    If i/r = 1, specifies register shift count.

Register field — Specifies a data register whose content is to be shifted.

— Continued —

LSL, LSR Logical Shift LSL, LSR

Instruction Format (Memory Shifts):

15	14	13	12	11	10	9	8	7	6	5 4 3	2 1 0
1	1	1	0	0	0	1	dr	1	1	Effective Address Mode	Register

Instruction Fields (Memory Shifts):

dr field — Specifies the direction of the shift:
  0 — shift right.
  1 — shift left.

Effective Address field — Specifies the operand to be shifted. Only memory alterable addressing modes are allowed as shown:

Addressing Mode	Mode	Register	Addressing Mode	Mode	Register
Dn	—	—	d(An, Xi)	110	register number
An	—	—	Abs.W	111	000
(An)	010	register number	Abs.L	111	001
(An)+	011	register number	d(PC)	—	—
−(An)	100	register number	d(PC, Xi)	—	—
d(An)	101	register number	Imm	—	—

MOVE   Move Data from Source to Destination   MOVE

Operation: (Source) → Destination

Assembler Syntax: MOVE <ea>, <ea>

Attributes: Size = (Byte, Word, Long)

Description: Move the content of the source to the destination location. The data is examined as it is moved, and the condition codes set accordingly. The size of the operation may be specified to be byte, word, or long.

Condition Codes:

X	N	Z	V	C
—	*	*	0	0

- N Set if the result is negative. Cleared otherwise.
- Z Set if the result is zero. Cleared otherwise.
- V Always cleared.
- C Always cleared.
- X Not affected.

Instruction Format:

15	14	13	12	11	10	9	8	7	6	5	4	3	2	1	0
0	0	Size		Destination Register			Destination Mode			Source Mode			Source Register		

Instruction Fields:

Size field — Specifies the size of the operand to be moved:
- 01 — byte operation.
- 11 — word operation.
- 10 — long operation.

Destination Effective Address field — Specifies the destination location. Only data alterable addressing modes are allowed as shown:

Addressing Mode	Mode	Register	Addressing Mode	Mode	Register
Dn	000	register number	d(An, Xi)	110	register number
An	—	—	Abs.W	111	000
(An)	010	register number	Abs.L	111	001
(An)+	011	register number	d(PC)	—	—
−(An)	100	register number	d(PC, Xi)	—	—
d(An)	101	register number	Imm	—	—

— Continued —

MOVE Move Data from Source to Destination MOVE

Instruction Fields: (Continued)

Source Effective Address field — Specifies the source operand. All addressing modes are allowed as shown:

Addressing Mode	Mode	Register	Addressing Mode	Mode	Register
Dn	000	register number	d(An, Xi)	110	register number
An*	001	register number	Abs.W	111	000
(An)	010	register number	Abs.L	111	001
(An)+	011	register number	d(PC)	111	010
−(An)	100	register number	d(PC, Xi)	111	011
d(An)	101	register number	Imm	111	100

*For byte size operation, address register direct is not allowed.

Notes:
1. MOVEA is used when the destination is an address register. Most assemblers automatically make this distinction.
2. MOVEQ can also be used for certain operations on data registers.

MOVE from CCR

Move from the Condition Code Register

MOVE from CCR

Operation: CCR → Destination

Assembler Syntax: MOVE CCR, <ea>

Attributes: Size = (Word)

Description: The content of the status register is moved to the destination location. The source operand is a word, but only the low order byte contains the condition codes. The upper byte is all zeros.

Condition Codes: Not affected.

Instruction Format:

15	14	13	12	11	10	9	8	7	6	5	4	3	2	1	0
0	1	0	0	0	0	1	0	1	1	\multicolumn{3}{c}{Effective Address Mode}		\multicolumn{3}{c}{Register}		

Instruction Fields:

Effective Address field — Specifies the destination location.
Only data alterable addressing modes are allowed as shown:

Addressing Mode	Mode	Register	Addressing Mode	Mode	Register
Dn	000	register number	d(An, Xi)	110	register number
An	—	—	Abs.W	111	000
(An)	010	register number	Abs.L	111	001
(An)+	011	register number	d(PC)	—	—
−(An)	100	register number	d(PC, Xi)	—	—
d(An)	101	register number	Imm	—	—

Note: MOVE to CCR is a word operation. AND, OR, and EOR to CCR are byte operations.

MOVE to CCR

Move to Condition Codes

MOVE to CCR

Operation: (Source) → CCR

Assembler Syntax: MOVE <ea>, CCR

Attributes: Size = (Word)

Description: The content of the source operand is moved to the condition codes. The source operand is a word, but only the low order byte is used to update the condition codes. The upper byte is ignored.

Condition Codes:

X	N	Z	V	C
*	*	*	*	*

- N Set the same as bit 3 of the source operand.
- Z Set the same as bit 2 of the source operand.
- V Set the same as bit 1 of the source operand.
- C Set the same as bit 0 of the source operand.
- X Set the same as bit 4 of the source operand.

Instruction Format:

15	14	13	12	11	10	9	8	7	6	5	4	3	2	1	0
0	1	0	0	0	1	0	0	1	1	\multicolumn{6}{c	}{Effective Address Mode | Register}

Instruction Fields:

Effective Address field — Specifies the location of the source operand. Only data addressing modes are allowed as shown:

Addressing Mode	Mode	Register	Addressing Mode	Mode	Register
Dn	000	register number	d(An, Xi)	110	register number
An	—	—	Abs.W	111	000
(An)	010	register number	Abs.L	111	001
(An)+	011	register number	d(PC)	111	010
−(An)	100	register number	d(PC, Xi)	111	011
d(An)	101	register number	Imm	111	100

Note: MOVE to CCR is a word operation. AND, OR, and EOR to CCR are byte operations.

MOVE to SR

Move to the Status Register (Privileged Instruction)

MOVE to SR

Operation: If supervisor state
then (Source) → SR
else TRAP

Assembler Syntax: MOVE <ea>, SR

Attributes: Size = (Word)

Description: The content of the source operand is moved to the status register. The source operand is a word and all bits of the status register are affected.

Condition Codes: Set according to the source operand.

Instruction Format:

15	14	13	12	11	10	9	8	7	6	5	4	3	2	1	0
0	1	0	0	0	1	1	0	1	1	\multicolumn{3}{c}{Effective Address Mode}	\multicolumn{3}{c}{Register}

Instruction Fields:

Effective Address field — Specifies the location of the source operand. Only data addressing modes are allowed as shown:

Addressing Mode	Mode	Register	Addressing Mode	Mode	Register
Dn	000	register number	d(An, Xi)	110	register number
An	—	—	Abs.W	111	000
(An)	010	register number	Abs.L	111	001
(An)+	011	register number	d(PC)	111	010
−(An)	100	register number	d(PC, Xi)	111	011
d(An)	101	register number	Imm	111	100

MOVE from SR

Move from the Status Register

MOVE from SR

Operation: SR → Destination

Assembler Syntax: MOVE SR, <ea>

Attributes: Size = (Word)

Description: The content of the status register is moved to the destination location. The operand size is a word.

Condition Codes: Not affected.

Instruction Format:

15	14	13	12	11	10	9	8	7	6	5	4	3	2	1	0
0	1	0	0	0	0	0	0	1	1	\multicolumn{3}{c}{Effective Address Mode}		\multicolumn{3}{c}{Register}		

Instruction Fields:

Effective Address field — Specifies the destination location. Only data alterable addressing modes are allowed as shown:

Addressing Mode	Mode	Register	Addressing Mode	Mode	Register
Dn	000	register number	d(An, Xi)	110	register number
An	—	—	Abs.W	111	000
(An)	010	register number	Abs.L	111	001
(An)+	011	register number	d(PC)	—	—
−(An)	100	register number	d(PC, Xi)	—	—
d(An)	101	register number	Imm	—	—

Note: A memory destination is read before it is written to.

MOVE from SR

**Move from the Status Register
(Privileged Instruction)**

MOVE from SR

Operation: If supervisor state
then SR → Destination
else TRAP

**Assembler
Syntax:** MOVE SR, <ea>

Attributes: Size = (Word)

Description: The content of the status register is moved to the destination location. The operand size is a word.

Condition Codes: Not affected.

Instruction Format:

15	14	13	12	11	10	9	8	7	6	5	4	3	2	1	0
0	1	0	0	0	0	0	0	1	1	\multicolumn{3}{c}{Effective Address Mode}	\multicolumn{3}{c}{Register}

Instruction Fields:
Effective Address field — Specifies the destination location. Only data alterable addressing modes are allowed as shown:

Addressing Mode	Mode	Register	Addressing Mode	Mode	Register
Dn	000	register number	d(An, Xi)	110	register number
An	—	—	Abs.W	111	000
(An)	010	register number	Abs.L	111	001
(An)+	011	register number	d(PC)	—	—
−(An)	100	register number	d(PC, Xi)	—	—
d(An)	101	register number	Imm	—	—

NOTE: Use the MOVE from CCR instruction to access the conditon codes.

MOVE USP

Move User Stack Pointer (Privileged Instruction)

MOVE USP

Operation: If supervisor state
then USP → An;
An → USP
else TRAP

Assembler MOVE USP, An
Syntax: MOVE An, USP

Attributes: Size = (Long)

Description: The contents of the user stack pointer are transferred to or from the specified address register.

Condition Codes: Not affected.

Instruction Format:

15	14	13	12	11	10	9	8	7	6	5	4	3	2	1	0
0	1	0	0	1	1	1	0	0	1	1	0	dr	\multicolumn{3}{c}{Register}

Instruction Fields:

dr field — Specifies the direction of transfer:
0 — transfer the address register to the USP.
1 — transfer the USP to the address register.

Register field — Specifies the address register to or from which the user stack pointer is to be transferred.

MOVEA Move Address MOVEA

Operation: (Source) → Destination

Assembler Syntax: MOVEA <ea>, An

Attributes: Size = (Word, Long)

Description: Move the content of the source to the destination address register. The size of the operation may be specified to be word or long. Word size source operands are sign extended to 32 bit quantities before the operation is done.

Condition Codes: Not affected.

Instruction Format:

15	14	13	12	11	10	9	8	7	6	5	4	3	2	1	0
0	0	\multicolumn{2}{c}{Size}	\multicolumn{3}{c}{Destination Register}	0	0	1	\multicolumn{3}{c}{Source Mode}	\multicolumn{3}{c}{Register}

Instruction Fields:

Size field — Specifies the size of the operand to be moved:
  11 — Word operation. The source operand is sign-extended to a long operand and all 32 bits are loaded into the address register.
  10 — Long operation.
Destination Register field — Specifies the destination address register.
Source Effective Address field — Specifies the location of the source operand. All addressing modes are allowed as shown:

Addressing Mode	Mode	Register	Addressing Mode	Mode	Register
Dn	000	register number	d(An, Xi)	110	register number
An	001	register number	Abs.W	111	000
(An)	010	register number	Abs.L	111	001
(An)+	011	register number	d(PC)	111	010
−(An)	100	register number	d(PC, Xi)	111	011
d(An)	101	register number	Imm	111	100

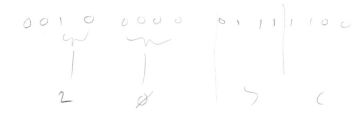

221

MOVEC

Move to/from Control Register (Privileged Instruction)

MOVEC

Operation: If supervisor state
then Rc → Rn, Rn → Rc
else TRAP

Assembler MOVEC Rc, Rn
Syntax: MOVEC Rn, Rc

Attributes: Size = (Long)

Description: Copy the contents of the specified control register to the specified general register or copy the contents of the specified general register to the specified control register. This is always a 32-bit transfer even though the control register may be implemented with fewer bits. Unimplemented bits are read as zeros.

Condition Codes: Not affected.

Instruction Format:

15	14	13	12	11	10	9	8	7	6	5	4	3	2	1	0
0	1	0	0	1	1	1	0	0	1	1	1	1	0	1	dr
A/D	Register			Control Register											

Instruction Fields:

dr field — Specifies the direction of the transfer:
  0—control register to general register.
  1—general register to control register.
A/D field — Specifies the type of general register:
  0—data register.
  1—address register.
Register field — Specifies the register number.
Control Register field — Specifies the control register.
Currently defined control registers are:

Binary	Hex	Name/Function
0000 0000 0000	000	Source Function Code (SFC) register.
0000 0000 0001	001	Destination Function Code (DFC) register.
1000 0000 0000	800	User Stack Pointer.
1000 0000 0001	801	Vector Base Register for exception vector table.

All other codes cause an illegal instruction exception.

MOVEM — Move Multiple Registers — MOVEM

Operation: Registers → Destination
(Source) → Registers

Assembler Syntax: MOVEM <register list>, <ea>
MOVEM <ea>, <register list>

Attributes: Size = (Word, Long)

Description: Selected registers are transferred to or from consecutive memory location starting at the location specified by the effective address. A register is transferred if the bit corresponding to that register is set in the mask field. The instruction selects how much of each register is transferred; either the entire long word can be moved or just the low order word. In the case of a word transfer to the registers, each word is sign-extended to 32 bits (also data registers) and the resulting long word loaded into the associated register.

MOVEM allows three forms of address modes: the control modes, the predecrement mode, or the postincrement mode. If the effective address is in one of the control modes, the registers are transferred starting at the specified address and up through higher addresses. The order of transfer is from data register 0 to data register 7, then from address register 0 to address register 7.

If the effective address is in the predecrement mode, only a register to memory operation is allowed. The registers are stored starting at the specified address minus two and down through lower addresses. The order of storing is from address register 7 to address register 0, then from data register 7 to data register 0. The decremented address register is updated to contain the address of the last word stored.

If the effective address is in the postincrement mode, only a memory to register operation is allowed. The registers are loaded starting at the specified address and up through higher addresses. The order of loading is the same as for the control mode addressing. The incremented address register is updated to contain the address of the last word loaded plus two.

Condition Codes: Not affected.

Instruction Format:

15	14	13	12	11	10	9	8	7	6	5 4 3	2 1 0
0	1	0	0	1	dr	0	0	1	Sz	Effective Address Mode	Register
Register List Mask											

— Continued —

MOVEM   Move Multiple Registers   MOVEM

Instruction Fields:

    dr field:

        Specifies the direction of the transfer:

        0 — register to memory

        1 — memory to register.

    Sz field — Specifies the size of the registers being transferred:

        0 — word transfer.

        1 — long transfer.

    Effective Address field — Specifies the memory address to or from which the registers are to be moved.

    For register to memory transfer, only control alterable addressing modes or the predecrement addressing mode are allowed as shown:

Addressing Mode	Mode	Register	Addressing Mode	Mode	Register
Dn	—	—	d(An, Xi)	110	register number
An	—	—	Abs.W	111	000
(An)	010	register number	Abs.L	111	001
(An)+	—	—	d(PC)	—	—
−(An)	100	register number	d(PC, Xi)	—	—
d(An)	101	register number	Imm	—	—

    For memory to register transfer, only control addressing modes or the postincrement addressing mode are allowed as shown:

Addressing Mode	Mode	Register	Addressing Mode	Mode	Register
Dn	—	—	d(An, Xi)	110	register number
An	—	—	Abs.W	111	000
(An)	010	register number	Abs.L	111	001
(An)+	011	register number	d(PC)	111	010
−(An)	—	—	d(PC, Xi)	111	011
d(An)	101	register number	Imm	—	—

    Register List Mask field — Specifies which registers are to be transferred. The low order bit corresponds to the first register to be transferred; the high bit corresponds to the last register to be transferred. Thus, both for control modes and for the postincrement mode addresses, the mask correspondence is

15	14	13	12	11	10	9	8	7	6	5	4	3	2	1	0
A7	A6	A5	A4	A3	A2	A1	A0	D7	D6	D5	D4	D3	D2	D1	D0

while for the predecrement mode addresses, the mask correspondence is

15	14	13	12	11	10	9	8	7	6	5	4	3	2	1	0
D0	D1	D2	D3	D4	D5	D6	D7	A0	A1	A2	A3	A4	A5	A6	A7

Note: An extra read bus cycle occurs for memory operands. This amounts to a memory word at one address higher than expected being addressed during operation.

MOVEP   Move Peripheral Data   MOVEP

Operation: (Source) → Destination

Assembler Syntax: MOVEP Dx, d(Ay)
MOVEP d(Ay), Dx

Attributes: Size = (Word, Long)

Description: Data is transferred between a data register and alternate bytes of memory, starting at the location specified and incrementing by two. The high order byte of the data register is transferred first and the low order byte is transferred last. The memory address is specified using the address register indirect plus displacement addressing mode. If the address is even, all the transfers are made on the high order half of the data bus; if the address is odd, all the transfers are made on the low order half of the data bus.

Example: Long transfer to/from an even address.

Byte organization in register

31 24	23 16	15 8	7 0
hi-order	mid-upper	mid-lower	low-order

Byte organization in memory (low address at top)

15 14 13 12 11 10 9 8	7 6 5 4 3 2 1 0
hi-order	
mid-upper	
mid-lower	
low-order	

Example: Word transfer to/from an odd address.

Byte organization in register

31 24	23 16	15 8	7 0
		hi-order	low-order

Byte organization in memory (low address at top)

15 14 13 12 11 10 9 8	7 6 5 4 3 2 1 0
	hi-order
	low-order

Condition Codes: Not affected.

— Continued —

MOVEP   Move Peripheral Data   MOVEP

Instruction Format:

15	14	13	12	11 10 9	8 7 6	5	4	3	2 1 0
0	0	0	0	Data Register	Op-Mode	0	0	1	Address Register
Displacement									

Instruction Fields:

Data Register field — Specifies the data register to or from which the data is to be transferred.

Op-Mode field — Specifies the direction and size of the operation:
- 100 — transfer word from memory to register.
- 101 — transfer long from memory to register.
- 110 — transfer word from register to memory.
- 111 — transfer long from register to memory.

Address Register field — Specifies the address register which is used in the address register indirect plus displacement addressing mode.

Displacement field — Specifies the displacement which is used in calculating the operand address.

MOVEQ   Move Quick   MOVEQ

Operation: Immediate Data → Destination

Assembler Syntax: MOVEQ #<data>, Dn

Attributes: Size = (Long)

Description: Move immediate data to a data register. The data is contained in an 8-bit field within the operation word. The data is sign-extended to a long operand and all 32 bits are transferred to the data register.

Condition Codes:

X	N	Z	V	C
—	*	*	0	0

- N   Set if the result is negative. Cleared otherwise.
- Z   Set if the result is zero. Cleared otherwise.
- V   Always cleared.
- C   Always cleared.
- X   Not affected.

Instruction Format:

15	14	13	12	11	10	9	8	7	6	5	4	3	2	1	0
0	1	1	1	Register			0	Data							

Instruction Fields:

Register field — Specifies the data register to be loaded.
Data field — 8 bits of data which are sign extended to a long operand.

MOVES — Move to/from Address Space (Privileged Instruction)

Operation: If supervisor state
then Rn → Destination \<DFC\>
Source \<SFC\> → Rn
else TRAP

Assembler Syntax: MOVES Rn, \<ea\>
MOVES \<ea\>, Rn

Attributes: Size = (Byte, Word, Long)

Description: Move the byte, word, or long operand from the specified general register to a location within the address space specified by the destination function code (DFC) register. Or, move the byte, word, or long operand from a location within the address space specified by the source function code (SFC) register to the specified general register.

If the destination is a data register, the source operand replaces the corresponding low-order bits of the that data register. If the destination is an address register, the source operand is sign-extended to 32 bits and then loaded into that address register.

Condition Codes: Not affected.

Instruction Format:

15	14	13	12	11	10	9	8	7	6	5	4	3	2	1	0
0	0	0	0	1	1	1	0	\multicolumn{2}{c}{Size}	\multicolumn{6}{c}{Effective Address}					
A/D	\multicolumn{3}{c}{Register}	dr	0	0	0	0	0	0	0	0	0	0	0

Instruction Fields:

Size field — Specifies the size of the operation:
  00—byte operation.
  01—word operation.
  10—long operation.

A/D field — Specifies the type of general register:
  0—data register.
  1—address register.
Register field — Specifies the register number.
dr field — Specifies the direction of the transfer:
  0—from \<ea\> to general register.
  1—from general register to \<ea\>.

—Continued—

MOVES Move to/from Address Space (Privileged Instruction) MOVES

Instruction Fields: (continued)

Effective Address field — Specifies the source or destination location within the alternate address space. Only alterable memory addressing modes are allowed as shown:

Addressing Mode	Mode	Register
Dn	—	—
An	—	—
(An)	010	register number
(An)+	011	register number
−(An)	100	register number
d(An)	101	register number

Addressing Mode	Mode	Register
d(An, Xi)	110	register number
Abs.W	111	000
Abs.L	111	001
d(PC)	—	—
d(PC, Xi)	—	—
Imm	—	—

MULS   Signed Multiply   MULS

Operation: (Source)*(Destination) → Destination

Assembler Syntax: MULS <ea>, Dn

Attributes: Size = (Word)

Description: Multiply two signed 16-bit operands yielding a 32-bit signed result. The operation is performed using signed arithmetic. A register operand is taken from the low order word; the upper word is unused. All 32 bits of the product are saved in the destination data register.

Condition Codes:

X	N	Z	V	C
—	*	*	0	0

- N Set if the result is negative. Cleared otherwise.
- Z Set if the result is zero. Cleared otherwise.
- V Always cleared.
- C Always cleared.
- X Not affected.

Instruction Format:

15	14	13	12	11	10	9	8	7	6	5	4	3	2	1	0
1	1	0	0	\multicolumn{3}{c}{Register}	1	1	1	\multicolumn{3}{c}{Effective Address Mode}	\multicolumn{3}{c}{Register}

Instruction Fields:

Register field — Specifies one of the data registers. This field always specifies the destination.

Effective Address field — Specifies the source operand. Only data addressing modes are allowed as shown:

Addressing Mode	Mode	Register	Addressing Mode	Mode	Register
Dn	000	register number	d(An, Xi)	110	register number
An	—	—	Abs.W	111	000
(An)	010	register number	Abs.L	111	001
(An)+	011	register number	d(PC)	111	010
−(An)	100	register number	d(PC, Xi)	111	011
d(An)	101	register number	Imm	111	100

MULU Unsigned Mulitply MULU

Operation: (Source) * (Destination) → Destination

Assembler Syntax: MULU <ea>, Dn

Attributes: Size = (Word)

Description: Multiply two unsigned 16-bit operands yielding a 32-bit unsigned result. The operation is performed using unsigned arithmetic. A register operand is taken from the low order word; the upper word is unused. All 32 bits of the product are saved in the destination data register.

Condition Codes:

X	N	Z	V	C
—	*	*	0	0

- N Set if the most significant bit of the result is set. Cleared otherwise.
- Z Set if the result is zero. Cleared otherwise.
- V Always cleared.
- C Always cleared.
- X Not affected.

Instruction Format:

15	14	13	12	11	10	9	8	7	6	5	4	3	2	1	0
1	1	0	0	\multicolumn{3}{c}{Register}	0	1	1	\multicolumn{3}{c}{Mode}	\multicolumn{3}{c}{Register}

Instruction Fields:

Register field — Specifies one of the data registers. This field always specifies the destination.

Effective Address field — Specifies the source operand. Only data addressing modes are allowed as shown:

Addressing Mode	Mode	Register	Addressing Mode	Mode	Register
Dn	000	register number	d(An, Xi)	110	register number
An	—	—	Abs.W	111	000
(An)	010	register number	Abs.L	111	001
(An)+	011	register number	d(PC)	111	010
−(An)	100	register number	d(PC, Xi)	111	011
d(An)	101	register number	Imm	111	100

NBCD   Negate Decimal with Extend   NBCD

Operation: $0 - (Destination)_{10} - X \rightarrow$ Destination

Assembler Syntax: NBCD <ea>

Attributes: Size = (Byte)

Description: The operand addressed as the destination and the extend bit are subtracted from zero. The operation is performed using decimal arithmetic. The result is saved in the destination location. This instruction produces the tens complement of the destination if the extend bit is clear, the nines complement if the extend bit is set. This is a byte operation only.

Condition Codes:

X	N	Z	V	C
*	U	*	U	*

N Undefined.
Z Cleared if the result is non-zero. Unchanged otherwise.
V Undefined.
C Set if a borrow (decimal) was generated. Cleared otherwise.
X Set the same as the carry bit.

NOTE

Normally the Z condition code bit is set via programming before the start of an operation. This allows successful tests for zero results upon completion of multiple-precision operations.

Instruction Format:

15	14	13	12	11	10	9	8	7	6	5	4	3	2	1	0
0	1	0	0	1	0	0	0	0	0	\multicolumn{3}{c}{Effective Address}			

| 15 | 14 | 13 | 12 | 11 | 10 | 9 | 8 | 7 | 6 | Mode | | | Register | | |

Instruction Fields:

Effective Address field — Specifies the destination operand. Only data alterable addressing modes are allowed as shown:

Addressing Mode	Mode	Register	Addressing Mode	Mode	Register
Dn	000	register number	d(An, Xi)	110	register number
An	—	—	Abs.W	111	000
(An)	010	register number	Abs.L	111	001
(An)+	011	register number	d(PC)	—	—
−(An)	100	register number	d(PC, Xi)	—	—
d(An)	101	register number	Imm	—	—

NEG   Negate   NEG

Operation: 0 − (Destination) → Destination

**Assembler
Syntax:** NEG <ea>

Attributes: Size = (Byte, Word, Long)

Description: The operand addressed as the destination is subtracted from zero. The result is stored in the destination location. The size of the operation may be specified to be byte, word, or long.

Condition Codes:

X	N	Z	V	C
*	*	*	*	*

N Set if the result is negative. Cleared otherwise.
Z Set if the result is zero. Cleared otherwise.
V Set if an overflow is generated. Cleared otherwise.
C Cleared if the result is zero. Set otherwise.
X Set the same as the carry bit.

Instruction Format:

15	14	13	12	11	10	9	8	7	6	5	4	3	2	1	0
0	1	0	0	0	1	0	0	Size		Effective Address					
										Mode			Register		

Instruction Fields:

Size field — Specifies the size of the operation:
    00 — byte operation.
    01 — word operation.
    10 — long operation.
Effective Address field — Specifies the destination operand. Only data alterable addressing modes are allowed as shown:

Addressing Mode	Mode	Register	Addressing Mode	Mode	Register
Dn	000	register number	d(An, Xi)	110	register number
An	—	—	Abs.W	111	000
(An)	010	register number	Abs.L	111	001
(An)+	011	register number	d(PC)	—	—
−(An)	100	register number	d(PC, Xi)	—	—
d(An)	101	register number	Imm	—	—

NEGX Negate with Extend NEGX

Operation: 0 − (Destination) − X → Destination

Assembler Syntax: NEGX <ea>

Attributes: Size = (Byte, Word, Long)

Description: The operand addressed as the destination and the extend bit are subtracted from zero. The result is stored in the destination location. The size of the operation may be specified to be byte, word, or long.

Condition Codes:

X	N	Z	V	C
*	*	*	*	*

- N Set if the result is negative. Cleared otherwise.
- Z Cleared if the result is non-zero. Unchanged otherwise.
- V Set if an overflow is generated. Cleared otherwise.
- C Set if a borrow is generated. Cleared otherwise.
- X Set the same as the carry bit.

NOTE

Normally the Z condition code bit is set via programming before the start of an operation. This allows successful tests for zero results upon completion of multiple-precision operations.

Instruction Format:

15	14	13	12	11	10	9	8	7	6	5	4	3	2	1	0
0	1	0	0	0	0	0	0	Size		Effective Address Mode			Register		

Instruction Fields:

Size field — Specifies the size of the operation:
- 00 — byte operation.
- 01 — word operation.
- 10 — long operation.

Effective Address field — Specifies the destination operand. Only data alterable addressing modes are allowed as shown:

Addressing Mode	Mode	Register	Addressing Mode	Mode	Register
Dn	000	register number	d(An, Xi)	110	register number
An	—	—	Abs.W	111	000
(An)	010	register number	Abs.L	111	001
(An)+	011	register number	d(PC)	—	—
−(An)	100	register number	d(PC, Xi)	—	—
d(An)	101	register number	Imm	—	—

NOP　　　　　　　　No Operation　　　　　　　　NOP

Operation: None

Assembler Syntax: NOP

Attributes: Unsized

Description: No operation occurs. The processor state, other than the program counter, is unaffected. Execution continues with the instruction following the NOP instruction.

Condition Codes: Not affected.

Instruction Format:

15	14	13	12	11	10	9	8	7	6	5	4	3	2	1	0
0	1	0	0	1	1	1	0	0	1	1	1	0	0	0	1

NOT

Logical Complement

NOT

Operation: ~(Destination) → Destination

Assembler Syntax: NOT <ea>

Attributes: Size = (Byte, Word, Long)

Description: The ones complement of the destination operand is taken and the result stored in the destination location. The size of the operation may be specified to be byte, word, or long.

Condition Codes:

X	N	Z	V	C
—	*	*	0	0

N Set if the result is negative. Cleared otherwise.
Z Set if the result is zero. Cleared otherwise.
V Always cleared.
C Always cleared.
X Not affected.

Instruction Format:

15	14	13	12	11	10	9	8	7	6	5	4	3	2	1	0
0	1	0	0	0	1	1	0	Size		Effective Address					
										Mode			Register		

Instruction Fields:

Size field — Specifies the size of the operation:
00 — byte operation.
01 — word operation.
10 — long operation.

Effective Address field — Specifies the destination operand. Only data alterable addressing modes are allowed as shown:

Addressing Mode	Mode	Register	Addressing Mode	Mode	Register
Dn	000	register number	d(An, Xi)	110	register number
An	—	—	Abs.W	111	000
(An)	010	register number	Abs.L	111	001
(An)+	011	register number	d(PC)	—	—
−(An)	100	register number	d(PC, Xi)	—	—
d(An)	101	register number	Imm	—	—

OR

Inclusive OR Logical

OR

Operation: (Source) v (Destination) → Destination

Assembler OR <ea>, Dn
Syntax: OR Dn, <ea>

Attributes: Size = (Byte, Word, Long)

Description: Inclusive OR the source operand to the destination operand and store the result in the destination location. The size of the operation may be specified to be byte, word, or long. The contents of an address register may not be used as an operand.

Condition Codes:

X	N	Z	V	C
—	*	*	0	0

N Set if the most significant bit of the result is set. Cleared otherwise.
Z Set if the result is zero. Cleared otherwise.
V Always cleared.
C Always cleared.
X Not affected.

Instruction Format:

15	14	13	12	11	10	9	8	7	6	5	4	3	2	1	0
1	0	0	0	Register			Op-Mode			Effective Address Mode			Register		

Instruction Fields:

Register field — Specifies any of the eight data registers.
Op-Mode field —

Byte	Word	Long	Operation
000	001	010	(<Dn>) v (<ea>) → <Dn>
100	101	110	(<ea>) v (<Dn>) → <ea>

Effective Address field —
If the location specified is a source operand then only data addressing modes are allowed as shown:

Addressing Mode	Mode	Register	Addressing Mode	Mode	Register
Dn	000	register number	d(An, Xi)	110	register number
An	—	—	Abs.W	111	000
(An)	010	register number	Abs.L	111	001
(An)+	011	register number	d(PC)	111	010
-(An)	100	register number	d(PC, Xi)	111	011
d(An)	101	register number	Imm	111	100

— Continued —

OR

Inclusive OR Logical

OR

Effective Address field (Continued)

If the location specified is a destination operand then only memory alterable addressing modes are allowed as shown:

Addressing Mode	Mode	Register	Addressing Mode	Mode	Register
Dn	—	—	d(An, Xi)	110	register number
An	—	—	Abs.W	111	000
(An)	010	register number	Abs.L	111	001
(An)+	011	register number	d(PC)	—	—
−(An)	100	register number	d(PC, Xi)	—	—
d(An)	101	register number	Imm	—	—

Notes:
1. If the destination is a data register, then it cannot be specified by using the destination <ea> mode, but must use the destination Dn mode instead.
2. ORI is used when the source is immediate data. Most assemblers automatically make this distinction.

ORI   Inclusive OR Immediate   ORI

Operation: Immediate Data v (Destination) → Destination

Assembler Syntax: ORI #<data>, <ea>

Attributes: Size = (Byte, Word, Long)

Description: Inclusive OR the immediate data to the destination operand and store the result in the destination location. The size of the operation may be specified to be byte, word, or long. The size of the immediate data matches the operation size.

Condition Codes:

X	N	Z	V	C
—	*	*	0	0

N Set if the most significant bit of the result is set. Cleared otherwise.
Z Set if the result is zero. Cleared otherwise.
V Always cleared.
C Always cleared.
X Not affected.

Instruction Format:

15	14	13	12	11	10	9	8	7	6	5	4	3	2	1	0
0	0	0	0	0	0	0	0	Size		Effective Address Mode | Register					
Word Data (16 bites)								Byte Data (8 bits)							
Long Data (32 bits, including previous word)															

Instruction Fields:

Size field — Specifies the size of the operation:
00 — byte operation.
01 — word operation.
10 — long operation.

Effective Address field — Specifies the destination operand. Only data alterable addressing modes are allowed as shown:

Addressing Mode	Mode	Register	Addressing Mode	Mode	Register
Dn	000	register number	d(An, Xi)	110	register number
An	—	—	Abs.W	111	000
(An)	010	register number	Abs.L	111	001
(An)+	011	register number	d(PC)	—	—
-(An)	100	register number	d(PC, Xi)	—	—
d(An)	101	register number	Imm	—	—

Immediate field — (Data immediately following the instruction):
If size = 00, then the data is the low order byte of the immediate word.
If size = 01, then the data is the entire immediate word.
If size = 10, then the data is the next two immediate words.

ORI to CCR

Inclusive OR Immediate to Condition Codes

ORI to CCR

Operation: (Source) v CCR → CCR

Assembler Syntax: ORI #xxx, CCR

Attributes: Size = (Byte)

Description: Inclusive OR the immediate operand with the condition codes and store the result in the low-order byte of the status register.

Condition Codes:

X	N	Z	V	C
*	*	*	*	*

- N Set if bit 3 of immediate operand is one. Unchanged otherwise.
- Z Set if bit 2 of immediate operand is one. Unchanged otherwise.
- V Set if bit 1 of immediate operand is one. Unchanged otherwise.
- C Set if bit 0 of immediate operand is one. Unchanged otherwise.
- X Set if bit 4 of immediate operand is one. Unchanged otherwise.

Instruction Format:

15	14	13	12	11	10	9	8	7	6	5	4	3	2	1	0
0	0	0	0	0	0	0	0	0	0	1	1	1	1	0	0
0	0	0	0	0	0	0	0	\multicolumn{8}{c}{Byte Data (8 bits)}

ORI to SR

Inclusive OR Immediate to the Status Register
(Privileged Instruction)

ORI to SR

Operation: If supervisor state
then (Source) v SR → SR
else TRAP

Assembler Syntax: ORI #xxx, SR

Attributes: Size = (Word)

Description: Inclusive OR the immediate operand with the contents of the status register and store the result in the status register. All bits of the status register are affected.

Condition Codes:

X	N	Z	V	C
*	*	*	*	*

N Set if bit 3 of immediate operand is one. Unchanged otherwise.
Z Set if bit 2 of immediate operand is one. Unchanged otherwise.
V Set if bit 1 of immediate operand is one. Unchanged otherwise.
C Set if bit 0 of immediate operand is one. Unchanged otherwise.
X Set if bit 4 of immediate operand is one. Unchanged otherwise.

Instruction Format:

15	14	13	12	11	10	9	8	7	6	5	4	3	2	1	0
0	0	0	0	0	0	0	0	0	1	1	1	1	1	0	0
Word Data (16 bits)																

PEA

Push Effective Address

Operation: Destination → −(SP)

Assembler Syntax: PEA <ea>

Attributes: Size = (Long)

Description: The effective address is computed and pushed onto the stack. A long word address is pushed onto the stack.

Condition Codes: Not affected.

Instruction Format:

15	14	13	12	11	10	9	8	7	6	5 4 3	2 1 0
0	1	0	0	1	0	0	0	0	1	Effective Address Mode	Register

Instruction Fields:

Effective Address field — Specifies the address to be pushed onto the stack. Only control addressing modes are allowed as shown:

Addressing Mode	Mode	Register	Addressing Mode	Mode	Register
Dn	—	—	d(An, Xi)	110	register number
An	—	—	Abs.W	111	000
(An)	010	register number	Abs.L	111	001
(An)+	—	—	d(PC)	111	010
−(An)	—	—	d(PC, Xi)	111	011
d(An)	101	register number	Imm	—	—

RESET

**Reset External Devices
(Privileged Instruction)**

RESET

Operation: If supervisor state
  then Assert RESET Line
  else TRAP

**Assembler
Syntax:** RESET

Attributes: Unsized

Description: The reset line is asserted causing all external devices to be reset. The processor state, other than the program counter, is unaffected and execution continues with the next instruction.

Condition Codes: Not affected.

Instruction Format:

15	14	13	12	11	10	9	8	7	6	5	4	3	2	1	0
0	1	0	0	1	1	1	0	0	1	1	1	0	0	0	0

ROL
ROR

Rotate (without Extend)

ROL
ROR

Operation: (Destination) Rotated by <count> → Destination

Assembler Syntax:
ROd Dx, Dy
ROd #<data>, Dy
ROd <ea>

Attributes: Size = (Byte, Word, Long)

Description: Rotate the bits of the operand in the direction specified. The extend bit is not included in the rotation. The shift count for the rotation of a register may be specified in two different ways:
1. Immediate — the shift count is specified in the instruction (shift range, 1-8).
2. Register — the shift count is contained in a data register specified in the instruction.

The size of the operation may be specified to be byte, word, or long. The content of memory may be rotated one bit only and the operand size is restricted to a word.

For ROL, the operand is rotated left; the number of positions shifted is the shift count. Bits shifted out of the high order bit go to both the carry bit and back into the low order bit. The extend bit is not modified or used.

ROL:

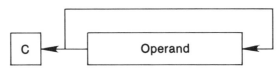

For ROR, the operand is rotated right; the number of position shifted is the shift count. Bits shifted out of the low order bit go to both the carry bit and back into the high order bit. The extend bit is not modified or used.

ROR:

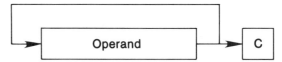

Condition Codes:

X	N	Z	V	C
—	*	*	0	*

N Set if the most significant bit of the result is set. Cleared otherwise.
Z Set if the result is zero. Cleared otherwise.
V Always cleared.
C Set according to the last bit shfited out of the operand. Cleared for a shift count of zero.
X Not affected.

— Continued —

ROL
ROR

Rotate (Without Extend)

ROL
ROR

Instruction Format (Register Rotate):

15	14	13	12	11 10 9	8	7 6	5	4	3	2 1 0
1	1	1	0	Count/Register	dr	Size	i/r	1	1	Register

Instruction Fields (Register Rotate):

Count/Register field —
  if i/r = 0, the rotate count is specified in this field. The values 0, 1-7 represent a range of 8, 1 to 7 respectively.
  If i/r = 1, the rotate count (modulo 64) is contained in the data register specified in this field.

dr field — Specifies the direction of the rotate:
  0 — rotate right.
  1 — rotate left.

Size field — Specifies the size of the operation:
  00 — byte operation.
  01 — word operation.
  10 — long operation.

i/r field —
  If i/r = 0, specifies immediate rotate count.
  If i/r = 1, specifies register rotate count.

Register field — Specifies a data register whose content is to be rotated.

Instruction Format (Memory Rotate):

15	14	13	12	11	10	9	8	7	6	5 4 3	2 1 0
1	1	1	0	0	1	1	dr	1	1	Effective Address Mode	Register

Instruction Fields (Memory Rotate):

dr field — Specifies the direction of the rotate:
  0 — rotate right
  1 — rotate left.

Effective Address field — Specifies the operand to be rotated. Only memory alterable addressing modes are allowed as shown:

Addressing Mode	Mode	Register	Addressing Mode	Mode	Register
Dn	—	—	d(An, Xi)	110	register number
An	—	—	Abs.W	111	000
(An)	010	register number	Abs.L	111	001
(An)+	011	register number	d(PC)	—	—
−(An)	100	register number	d(PC, Xi)	—	—
d(An)	101	register number	Imm	—	—

ROXL
ROXR

Rotate with Extend

ROXL
ROXR

Operation: (Destination) Rotated by <count> → Destination

Assembler Syntax:
ROXd Dx, Dy
ROXd #<data>, Dy
ROXd <ea>

Attributes: Size = (Byte, Word, Long)

Description: Rotate the bits of the destination operand in the direction specified. The extend bit is included in the rotation. The shift count for the rotation of a register may be specified in two different ways:
1. Immediate — the shift count is specified in the instruction (shift range, 1-8).
2. Register — the shift count is contained in a data register specified in the instruction.

The size of the operation may be specified to be byte, word, or long. The content of memory may be rotated one bit only and the operand size is restricted to a word.

For ROXL, the operand is rotated left; the number of positions shifted is the shift count. Bits shifted out of the high order bit go to both the carry and extend bits; the previous value of the extend bit is shifted into the low order bit.

ROXL:

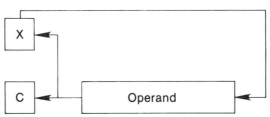

For ROXR, the operand is rotated right; the number of positions shifted is the shift count. Bits shifted out of the low order bit go to both the carry and extend bits; the previous value of the extend bit is shifted into the high order bit.

ROXR:

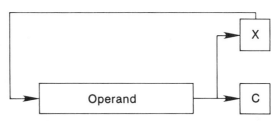

— Continued —

ROXL
ROXR

Rotate with Extend

ROXL
ROXR

Condition Codes:

X	N	Z	V	C
*	*	*	0	*

    N   Set if the most significant bit of the result is set. Cleared otherwise.
    Z   Set if the result is zero. Cleared otherwise.
    V   Always cleared.
    C   Set according to the last bit shifted out of the operand. Set to the value of the extend bit for a shift count of zero.
    X   Set according to the last bit shifted out of the operand. Unaffected for a shift count of zero.

Instruction Format (Register Rotate):

15	14	13	12	11 10 9	8	7 6	5	4	3	2 1 0
1	1	1	0	Count/Register	dr	Size	i/r	1	0	Register

Instruction Fields (Register Rotate):

    Count/Register field:
        If i/r = 0, the rotate count is specified in this field. The values 0, 1-7 represent range of 8, 1 to 7 respectively.
        If i/r = 1, the rotate count (modulo 64) is contained in the data register specified in this field.
    dr field — Specifies the direction of the rotate:
        0 — rotate right.
        1 — rotate left.
    Size field — Specifies the size of the operation:
        00 — byte operation.
        01 — word operation.
        10 — long operation.
    i/r field —
        If i/r = 0, specifies immediate rotate count.
        If i/r = 1, specifies register rotate count.
    Register field — Specifies a data register whose content is to be rotated.

— Continued —

ROXL
ROXR

Rotate with Extend

ROXL
ROXR

Instruction Format (Memory Rotate):

15	14	13	12	11	10	9	8	7	6	5	4	3	2	1	0
1	1	1	0	0	1	0	dr	1	1	\multicolumn{6}{c}{Effective Address}

| | | | | | | | | | | Mode | | | Register | | |

Instruction Fields (Memory Rotate):

dr field — Specifies the direction of the rotate:
    0 — rotate right.
    1 — rotate left.

Effective Address field — Specifies the operand to be rotated. Only memory alterable addressing modes are allowed as shown:

Addressing Mode	Mode	Register	Addressing Mode	Mode	Register
Dn	—	—	d(An, Xi)	110	register number
An	—	—	Abs.W	111	000
(An)	010	register number	Abs.L	111	001
(An)+	011	register number	d(PC)	—	—
−(An)	100	register number	d(PC, Xi)	—	—
d(An)	101	register number	Imm	—	—

RTD

RTD

Return and Deallocate Parameters

Operation: (SP)+ → PC; SP + d → SP

Assembler Syntax: RTD #<displacement>

Attributes: Unsized

Description: The program counter is pulled from the stack. The previous program counter value is lost. After the program counter is read from the stack, the displacement value is sign-extended to 32 bits and added to the stack pointer.

Condition Codes: Not affected.

Instruction Format:

15	14	13	12	11	10	9	8	7	6	5	4	3	2	1	0
0	1	0	0	1	1	1	0	0	1	1	1	0	1	0	0
Displacement																

Instruction Field:

Displacement field — Specifies the twos complement integer which is to be sign-extended and added to the stack pointer.

RTE

**Return from Exception
(Privileged Instruction)**

Operation: If supervisor state
then (SP) + → SR; (SP) + → PC
else TRAP

**Assembler
Syntax:** RTE

Attributes: Unsized

Description: The status register and program counter are pulled from the system stack. The previous status register and program counter are lost. All bits in the status register are affected.

Condition Codes: Set according to the content of the word on the stack.

Instruction Format:

15	14	13	12	11	10	9	8	7	6	5	4	3	2	1	0
0	1	0	0	1	1	1	0	0	1	1	1	0	0	1	1

RTE

**Return from Exception
(Privileged Instruction)**

RTE

Operation: If supervisor state
 then (SP) + → SR; (SP) + → PC
 If (SP) + = long format
  then full restore
 else TRAP

**Assembler
Syntax:** RTE

Attributes: Unsized

Description: The status register and program counter are pulled from the system stack. The previous status register and program counter are lost. The vector offset word is also pulled from the stack and the format field is examined to determine the amount of information to be restored.

Condition Codes: Set according to the content of the word on the stack.

Instruction Format:

15	14	13	12	11	10	9	8	7	6	5	4	3	2	1	0
0	1	0	0	1	1	1	0	0	1	1	1	0	0	1	1

Vector Offset Word Format:

15 12	11	10	9 0
Format	0	0	Vector Offset

Vector Offset Word Format Fields:

Format Field: — Specifies the amount of information to be restored.
 0000 — Short. Four words are to be removed from the top of the stack.
 1000 — Long. Twenty-nine words are to be removed from the top of the stack.
 Any Other
  Pattern — Error. The processor takes the format error exception.

RTR Return and Restore Condition Codes RTR

Operation: (SP)+ → CC; (SP)+ → PC

**Assembler
Syntax:** RTR

Attributes: Unsized

Description: The condition codes and program counter are pulled from the stack. The previous condition codes and program counter are lost. The supervisor portion of the status register is unaffected.

Condition Codes: Set according to the content of the word on the stack.

Instruction Format:

15	14	13	12	11	10	9	8	7	6	5	4	3	2	1	0
0	1	0	0	1	1	1	0	0	1	1	1	0	1	1	1

RTS   Return from Subroutine   RTS

Operation: (SP)+ → PC

Assembler Syntax: RTS

Attributes: Unsized

Description: The program counter is pulled from the stack. The previous program counter is lost.

Condition Codes: Not affected.

Instruction Format:

15	14	13	12	11	10	9	8	7	6	5	4	3	2	1	0
0	1	0	0	1	1	1	0	0	1	1	1	0	1	0	1

SBCD Subtract Decimal with Extend SBCD

Operation: $(Destination)_{10} - (Source)_{10} - X \rightarrow Destination$

Assembler SBCD Dy, Dx
Syntax: SBCD −(Ay), −(Ax)

Attributes: Size = (Byte)

Description: Subtract the source operand from the destination operand along with the extend bit and store the result in the destination location. The subtraction is performed using binary coded decimal arithmetic. The operands may be addressed in two different ways:
1. Data register to data register: The operands are contained in the data registers specified in the instruction.
2. Memory to memory: The operands are addressed with the predecrement addressing mode using the address registers specified in the instruction.

This operation is a byte operation only.

Condition Codes:

X	N	Z	V	C
*	U	*	U	*

N Undefined.
Z Cleared if the result is non-zero. Unchanged otherwise.
V Undefined.
C Set if a borrow (decimal) is generated. Cleared otherwise.
X Set the same as the carry bit.

NOTE
Normally the Z condition code bit is set via programming before the start of an operation. This allows successful tests for zero results upon completion of multiple-precision operations.

Instruction Format:

15	14	13	12	11	10	9	8	7	6	5	4	3	2	1	0
1	0	0	0	Register Rx			1	0	0	0	0	R/M	Register Ry		

Instruction Fields:

Register Rx field — Specifies the destination register:
If R/M = 0, specifies a data register.
If R/M = 1, specifies an address register for the prececrement addressing mode.

R/M field — Specifies the operand addressing mode:
0 — The operation is data register to data register.
1 — The operation is memory to memory.

Register Ry field — Specifies the source register:
If R/M = 0, specifies a data register.
If R/M = 1, specifies an address register for the predecrement addressing mode.

Scc

Scc   Set According to Condition   **Scc**

Operation: If (Condition True)
then 1s → Destination
else 0s → Destination

**Assembler
Syntax:** Scc <ea>

Attributes: Size = (Byte)

Description: The specified condition code is tested; if the condition is true, the byte specified by the effective address is set to TRUE (all ones), otherwise that byte is set to FALSE (all zeroes). "cc" may specify the following conditions:

CC	carry clear	0100	$\overline{C}$		LS	low or same	0011	$C+Z$
CS	carry set	0101	C		LT	less than	1101	$N\cdot\overline{V}+\overline{N}\cdot V$
EQ	equal	0111	Z		MI	minus	1011	N
F	false	0001	0		NE	not equal	0110	$\overline{Z}$
GE	greater or equal	1100	$N\cdot V+\overline{N}\cdot\overline{V}$		PI	plus	1010	$\overline{N}$
GT	greater than	1110	$N\cdot V\cdot\overline{Z}+\overline{N}\cdot\overline{V}\cdot\overline{Z}$		T	true	0000	1
HI	high	0010	$\overline{C}\cdot\overline{Z}$		VC	overflow clear	1000	$\overline{V}$
LE	less or equal	1111	$Z+N\cdot\overline{V}+\overline{N}\cdot V$		VS	overflow set	1001	V

Condition Codes: Not affected.

Instruction Format:

15	14	13	12	11	10	9	8	7	6	5	4	3	2	1	0
0	1	0	1	\multicolumn{4}{c}{Condition}	1	1	\multicolumn{3}{c}{Mode}	\multicolumn{3}{c}{Register}

Effective Address: Mode | Register

Instruction Fields:

    Condition field — One of sixteen conditions discussed in description.
    Effective Address field — Specifies the location in which the true/false byte is to be stored. Only data alterable addressing modes are allowed as shown:

Addressing Mode	Mode	Register	Addressing Mode	Mode	Register
Dn	000	register number	d(An, Xi)	110	register number
An	—	—	Abs.W	111	000
(An)	010	register number	Abs.L	111	001
(An)+	011	register number	d(PC)	—	—
−(An)	100	register number	d(PC, Xi)	—	—
d(An)	101	register number	Imm	—	—

Notes:
1. A memory destination is read before being written to.
2. An arithmetic one and zero result may be generated by following the Scc instruction with a NEG instruction.

STOP

**Load Status Register and Stop
(Privileged Instruction)**

Operation: If supervisor state
then Immediate Data → SR; STOP
else TRAP

**Assembler
Syntax:** STOP #xxx

Attributes: Unsized

Description: The immediate operand is moved into the entire status register; the program counter is advanced to point to the next instruction and the processor stops fetching and executing instructions. Execution of instructions resumes when a trace, interrupt, or reset exception occurs. A trace exception will occur if the trace state is on when the STOP instruction is executed. If an interrupt request arrives whose priority is higher than the current processor priority, an interrupt exception occurs, otherwise the interrupt request has no effect. If the bit of the immediate data corresponding to the S-bit is off, execution of the instruction will cause a privilege violation. External reset will always initiate reset exception processing.

Condition Codes: Set according to the immediate operand.

Instruction Format:

15	14	13	12	11	10	9	8	7	6	5	4	3	2	1	0
0	1	0	0	1	1	1	0	0	1	1	1	0	0	1	0
							Immediate Data								

Instruction Fields:

Immediate field — Specifies the data to be loaded into the status register.

SUB　　　Subtract Binary　　　SUB

Operation: (Destination) − (Source) → Destination

Assembler SUB <ea>, Dn
Syntax: SUB Dn, <ea>

Attributes: Size = (Byte, Word, Long)

Description: Subtract the source operand from the destination operand and store the result in the destination. The size of the operation may be specified to be byte, word, or long. The mode of the instruction indicates which operand is the source and which is the destination as well as the operand size.

Condition Codes:

X	N	Z	V	C
*	*	*	*	*

N   Set if the result is negative. Cleared otherwise.
Z   Set if the result is zero. Cleared otherwise.
V   Set if an overflow is generated. Cleared otherwise.
C   Set if a borrow is generated. Cleared otherwise.
X   Set the same as the carry bit.

Instruction Format:

15	14	13	12	11	10	9	8	7	6	5	4	3	2	1	0
1	0	0	1	Register			Op-Mode			Effective Address					
										Mode			Register		

Instruction Fields:

Register field — Specifies any of the eight data registers.
Op-Mode field —

Byte	Word	Long	Operation
000	001	010	(<Dn>) − (<ea>) → <Dn>
100	101	110	(<ea>) − (<Dn>) → <ea>

Effective Address field — Determines addressing mode:
If the location specified is a source operand, then all addressing modes are allowed as shown:

Addressing Mode	Mode	Register	Addressing Mode	Mode	Register
Dn	000	register number	d(An, Xi)	110	register number
An*	001	register number	Abs.W	111	000
(An)	010	register number	Abs.L	111	001
(An)+	011	register number	d(PC)	111	010
−(An)	100	register number	d(PC, Xi)	111	011
d(An)	101	register number	Imm	111	100

*For byte size operation, address register direct is not allowed.

— Continued —

SUB Subtract Binary SUB

Effective Address field (Continued)

If the location specified is a destination operand, then only alterable memory addressing modes are allowed as shown:

Addressing Mode	Mode	Register	Addressing Mode	Mode	Register
Dn	—	—	d(An, Xi)	110	register number
An	—	—	Abs.W	111	000
(An)	010	register number	Abs.L	111	001
(An)+	011	register number	d(PC)	—	—
−(An)	100	register number	d(PC, Xi)	—	—
d(An)	101	register number	Imm	—	—

Notes:
1. If the destination is a data register, then it cannot be specified by using the destination <ea> mode, but must use the destination Dn mode instead.
2. SUBA is used when the destination is an address register. SUBI and SUBQ are used when the source is immediate data. Most assemblers automatically make this distinction.

SUBA Subtract Address SUBA

Operation: (Destination) − (Source) → Destination

**Assembler
Syntax:** SUBA <ea>, An

Attributes: Size = (Word, Long)

Description: Subtract the source operand from the destination address register and store the result in the address register. The size of the operation may be specified to be word or long. Word size source operands are sign extended to 32 bit quantities before the operation is done.

Condition Codes: Not affected.

Instruction Format:

15	14	13	12	11 10 9	8 7 6	5 4 3	2 1 0
1	0	0	1	Register	Op-Mode	Effective Address Mode	Register

Instruction Fields:

Register field — Specifies any of the eight address registers. This is always the destination.

Op-Mode field — Specifies the size of the operation:

011 — Word operation. The source operand is sign-extended to a long operand and the operation is performed on the address register using all 32 bits.

111 — Long operations.

Effective Address field — Specifies the source operand. All addressing modes are allowed as shown:

Addressing Mode	Mode	Register	Addressing Mode	Mode	Register
Dn	000	register number	d(An, Xi)	110	register number
An	001	register number	Abs.W	111	000
(An)	010	register number	Abs.L	111	001
(An)+	011	register number	d(PC)	111	010
−(An)	100	register number	d(PC, Xi)	111	011
d(An)	101	register number	Imm	111	100

SUBI   Subtract Immediate   SUBI

Operation: (Destination) − Immediate Data → Destination

Assembler Syntax: SUBI #<data>, <ea>

Attributes: Size = (Byte, Word, Long)

Description: Subtract the immediate data from the destination operand and store the result in the destination location. The size of the operation may be specified to be byte, word, or long. The size of the immediate data matches the operation size.

Condition Codes:

X	N	Z	V	C
*	*	*	*	*

- N Set if the result is negative. Cleared otherwise.
- Z Set if the result is zero. Cleared otherwise.
- V Set if an overflow is generated. Cleared otherwise.
- C Set if a borrow is generated. Cleared otherwise.
- X Set the same as the carry bit.

Instruction Format:

15	14	13	12	11	10	9	8	7	6	5	4	3	2	1	0
0	0	0	0	0	1	0	0	Size		Effective Address					
										Mode			Register		
Word Data (16 bits)								Byte Data (8 bits)							
Long Data (32 bits, including previous word)															

Instruction Fields:

Size field — Specifies the size of the operation.
- 00 — byte operation.
- 01 — word operation.
- 10 — long operation.

Effective Address field — Specifies the destination operand. Only data alterable addressing modes are allowed as shown:

Addressing Mode	Mode	Register	Addressing Mode	Mode	Register
Dn	000	register number	d(An, Xi)	110	register number
An	—	—	Abs.W	111	000
(An)	010	register number	Abs.L	111	001
(An)+	011	register number	d(PC)	—	—
−(An)	100	register number	d(PC, Xi)	—	—
d(An)	101	register number	Imm	—	—

Immediate field — (Data immediately following the instruction)
- If size = 00, then the data is the low order byte of the immediate word.
- If size = 01, then the data is the entire immediate word.
- If size = 10, then the data is the next two immediate words.

SUBQ Subtract Quick SUBQ

Operation: (Destination) − Immediate Data → Destination

Assembler Syntax: SUBQ #<data>, <ea>

Attributes: Size = (Byte, Word, Long)

Description: Subtract the immediate data from the destination operand. The data range is from 1-8. The size of the operation may be specified to be byte, word, or long. Word and long operations are also allowed on the address registers and the condition codes are not affected. Word size source operands are sign extended to 32 bit quantities before the operation is done.

Condition Codes:

X	N	Z	V	C
*	*	*	*	*

N Set if the result is negative. Cleared otherwise.
Z Set if the result is zero. Cleared otherwise.
V Set if an overflow is generated. Cleared otherwise.
C Set if a borrow is generated. Cleared otherwise.
X Set the same as the carry bit.

The condition codes are not affected if a subtraction from an address register is made.

Instruction Format:

15	14	13	12	11	10	9	8	7	6	5	4	3	2	1	0
0	1	0	1	Data			1	Size		Effective Address				
										Mode			Register		

Instruction Fields:

Data field — Three bits of immediate data, 0, 1-7 representing a range of 8, 1 to 7 respectively.

Size field — Specifies the size of the operation:
00 — byte operation.
01 — word operation.
10 — long operation.

Effective Address field — Specifies the destination location. Only alterable addressing modes are allowed as shown:

Addressing Mode	Mode	Register	Addressing Mode	Mode	Register
Dn	000	register number	d(An, Xi)	110	register number
An*	001	register number	Abs.W	111	000
(An)	010	register number	Abs.L	111	001
(An)+	011	register number	d(PC)	—	—
−(An)	100	register number	d(PC, Xi)	—	—
d(An)	101	register number	Imm	—	—

*Word and Long only.

SUBX Subtract with Extend SUBX

Operation: (Destination) − (Source) − X → Destination

Assembler SUBX Dy, Dx
Syntax: SUBX −(Ay), −(Ax)

Attributes: Size = (Byte, Word, Long)

Description: Subtract the source operand from the destination operand along with the extend bit and store the result in the destination location. The operands may be addressed in two different ways:
1. Data register to data register: The operands are contained in data registers specified in the instruction.
2. Memory to memory. The operands are contained in memory and addressed with the predecrement addressing mode using the address registers specified in the instruction.

The size of the operation may be specified to be byte, word, or long.

Condition Codes:

X	N	Z	V	C
*	*	*	*	*

N Set if the result is negative. Cleared otherwise.
Z Cleared if the result is non-zero. Unchanged otherwise.
V Set if an overflow is generated. Cleared otherwise.
C Set if a carry is generated. Cleared otherwise.
X Set the same as the carry bit.

NOTE

Normally the Z condition code bit is set via programming before the start of an operation. This allows successful tests for zero results upon completion of multiple-precision operations.

Instruction Format:

15	14	13	12	11	10	9	8	7	6	5	4	3	2	1	0
1	0	0	1	Register Rx			1	Size		0	0	R/M	Register Ry		

— Continued —

SUBX   Subtract with Extend   SUBX

Instruction Fields:
- Register Rx field — Specifies the destination register:
  - If R/M = 0, specifies a data register.
  - If R/M = 1, specifies an address register for the predecrement addressing mode.
- Size field — Specifies the size of the operation:
  - 00 — byte operation.
  - 01 — word operation.
  - 10 — long operation.
- R/M field — Specifies the operand addressing mode:
  - 0 — The operation is data register to data register.
  - 1 — The operation is memory to memory.
- Register Ry field — Specifies the source register:
  - If R/M = 0, specifies a data register.
  - If R/M = 1, specifies an address register for the predecrement addressing mode.

SWAP   Swap Register Halves   SWAP

Operation: Register [31:16] ↔ Register [15:0]

Assembler Syntax: SWAP Dn

Attributes: Size = (Word)

Description: Exchange the 16-bit halves of a data register.

Condition Codes:

X	N	Z	V	C
—	*	*	0	0

N Set if the most significant bit of the 32-bit result is set. Cleared otherwise.
Z Set if the 32-bit result is zero. Cleared otherwise.
V Always cleared.
C Always cleared.
X Not affected.

Instruction Format:

15	14	13	12	11	10	9	8	7	6	5	4	3	2	1	0
0	1	0	0	1	0	0	0	0	1	0	0	0	Register		

Instruction Fields:

Register field — Specifies the data register to swap.

TAS   Test and Set an Operand   TAS

Operation: (Destination) Tested → CC; 1 → bit 7 OF Destination

Assembler Syntax: TAS <ea>

Attributes: Size = (Byte)

Description: Test and set the byte operand addressed by the effective address field. The current value of the operand is tested and N and Z are set accordingly. The high order bit of the operand is set. The operation is indivisible (using a read-modify-write memory cycle) to allow synchronization of several processors.

Condition Codes:

X	N	Z	V	C
—	*	*	0	0

- N   Set if the most significant bit of the operand was set. Cleared otherwise.
- Z   Set if the operand was zero. Cleared otherwise.
- V   Always cleared.
- C   Always cleared.
- X   Not affected.

Instruction Format:

15	14	13	12	11	10	9	8	7	6	5	4	3	2	1	0
0	1	0	0	1	0	1	0	1	1	\multicolumn{3}{c}{Effective Address}			

(Bits 5-3: Mode, Bits 2-0: Register)

Instruction Fields:

Effective Address field — Specifies the location of the tested operand. Only data alterable addressing modes are allowed as shown:

Addressing Mode	Mode	Register	Addressing Mode	Mode	Register
Dn	000	register number	d(An, Xi)	110	register number
An	—	—	Abs.W	111	000
(An)	010	register number	Abs.L	111	001
(An)+	011	register number	d(PC)	—	—
−(An)	100	register number	d(PC, Xi)	—	—
d(An)	101	register number	Imm	—	—

Note: Bus error retry is inhibited on the read portion of the TAS read-modify-write bus cycle to ensure system integrity. The bus error exception is always taken.

TRAP   Trap   TRAP

Operation: PC $\rightarrow$ $-$(SSP); SR $\rightarrow$ $-$(SSP); (Vector) $\rightarrow$ PC

Assembler Syntax: TRAP #<vector>

Attributes: Unsized

Description: The processor initiates exception processing. The vector number is generated to reference the TRAP instruction exception vector specified by the low order four bits of the instruction. Sixteen TRAP instruction vectors are available.

Condition Codes: Not affected.

Instruction Format:

15	14	13	12	11	10	9	8	7	6	5	4	3	2	1	0
0	1	0	0	1	1	1	0	0	1	0	0	\multicolumn{4}{c}{Vector}

Instruction Fields:

     Vector field — Specifies which trap vector contains the new program counter to be loaded.

TRAPV

Trap on Overflow

TRAPV

Operation: If V then TRAP

Assembler Syntax: TRAPV

Attributes: Unsized

Description: If the overflow condition is on, the processor initiates exception processing. The vector number is generated to reference the TRAPV exception vector. If the overflow condition is off, no operation is performed and execution continues with the next instruction in sequence.

Condition Codes: Not affected.

Instruction Format:

15	14	13	12	11	10	9	8	7	6	5	4	3	2	1	0
0	1	0	0	1	1	1	0	0	1	1	1	0	1	1	0

TST   Test an Operand   TST

Operation: (Destination) Tested → CC

Assembler Syntax: TST <ea>

Attributes: Size = (Byte, Word, Long)

Description: Compare the operand with zero. No results are saved; however, the condition codes are set according to results of the test. The size of the operation may be specified to be byte, word, or long.

Condition Codes:

X	N	Z	V	C
—	*	*	0	0

N   Set if the operand is negative. Cleared otherwise.
Z   Set if the operand is zero. Cleared otherwise.
V   Always cleared.
C   Always cleared.
X   Not affected.

Instruction Format:

15	14	13	12	11	10	9	8	7	6	5	4	3	2	1	0
0	1	0	0	1	0	1	0	Size		Effective Address Mode			Register		

Instruction Fields:

Size field — Specifies the size of the operation:
  00 — byte operation.
  01 — word operation.
  10 — long operation.

Effective Address field — Specifies the destination operand. Only data alterable addressing modes are allowed as shown:

Addressing Mode	Mode	Register	Addressing Mode	Mode	Register
Dn	000	register number	d(An, Xi)	110	register number
An	—	—	Abs.W	111	000
(An)	010	register number	Abs.L	111	001
(An)+	011	register number	d(PC)	—	—
−(An)	100	register number	d(PC, Xi)	—	—
d(An)	101	register number	Imm	—	—

UNLK Unlink UNLK

Operation: An → SP; (SP) + → An

**Assembler
Syntax:** UNLK An

Attributes: Unsized

Description: The stack pointer is loaded from the specified address register. The address register is then loaded with the long word pulled from the top of the stack.

Condition Codes: Not affected.

Instruction Format:

15	14	13	12	11	10	9	8	7	6	5	4	3	2	1	0
0	1	0	0	1	1	1	0	0	1	0	1	1	Register		

Instruction Fields:

Register field — specifies the address register through which the unlinking is to be done.

Appendix C
INSTRUCTION FORMAT SUMMARY

C.1 INTRODUCTION

This appendix provides a summary of the first word in each instruction of the instruction set. Table C-1 is an operation code (op-code) map which illustrates how bits 15 through 12 are used to specify the operations. The remaining paragraph groups the instructions according to the op-code map.

Table C-1. Operation Code Map

Bits 15 through 12	Operation	Bits 15 through 12	Operation
0000	Bit Manipulation/MOVEP/Immediate	1000	OR/DIV/SBCD
0001	Move Byte	1001	SUB/SUBX
0010	Move Long	1010	(Unassigned)
0011	Move Word	1011	CMP/EOR
0100	Miscellaneous	1100	AND/MUL/ABCD/EXG
0101	ADDQ/SUBQ/Scc/DBcc	1101	ADD/ADDX
0110	Bcc/BSR	1110	Shift/Rotate
0111	MOVEQ	1111	(Unassigned)

Table C-2. Effective Address Encoding Summary

Addressing Mode	Mode	Register
Data Register Direct	000	register number
Address Register Direct	001	register number
Address Register Indirect	010	register number
Address Register Indirect with Postincrement	011	register number
Address Register Indirect with Predecrement	100	register number
Address Register Indirect with Displacement	101	register number
Address Register Indirect with Index	110	register number
Absolute Short	111	000
Absolute Long	111	001
Program Counter with Displacement	111	010
Program Counter with Index	111	011
Immediate or Status Register	111	100

Table C-3. Conditional Tests

Mnemonic	Condition	Encoding	Test
T	true	0000	1
F	false	0001	0
HI	high	0010	$\overline{C}\cdot\overline{Z}$
LS	low or same	0011	$C+Z$
CC(HS)	carry clear	0100	$\overline{C}$
CS(LO)	carry set	0101	C
NE	not equal	0110	$\overline{Z}$
EQ	equal	0111	Z
VC	overflow clear	1000	$\overline{V}$
VS	overflow set	1001	V
PL	plus	1010	$\overline{N}$
MI	minus	1011	N
GE	greater or equal	1100	$N\cdot V + \overline{N}\cdot\overline{V}$
LT	less than	1101	$N\cdot\overline{V} + \overline{N}\cdot V$
GT	greater than	1110	$N\cdot V\cdot\overline{Z} + \overline{N}\cdot\overline{V}\cdot\overline{Z}$
LE	less or equal	1111	$Z + N\cdot\overline{V} + \overline{N}\cdot V$

OR Immediate

15	14	13	12	11	10	9	8	7	6	5	4	3	2	1	0
0	0	0	0	0	0	0	0	Size		Effective Address					
										Mode			Register		

Size field: 00 = byte
01 = word
10 = long

OR Immediate to CCR

15	14	13	12	11	10	9	8	7	6	5	4	3	2	1	0
0	0	0	0	0	0	0	0	0	0	1	1	1	1	0	0

OR Immediate to SR

15	14	13	12	11	10	9	8	7	6	5	4	3	2	1	0
0	0	0	0	0	0	0	0	0	1	1	1	1	1	0	0

Dynamic Bit

15	14	13	12	11 10 9	8	7 6	5 4 3	2 1 0
0	0	0	0	Data Register	1	Type	Effective Address Mode	Register

Type field: 00 = TST
 01 = CHG
 10 = CLR
 11 = SET

MOVEP

15	14	13	12	11 10 9	8 7 6	5	4	3	2 1 0
0	0	0	0	Data Register	Op-Mode	0	0	1	Address Register

Op-Mode field: 100 = transfer word from memory to register
 101 = transfer long from memory to register
 110 = transfer word from register to memory
 111 = transfer long from register to memory

AND Immediate

15	14	13	12	11	10	9	8	7 6	5 4 3	2 1 0
0	0	0	0	0	0	1	0	Size	Effective Address Mode	Register

Size field: 00 = byte
 01 = word
 10 = long

AND Immediate to CCR

15	14	13	12	11	10	9	8	7	6	5	4	3	2	1	0
0	0	0	0	0	0	1	0	0	0	1	1	1	1	0	0

AND Immediate to SR

15	14	13	12	11	10	9	8	7	6	5	4	3	2	1	0
0	0	0	0	0	0	1	0	0	1	1	1	1	1	0	0

SUB Immediate

15	14	13	12	11	10	9	8	7	6	5	4	3	2	1	0
0	0	0	0	0	1	0	0	Size		Effective Address					
										Mode			Register		

Size field: 00 = byte
01 = word
10 = long

ADD Immediate

15	14	13	12	11	10	9	8	7	6	5	4	3	2	1	0
0	0	0	0	0	1	1	0	Size		Effective Address					
										Mode			Register		

Size field: 00 = byte
01 = word
10 = long

Static Bit

15	14	13	12	11	10	9	8	7	6	5	4	3	2	1	0
0	0	0	0	1	0	0	0	Type		Effective Address					
										Mode			Register		

Type field: 00 = TST
01 = CHG
10 = CLR
11 = SET

EOR Immediate

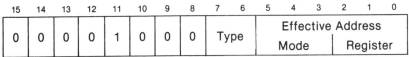

15	14	13	12	11	10	9	8	7	6	5	4	3	2	1	0
0	0	0	0	1	0	1	0	Size		Effective Address					
										Mode			Register		

Size field: 00 = byte
01 = word
10 = long

EOR Immediate to CCR

15	14	13	12	11	10	9	8	7	6	5	4	3	2	1	0
0	0	0	0	1	0	1	0	0	0	1	1	1	1	0	0

EOR Immediate to SR

15	14	13	12	11	10	9	8	7	6	5	4	3	2	1	0
0	0	0	0	1	0	1	0	0	1	1	1	1	1	0	0

CMP Immediate

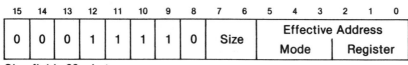

Size field: 00 = byte
01 = word
10 = word

MOVES   MC68010

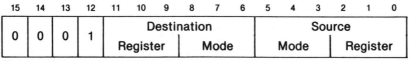

Size field: 00 = byte
01 = word
10 = long

MOVE Byte

15	14	13	12	11	10	9	8	7	6	5	4	3	2	1	0
0	0	0	1	\multicolumn{3}{Destination}				\multicolumn{3}{Source}			
				Register			Mode			Mode			Register		

Note register and mode locations

MOVEA Long

14	14	13	12	11 10 9	8	7	6	5 4 3	2 1 0
0	0	1	0	Destination Register	0	0	1	Source Mode	Register

MOVE Long

15	14	13	12	11 10 9	8 7 6	5 4 3	2 1 0
0	0	1	0	Destination Register	Mode	Source Mode	Register

Note register and mode locations

MOVEA Word

15	14	13	12	11 10 9	8	7	6	5 4 3	2 1 0
0	0	1	1	Destination Register	0	0	1	Source Mode	Register

MOVE Word

15	14	13	12	11 10 9	8 7 6	5 4 3	2 1 0
0	0	1	1	Destination Register	Mode	Source Mode	Register

Note register and mode locations

NEGX

15	14	13	12	11	10	9	8	7	6	5	4	3	2	1	0
0	1	0	0	0	0	0	0	Size		Effective Address					
										Mode			Register		

Size field: 00 = byte
01 = word
10 = long

MOVE from SR

15	14	13	12	11	10	9	8	7	6	5	4	3	2	1	0
0	1	0	0	0	0	0	0	1	1	Effective Address					
										Mode			Register		

CHK

15	14	13	12	11	10	9	8	7	6	5	4	3	2	1	0
0	1	0	0	Data Register			1	1	0	Effective Address					
										Mode			Register		

LEA

15	14	13	12	11	10	9	8	7	6	5	4	3	2	1	0
0	1	0	0	Address Register			1	1	1	Effective Address					
										Mode			Register		

CLR

15	14	13	12	11	10	9	8	7	6	5	4	3	2	1	0
0	1	0	0	0	0	1	0	Size		Effective Address					
										Mode			Register		

Size field: 00 = byte
01 = word
10 = long

MOVE from CCR   MC68010

15	14	13	12	11	10	9	8	7	6	5	4	3	2	1	0
0	1	0	0	0	0	1	0	1	1	\multicolumn{3}{c}{Effective Address Mode}	\multicolumn{3}{c}{Register}			

NEG

15	14	13	12	11	10	9	8	7	6	5	4	3	2	1	0
0	1	0	0	0	1	0	0	Size		Effective Address Mode			Register		

Size field: 00 = byte
01 = word
10 = long

MOVE to CCR

15	14	13	12	11	10	9	8	7	6	5	4	3	2	1	0
0	1	0	0	0	1	0	0	1	1	Effective Address Mode			Register		

NOT

15	14	13	12	11	10	9	8	7	6	5	4	3	2	1	0
0	1	0	0	0	1	1	0	Size		Effective Address Mode			Register		

Size field: 00 = byte
01 = word
10 = long

MOVE to SR

15	14	13	12	11	10	9	8	7	6	5	4	3	2	1	0
0	1	0	0	0	1	1	0	1	1	Effective Address Mode			Register		

NBCD

15	14	13	12	11	10	9	8	7	6	5	4	3	2	1	0
0	1	0	0	1	0	0	0	0	0	\multicolumn{6}{c}{Effective Address}

15	14	13	12	11	10	9	8	7	6	5	4	3	2	1	0
0	1	0	0	1	0	0	0	0	0	Mode			Register		

SWAP

15	14	13	12	11	10	9	8	7	6	5	4	3	2	1	0
0	1	0	0	1	0	0	0	1	0	0	0	Data Register			

PEA

15	14	13	12	11	10	9	8	7	6	5	4	3	2	1	0
0	1	0	0	1	0	0	0	0	1	Mode			Register		

(Effective Address)

EXT Word

15	14	13	12	11	10	9	8	7	6	5	4	3	2	1	0
0	1	0	0	1	0	0	0	1	0	0	0	0	Data Register		

MOVEM Registers to EA

15	14	13	12	11	10	9	8	7	6	5	4	3	2	1	0
0	1	0	0	1	0	0	0	1	Sz	Mode			Register		

(Effective Address)

Sz field: 0 = word transfer
1 = long transfer

EXT Long

15	14	13	12	11	10	9	8	7	6	5	4	3	2	1	0
0	1	0	0	1	0	0	0	1	1	0	0	0	\multicolumn{3}{	c	}{Data Register}

TST

15	14	13	12	11	10	9	8	7	6	5	4	3	2	1	0
0	1	0	0	1	0	1	0	\multicolumn{2}{	c	}{Size}	\multicolumn{3}{	c	}{Effective Address Mode}	\multicolumn{3}{	c	}{Register}

Size field: 00 = byte
             01 = word
             10 = long

TAS

15	14	13	12	11	10	9	8	7	6	5	4	3	2	1	0
0	1	0	0	1	0	1	0	1	1	\multicolumn{3}{	c	}{Effective Address Mode}	\multicolumn{3}{	c	}{Register}

ILLEGAL

15	14	13	12	11	10	9	8	7	6	5	4	3	2	1	0
0	1	0	0	1	0	1	0	1	1	1	1	1	1	0	0

MOVEM EA to Registers

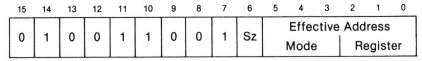

Sz field: 0 = word transfer
           1 = long transfer

TRAP

15	14	13	12	11	10	9	8	7	6	5	4	3	2	1	0
0	1	0	0	1	1	1	0	0	1	0	0	Vector			

LINK

15	14	13	12	11	10	9	8	7	6	5	4	3	2	1	0
0	1	0	0	1	1	1	0	0	1	0	1	0	Address Register		

UNLK

15	14	13	12	11	10	9	8	7	6	5	4	3	2	1	0
0	1	0	0	1	1	1	0	0	1	0	1	1	Address Register		

MOVE to USP

15	14	13	12	11	10	9	8	7	6	5	4	3	2	1	0
0	1	0	0	1	1	1	0	0	1	1	0	0	Address Register		

MOVE from USP

15	14	13	12	11	10	9	8	7	6	5	4	3	2	1	0
0	1	0	0	1	1	1	0	0	1	1	0	1	Address Register		

RESET

15	14	13	12	11	10	9	8	7	6	5	4	3	2	1	0
0	1	0	0	1	1	1	0	0	1	1	1	0	0	0	0

NOP

15	14	13	12	11	10	9	8	7	6	5	4	3	2	1	0
0	1	0	0	1	1	1	0	0	1	1	1	0	0	0	1

STOP

15	14	13	12	11	10	9	8	7	6	5	4	3	2	1	0
0	1	0	0	1	1	1	0	0	1	1	1	0	0	1	0

RTE

15	14	13	12	11	10	9	8	7	6	5	4	3	2	1	0
0	1	0	0	1	1	1	0	0	1	1	1	0	0	1	1

RTD MC68010

15	14	13	12	11	10	9	8	7	6	5	4	3	2	1	0
0	1	0	0	1	1	1	0	0	1	1	1	0	1	0	0

RTS

15	14	13	12	11	10	9	8	7	6	5	4	3	2	1	0
0	1	0	0	1	1	1	0	0	1	1	1	0	1	0	1

TRAPV

15	14	13	12	11	10	9	8	7	6	5	4	3	2	1	0
0	1	0	0	1	1	1	0	0	1	1	1	0	1	1	0

RTR

15	14	13	12	11	10	9	8	7	6	5	4	3	2	1	0
0	1	0	0	1	1	1	0	0	1	1	1	0	1	1	1

MOVEC MC68010

15	14	13	12	11	10	9	8	7	6	5	4	3	2	1	0
0	1	0	0	1	1	1	0	0	1	1	1	1	0	1	dr

dr field: 0 = control register to general register
1 = general register to control register

JSR

15	14	13	12	11	10	9	8	7	6	5 4 3	2 1 0
										Effective Address	
0	1	0	0	1	1	1	0	1	0	Mode	Register

JMP

15	14	13	12	11	10	9	8	7	6	5 4 3	2 1 0
										Effective Mode	
0	1	0	0	1	1	1	0	1	1	Mode	Register

ADDQ

15	14	13	12	11	10	9	8	7	6	5	4	3	2	1	0
0	1	0	1	Data			0	Size		Effective Address					
										Mode			Register		

Data field: Three bits of immediate data, 0, 1-7 representing a range of 8, 1 to 7 respectively.

Size field: 00 = byte
01 = word
10 = long

Scc

15	14	13	12	11	10	9	8	7	6	5	4	3	2	1	0
0	1	0	1	Condition				1	1	Effective Address					
										Mode			Register		

Condition field:
0000 = true   1000 = overflow clear
0001 = false   1001 = overflow set
0010 = high   1010 = plus
0011 = low or same 1011 = minus
0100 = carry clear 1100 = greater or equal
0101 = carry set   1101 = less than
0110 = not equal   1110 = greater than
0111 = equal   1111 = less or equal

DBcc

15	14	13	12	11	10	9	8	7	6	5	4	3	2	1	0
0	1	0	1	Condition				1	1	0	0	1	Data Register		

Condition field:
0000 = true   1000 = overflow clear
0001 = false   1001 = overflow set
0010 = high   1010 = plus
0011 = low or same 1011 = minus
0100 = carry clear 1100 = greater or equal
0101 = carry set   1101 = less than
0110 = not equal   1110 = greater than
0111 = equal   1111 = less or equal

SUBQ

15	14	13	12	11	10	9	8	7	6	5	4	3	2	1	0
0	1	0	1	Data			1	Size		Effective Address					
										Mode			Register		

Data field: Three bits of immediate data, 0, 1-7 representing a range of 8, 1 to 7 respectively.
Size field: 00 = byte
01 = word
10 = long

Bcc

15	14	13	12	11	10	9	8	7	6	5	4	3	2	1	0
0	1	1	0	Condition				8-Bit Displacement							

Condition field: 0010 = high   1001 = overflow set
0011 = low or same   1010 = plus
0100 = carry clear   1011 = minus
0101 = carry set   1100 = greater or equal
0110 = not equal   1101 = less than
0111 = equal   1110 = greater than
1000 = overflow clear 1111 = less or equal

BRA

15	14	13	12	11	10	9	8	7	6	5	4	3	2	1	0
0	1	1	0	0	0	0	0	8-Bit Displacement							

BSR

15	14	13	12	11	10	9	8	7	6	5	4	3	2	1	0
0	1	1	0	0	0	0	1	8-Bit Displacement							

MOVEQ

15	14	13	12	11	10	9	8	7	6	5	4	3	2	1	0
0	1	1	1	\multicolumn{3}{c}{Data Register}	0	\multicolumn{8}{c}{Data}

Data field: Data is sign extended to a long operand and all 32 bits are transferred to the data register.

OR

15	14	13	12	11	10	9	8	7	6	5	4	3	2	1	0
1	0	0	0	Data Register			Op-Mode			Effective Address			
										Mode			Register		

Op-Mode field:

Byte	Word	Long	Operation
000	001	010	$(<Dn>) \vee (<ea>) \rightarrow Dn$
100	101	110	$(<ea>) \vee (<Dn>) \rightarrow ea$

DIVU

15	14	13	12	11	10	9	8	7	6	5	4	3	2	1	0
1	0	0	0	Data Register			0	1	1	Effective Address			
										Mode			Register		

SBCD

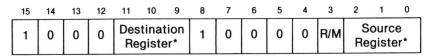

R/M field: 0 = data register to data register
  1 = memory to memory
*If R/M = 0, specifies a data register.
 If R/M = 1, specifies an address register for the predecrement addressing mode.

DIVS

15	14	13	12	11 10 9	8	7	6	5 4 3	2 1 0
								Effective Address	
1	0	0	0	Data Register	1	1	1	Mode	Register

SUB

15	14	13	12	11 10 9	8 7 6	5 4 3	2 1 0
						Effective Address	
1	0	0	1	Data Register	Op-Mode	Mode	Register

Op-Mode field:

Byte	Word	Long	Operation
000	001	010	(<Dn>)−(<ea>) →Dn
100	101	110	(<ea>)−(<Dn>) →ea

SUBA

15	14	13	12	11 10 9	8 7 6	5 4 3	2 1 0
						Effective Address	
1	0	0	1	Data Register	Op-Mode	Mode	Register

Op-Mode field:

Word	Long	Operation
011	111	(<ea>)−(<An>) →An

SUBX

15	14	13	12	11 10 9	8	7 6 5	4 3	2 1 0
1	0	0	1	Destination Register*	1	Size	0 0 R/M	Source Register*

Size field: 00 = byte
           01 = word
           10 = long
R/M field: 0 = data register to data register
           1 = memory to memory
*If R/M = 0, specifies a data register.
 If R/M = 1, specifies an address register for the predecrement addressing mode.

CMP

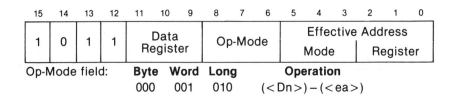

Op-Mode field:

Byte	Word	Long	Operation
000	001	010	(<Dn>)−(<ea>)

CMPA

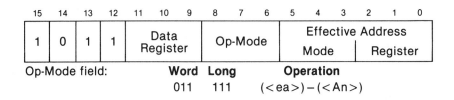

Op-Mode field:

Word	Long	Operation
011	111	(<ea>)−(<An>)

EOR

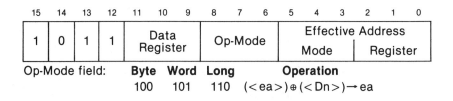

Op-Mode field:

Byte	Word	Long	Operation
100	101	110	(<ea>)⊕(<Dn>)→ea

CMPM

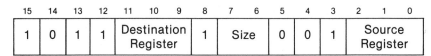

Size field: 00 = byte
            01 = word
            10 = long

AND

15	14	13	12	11 10 9	8 7 6	5 4 3	2 1 0
1	1	0	0	Data Register	Op-Mode	Effective Address Mode	Register

Op-Mode field:

Byte	**Word**	**Long**	**Operation**
000	001	010	$(<Dn>)\Lambda(<ea>) \rightarrow Dn$
100	101	110	$(<ea>)\Lambda(<Dn>) \rightarrow ea$

MULU

15	14	13	12	11 10 9	8	7	6	5 4 3	2 1 0
1	1	0	0	Data Register	0	1	1	Effective Address Mode	Register

ABCD

15	14	13	12	11 10 9	8	7	6	5	4	3	2 1 0
1	1	0	0	Destination Register*	1	0	0	0	0	R/M	Source Register*

R/M field: 0 = data register to data register
1 = memory to memory

*If R/M = 0, specifies a data register.
If R/M = 1, specifies an address register for the predecrement addressing mode.

EXG Data Registers

15	14	13	12	11 10 9	8	7	6	5	4	3	2 1 0
1	1	0	0	Data Register	1	0	1	0	0	0	Data Register

EXG Address Registers

15	14	13	12	11 10 9	8	7	6	5	4	3	2 1 0
1	1	0	0	Address Register	1	0	1	0	0	1	Address Register

EXG Data Register and Address Register

15	14	13	12	11 10 9	8	7	6	5	4	3	2 1 0
1	1	0	0	Data Register	1	1	0	0	0	1	Address Register

MULS

15	14	13	12	11 10 9	8	7	6	5 4 3	2 1 0
1	1	0	0	Data Register	1	1	1	Effective Address Mode	Register

ADD

15	14	13	12	11 10 9	8 7 6	5 4 3	2 1 0
1	1	0	1	Data Register	Op-Mode	Effective Address Mode	Register

Op-Mode field:

Byte	Word	Long	Operation
000	001	010	(<Dn>)+(<ea>)→Dn
100	101	110	(<ea>)+(<Dn>)→ea

ADDA

15	14	13	12	11 10 9	8 7 6	5 4 3	2 1 0
1	1	0	1	Data Register	Op-Mode	Effective Address Mode	Register

Op-Mode field:

Word	Long	Operation
011	111	(<ea>)+(<An>)→An

ADDX

15	14	13	12	11 10 9	8	7 6 5	4 3		2 1 0
1	1	0	1	Destination Register*	1	Size	0 0	R/M	Source Register*

Size field: 00 = byte
           01 = word
           10 = long
R/M field: 0 = data register to data register
            1 = memory to memory
*If R/M = 0, specifies a data register.
 If R/M = 1, specifies an address register for the predecrement addressing mode.

SHIFT/ROTATE — Register

15	14	13	12	11 10 9	8	7 6	5	4 3	2 1 0
1	1	1	0	Count/Register	dr	Size	i/r	Type	Data Register

Count/Register field: If i/r field = 0, specifies shift count
                    If i/r field = 1, specifies a data register that contains the shift count
dr field: 0 = right
          1 = left
Size field: 00 = byte
           01 = word
           10 = long
i/r field: 0 = immediate shift count
          1 = register shift count
Type field: 00 = arithmetic shift
            01 = logical shift
            10 = rotate with extend
            11 = rotate

SHIFT/ROTATE — Memory

15	14	13	12	11	10 9	8	7	6	5 4 3	2 1 0
1	1	1	0	0	Type	dr	1	1	Effective Address Mode	Register

Type field: 00 = arithmetic shift
            01 = logical shift
            10 = rotate with extend
            11 = rotate
dr field: 0 = right
          1 = left

Appendix D
MC68000 INSTRUCTION EXECUTION TIMES

D.1 INTRODUCTION

This Appendix contains listings of the instruction execution times in terms of external clock (CLK) periods. In this data, it is assumed that both memory read and write cycle times are four clock periods. A longer memory cycle will cause the generation of wait states which must be added to the total instruction time.

The number of bus read and write cycles for each instruction is also included with the timing data. This data is enclosed in parenthesis following the number of clock periods and is shown as: (r/w) where r is the number of read cycles and w is the number of write cycles included in the clock period number. Recalling that either a read or write cycle requires four clock periods, a timing number given as 18(3/1) relates to 12 clock periods for the three read cycles, plus 4 clock periods for the one write cycle, plus 2 cycles required for some internal function of the processor.

NOTE

The number of periods includes instruction fetch and all applicable operand fetches and stores.

D.2 OPERAND EFFECTIVE ADDRESS CALCULATION TIMING

Table D-1 lists the number of clock periods required to compute an instruction's effective address. It includes fetching of any extension words, the address computation, and fetching of the memory operand. The number of bus read and write cycles is shown in parenthesis as (r/w). Note there are no write cycles involved in processing the effective address.

Table D-1. Effective Address Calculation Times

Addressing Mode		Byte, Word	Long
Register			
Dn	Data Register Direct	0(0/0)	0(0/0)
An	Address Register Direct	0(0/0)	0(0/0)
Memory			
(An)	Address Register Indirect	4(1/0)	8(2/0)
(An)+	Address Register Indirect with Postincrement	4(1/0)	8(2/0)
-(An)	Address Register Indirect with Predecrement	6(1/0)	10(2/0)
d(An)	Address Register Indirect with Displacement	8(2/0)	12(3/0)
d(An, ix)*	Address Register Indirect with Index	10(2/0)	14(3/0)
xxx.W	Absolute Short	8(2/0)	12(3/0)
xxx.L	Absolute Long	12(3/0)	16(4/0)
d(PC)	Program Counter with Displacement	8(2/0)	12(3/0)
d(PC, ix)*	Program Counter with Index	10(2/0)	14(3/0)
#xxx	Immediate	4(1/0)	8(2/0)

*The size of the index register (ix) does not affect execution time.

D.3 MOVE INSTRUCTION EXECUTION TIMES

Tables D-2 and D-3 indicate the number of clock periods for the move instruction. This data includes instruction fetch, operand reads, and operand writes. The number of bus read and write cycles is shown in parenthesis as (r/w).

Table D-2. Move Byte and Word Instruction Execution Times

Source	Destination								
	Dn	An	(An)	(An)+	−(An)	d(An)	d(An, ix)*	xxx.W	xxx.L
Dn	4(1/0)	4(1/0)	8(1/1)	8(1/1)	8(1/1)	12(2/1)	14(2/1)	12(2/1)	16(3/1)
An	4(1/0)	4(1/0)	8(1/1)	8(1/1)	8(1/1)	12(2/1)	14(2/1)	12(2/1)	16(3/1)
(An)	8(2/0)	8(2/0)	12(2/1)	12(2/1)	12(2/1)	16(3/1)	18(3/1)	16(3/1)	20(4/1)
(An)+	8(2/0)	8(2/0)	12(2/1)	12(2/1)	12(2/1)	16(3/1)	18(3/1)	16(3/1)	20(4/1)
−(An)	10(2/0)	10(2/0)	14(2/1)	14(2/1)	14(2/1)	18(3/1)	20(3/1)	18(3/1)	22(4/1)
d(An)	12(3/0)	12(3/0)	16(3/1)	16(3/1)	16(3/1)	20(4/1)	22(4/1)	20(4/1)	24(5/1)
d(An, ix)*	14(3/0)	14(3/0)	18(3/1)	18(3/1)	18(3/1)	22(4/1)	24(4/1)	22(4/1)	26(5/1)
xxx.W	12(3/0)	12(3/0)	16(3/1)	16(3/1)	16(3/1)	20(4/1)	22(4/1)	20(4/1)	24(5/1)
xxx.L	16(4/0)	16(4/0)	20(4/1)	20(4/1)	20(4/1)	24(5/1)	26(5/1)	24(5/1)	28(6/1)
d(PC)	12(3/0)	12(3/0)	16(3/1)	16(3/1)	16(3/1)	20(4/1)	22(4/1)	20(4/1)	24(5/1)
d(PC, ix)*	14(3/0)	14(3/0)	18(3/1)	18(3/1)	18(3/1)	22(4/1)	24(4/1)	22(4/1)	26(5/1)
#xxx	8(2/0)	8(2/0)	12(2/1)	12(2/1)	12(2/1)	16(3/1)	18(3/1)	16(3/1)	20(4/1)

*The size of the index register (ix) does not affect execution time.

Table D-3. Move Long Instruction Execution Times

Source	Destination								
	Dn	An	(An)	(An)+	−(An)	d(An)	d(An, ix)*	xxx.W	xxx.L
Dn	4(1/0)	4(1/0)	12(1/2)	12(1/2)	12(1/2)	16(2/2)	18(2/2)	16(2/2)	20(3/2)
An	4(1/0)	4(1/0)	12(1/2)	12(1/2)	12(1/2)	16(2/2)	18(2/2)	16(2/2)	20(3/2)
(An)	12(3/0)	12(3/0)	20(3/2)	20(3/2)	20(3/2)	24(4/2)	26(4/2)	24(4/2)	28(5/2)
(An)+	12(3/0)	12(3/0)	20(3/2)	20(3/2)	20(3/2)	24(4/2)	26(4/2)	24(4/2)	28(5/2)
−(An)	14(3/0)	14(3/0)	22(3/2)	22(3/2)	22(3/2)	26(4/2)	28(4/2)	26(4/2)	30(5/2)
d(An)	16(4/0)	16(4/0)	24(4/2)	24(4/2)	24(4/2)	28(5/2)	30(5/2)	28(5/2)	32(6/2)
d(An, ix)*	18(4/0)	18(4/0)	26(4/2)	26(4/2)	26(4/2)	30(5/2)	32(5/2)	30(5/2)	34(6/2)
xxx.W	16(4/0)	16(4/0)	24(4/2)	24(4/2)	24(4/2)	28(5/2)	30(5/2)	28(5/2)	32(6/2)
xxx.L	20(5/0)	20(5/0)	28(5/2)	28(5/2)	28(5/2)	32(6/2)	34(6/2)	32(6/2)	36(7/2)
d(PC)	16(4/0)	16(4/0)	24(4/2)	24(4/2)	24(4/2)	28(5/2)	30(5/2)	28(5/2)	32(5/2)
d(PC, ix)*	18(4/0)	18(4/0)	26(4/2)	26(4/2)	26(4/2)	30(5/2)	32(5/2)	30(5/2)	34(6/2)
#xxx	12(3/0)	12(3/0)	20(3/2)	20(3/2)	20(3/2)	24(4/2)	26(4/2)	24(4/2)	28(5/2)

*The size of the index register (ix) does not affect execution time.

D.4 STANDARD INSTRUCTION EXECUTION TIMES

The number of clock periods shown in Table D-4 indicates the time required to perform the operations, store the results, and read the next instruction. The number of bus read and write cycles is shown in parenthesis as (r/w). The number of clock periods and the number of read and write cycles must be added respectively to those of the effective address calculation where indicated.

In Table D-4 the headings have the following meanings: An = address register operand, Dn = data register operand, ea = an operand specified by an effective address, and M = memory effective address operand.

Table D-4. Standard Instruction Execution Times

Instruction	Size	op<ea>, An†	op<ea>, Dn	op Dn, <M>
ADD	Byte, Word	8(1/0) +	4(1/0) +	8(1/1) +
	Long	6(1/0) + **	6(1/0) + **	12(1/2) +
AND	Byte, Word	—	4(1/0) +	8(1/1) +
	Long	—	6(1/0) + **	12(1/2) +
CMP	Byte, Word	6(1/0) +	4(1/0) +	—
	Long	6(1/0) +	6(1/0) +	—
DIVS	—	—	158(1/0) + *	—
DIVU	—	—	140(1/0) + *	—
EOR	Byte, Word	—	4(1/0) ***	8(1/1) +
	Long	—	8(1/0) ***	12(1/2) +
MULS	—	—	70(1/0) + *	—
MULU	—	—	70(1/0) + *	—
OR	Byte, Word	—	4(1/0) +	8(1/1) +
	Long	—	6(1/0) + **	12(1/2) +
SUB	Byte, Word	8(1/0) +	4(1/0) +	8(1/1) +
	Long	6(1/0) + **	6(1/0) + **	12(1/2) +

NOTES:
+ add effective address calculation time
† word or long only
* indicates maximum value
** The base time of six clock periods is increased to eight if the effective address mode is register direct or immediate (effective address time should also be added).
*** Only available effective address mode is data register direct.
DIVS, DIVU — The divide algorithm used by the MC68000 provides less than 10% difference between the best and worst case timings.
MULS, MULU — The multiply algorithm requires $38 + 2n$ clocks where n is defined as:
  MULU: n = the number of ones in the <ea>
  MULS: n = concatanate the <ea> with a zero as the LSB; n is the resultant number of 10 or 01 patterns in the 17-bit source; i.e., worst case happens when the source is $5555.

D.5 IMMEDIATE INSTRUCTION EXECUTION TIMES

The number of clock periods shown in Table D-5 includes the time to fetch immediate operands, perform the operations, store the results, and read the next operation. The number of bus read and write cycles is shown in parenthesis as (r/w). The number of clock periods and the number of read and write cycles must be added respectively to those of the effective address calculation where indicated.

In Table D-5, the headings have the following meanings: # = immediate operand, Dn = data register operand, An = address register operand, and M = memory operand. SR = status register.

Table D-5. Immediate Instruction Execution Times

Instruction	Size	op #, Dn	op #, An	op #, M
ADDI	Byte, Word	8(2/0)	—	12(2/1)+
	Long	16(3/0)	—	20(3/2)+
ADDQ	Byte, Word	4(1/0)	8(1/0)*	8(1/1)+
	Long	8(1/0)	8(1/0)	12(1/2)+
ANDI	Byte, Word	8(2/0)	—	12(2/1)+
	Long	16(3/0)	—	20(3/1)+
CMPI	Byte, Word	8(2/0)	—	8(2/0)+
	Long	14(3/0)	—	12(3/0)+
EORI	Byte, Word	8(2/0)	—	12(2/1)+
	Long	16(3/0)	—	20(3/2)+
MOVEQ	Long	4(1/0)	—	—
ORI	Byte, Word	8(2/0)	—	12(2/1)+
	Long	16(3/0)	—	20(3/2)+
SUBI	Byte, Word	8(2/0)	—	12(2/1)+
	Long	16(3/0)	—	20(3/2)+
SUBQ	Byte, Word	4(1/0)	8(1/0)*	8(1/1)+
	Long	8(1/0)	8(1/0)	12(1/2)+

+ add effective address calculation time
* word only

D.6 SINGLE OPERAND INSTRUCTION EXECUTION TIMES

Table D-6 indicates the number of clock periods for the single operand instructions. The number of bus read and write cycles is shown in parenthesis as (r/w). The number of clock periods and the number of read and write cycles must be added respectively to those of the effective address calculation where indicated.

Table D-6. Single Operand Instruction Execution Times

Instruction	Size	Register	Memory
CLR	Byte, Word	4(1/0)	8(1/1)+
	Long	6(1/0)	12(1/2)+
NBCD	Byte	6(1/0)	8(1/1)+
NEG	Byte, Word	4(1/0)	8(1/1)+
	Long	6(1/0)	12(1/2)+
NEGX	Byte, Word	4(1/0)	8(1/1)+
	Long	6(1/0)	12(1/2)+
NOT	Byte, Word	4(1/0)	8(1/1)+
	Long	6(1/0)	12(1/2)+
S_{CC}	Byte, False	4(1/0)	8(1/1)+
	Byte, True	6(1/0)	8(1/1)+
TAS	Byte	4(1/0)	10(1/1)+
TST	Byte, Word	4(1/0)	4(1/0)+
	Long	4(1/0)	4(1/0)+

+ add effective address calculation time

D.7 SHIFT/ROTATE INSTRUCTION EXECUTION TIMES

Table D-7 indicates the number of clock periods for the shift and rotate instructions. The number of bus read and write cycles is shown in parenthesis as (r/w). The number of clock periods and the number of read and write cycles must be added respectively to those of the effective address calculation where indicated.

Table D-7. Shift/Rotate Instruction Execution Times

Instruction	Size	Register	Memory
ASR, ASL	Byte, Word	6 + 2n(1/0)	8(1/1)+
	Long	8 + 2n(1/0)	—
LSR, LSL	Byte, Word	6 + 2n(1/0)	8(1/1)+
	Long	8 + 2n(1/0)	—
ROR, ROL	Byte, Word	6 + 2n(1/0)	8(1/1)+
	Long	8 + 2n(1/0)	—
ROXR, ROXL	Byte, Word	6 + 2n(1/0)	8(1/1)+
	Long	8 + 2n(1/0)	—

+ add effective address calculation time
n is the shift count

D.8 BIT MANIPULATION INSTRUCTION EXECUTION TIMES

Table D-8 indicates the number of clock periods required for the bit manipulation instructions. The number of bus read and write cycles is shown in parenthesis as (r/w). The number of clock periods and the number of read and write cycles must be added respectively to those of the effective address calculation where indicated.

Table D-8. Bit Manipulation Instruction Execution Times

Instruction	Size	Dynamic		Static	
		Register	Memory	Register	Memory
BCHG	Byte	—	8(1/1) +	—	12(2/1) +
	Long	8(1/0) *	—	12(2/0) *	—
BCLR	Byte	—	8(1/1) +	—	12(2/1) +
	Long	10(1/0) *	—	14(2/0) *	—
BSET	Byte	—	8(1/1) +	—	12(2/1) +
	Long	8(1/0) *	—	12(2/0) *	—
BTST	Byte	—	4(1/0) +	—	8(2/0) +
	Long	6(1/0)	—	10(2/0)	—

+ add effective address calculation time
* indicates maximum value

D.9 CONDITIONAL INSTRUCTION EXECUTION TIMES

Table D-9 indicates the number of clock periods required for the conditional instructions. The number of bus read and write cycles is indicated in parenthesis as (r/w). The number of clock periods and the number of read and write cycles must be added respectively to those of the effective address calculation where indicated.

Table D-9. Conditional Instruction Execution Times

Instruction	Displacement	Branch Taken	Branch Not Taken
B_{CC}	Byte	10(2/0)	8(1/0)
	Word	10(2/0)	12(2/0)
BRA	Byte	10(2/0)	—
	Word	10(2/0)	—
BSR	Byte	18(2/2)	—
	Word	18(2/2)	—
DB_{CC}	CC true	—	12(2/0)
	CC false	10(2/0)	14(3/0)

+ add effective address calculation time
* indicates maximum value

D.10 JMP, JSR, LEA, PEA, AND MOVEM INSTRUCTION EXECUTION TIMES

Table D-10 indicates the number of clock periods required for the jump, jump-to-subroutine, load effective address, push effective address, and move multiple registers instructions. The number of bus read and write cycles is shown in parenthesis as (r/w).

Table D-10. JMP, JSR, LEA, PEA, and MOVEM Instruction Execution Times

Instr	Size	(An)	(An)+	−(An)	d(An)	d(An, ix)+	xxx.W	xxx.L	d(PC)	d(PC, ix)*
JMP	—	8(2/0)	—	—	10(2/0)	14(3/0)	10(2/0)	12(3/0)	10(2/0)	14(3/0)
JSR	—	16(2/2)	—	—	18(2/2)	22(2/2)	18(2/2)	20(3/2)	18(2/2)	22(2/2)
LEA	—	4(1/0)	—	—	8(2/0)	12(2/0)	8(2/0)	12(3/0)	8(2/0)	12(2/0)
PEA	—	12(1/2)	—	—	16(2/2)	20(2/2)	16(2/2)	20(3/2)	16(2/2)	20(2/2)
MOVEM M→R	Word	12+4n (3+n/0)	12+4n (3+n/0)	—	16+4n (4+n/0)	18+4n (4+n/0)	16+4n (4+n/0)	20+4n (5+n/0)	16+4n (4+n/0)	18+4n (4+n/0)
	Long	12+8n (3+2n/0)	12+8n (3+2n/0)	—	16+8n (4+2n/0)	18+8n (4+2n/0)	16+8n (4+2n/0)	20+8n (5+2n/0)	16+8n (4+2n/0)	18+8n (4+2n/0)
MOVEM R→M	Word	8+4n (2/n)	—	8+4n (2/n)	12+4n (3/n)	14+4n (3/n)	12+4n (3/n)	16+4n (4/n)	—	—
	Long	8+8n (2/2n)	—	8+8n (2/2n)	12+8n (3/2n)	14+8n (3/2n)	12+8n (3/2n)	16+8n (4/2n)	—	—

n is the number of registers to move
*is the size of the index register (ix) does not affect the instruction's execution time

D 11 MULTI-PRECISION INSTRUCTION EXECUTION TIMES

Table D-11 indicates the number of clock periods for the multi-precision instructions. The number of clock periods includes the time to fetch both operands, peform the operations, store the results, and read the next instructions. The number of read and write cycles is shown in parenthesis as (r/w).

In Table D-11, the headings have the following meanings: Dn = data register operand and M = memory operand.

Table D-11. Multi-Precision Instruction Execution Times

Instruction	Size	op Dn, Dn	op M, M
ADDX	Byte, Word	4(1/0)	18(3/1)
	Long	8(1/0)	30(5/2)
CMPM	Byte, Word	—	12(3/0)
	Long	—	20(5/0)
SUBX	Byte, Word	4(1/0)	18(3/1)
	Long	8(1/0)	30(5/2)
ABCD	Byte	6(1/0)	18(3/1)
SBCD	Byte	6(1/0)	18(3/1)

D.12 MISCELLANEOUS INSTRUCTION EXECUTION TIMES

Tables D-12 and D-13 indicate the number of clock periods for the following miscellaneous instructions. The number of bus read and write cycles is shown in parenthesis as (r/w). The number of clock periods plus the number of read and write cycles must be added to those of the effective address calculation where indicated.

Table D-12. Miscellaneous Instruction Execution Times

Instruction	Size	Register	Memory
ANDI to CCR	Byte	20(3/0)	—
ANDI to SR	Word	20(3/0)	—
CHK	—	10(1/0)+	—
EORI to CCR	Byte	20(3/0)	—
EORI to SR	Word	20(3/0)	—
ORI to CCR	Byte	20(3/0)	—
ORI to SR	Word	20(3/0)	—
MOVE from SR	—	6(1/0)	8(1/1)+
MOVE to CCR	—	12(2/0)	12(2/0)+
MOVE to SR	—	12(2/0)	12(2/0)+
EXG	—	6(1/0)	—
EXT	Word	4(1/0)	—
EXT	Long	4(1/0)	—
LINK	—	16(2/2)	—
MOVE from USP	—	4(1/0)	—
MOVE to USP	—	4(1/0)	—
NOP	—	4(1/0)	—
RESET	—	132(1/0)	—
RTE	—	20(5/0)	—
RTR	—	20(5/0)	—
RTS	—	16(4/0)	—
STOP	—	4(0/0)	—
SWAP	—	4(1/0)	—
TRAPV	—	4(1/0)	—
UNLK	—	12(3/0)	—

+ add effective address calculation time

Table D-13. Move Peripheral Instruction Execution Times

Instruction	Size	Register → Memory	Memory → Register
MOVEP	Word	16(2/2)	16(4/0)
MOVEP	Long	24(2/4)	24(6/0)

D.13 EXCEPTION PROCESSING EXECUTION TIMES

Table D-14 indicates the number of clock periods for exception processing. The number of clock periods includes the time for all stacking, the vector fetch, and the fetch of the first two instruction words of the handler routine. The number of bus read and write cycles is shown in parenthesis as (r/w).

Table D-14. Exception Processing Execution Times

Exception	Periods
Address Error	50(4/7)
Bus Error	50(4/7)
CHK Instruction	44(5/4) +
Divide by Zero	42(5/4)
Illegal Instruction	34(4/3)
Interrupt	44(5/3)*
Privilege Violation	34(4/3)
$\overline{RESET}$**	40(6/0)
Trace	34(4/3)
TRAP Instruction	38(4/4)
TRAPV Instruction	34(4/3)

+ add effective address calculation time

* The interrupt acknowledge cycle is assumed to take four clock periods.

** Indicates the time from when $\overline{RESET}$ and $\overline{HALT}$ are first sampled as negated to when instruction execution starts.

Appendix E
MC68000 INSTRUCTION EXECUTION TIMES

E.1 INTRODUCTION

This Appendix contains listings of the instruction execution times in terms of external clock (CLK) periods. In this data, it is assumed that both memory read and write cycle times are four clock periods. A longer memory cycle will cause the generation of wait states which must be added to the total instruction time.

The number of bus read and write cycles for each instruction is also included with the timing data. This data is enclosed in parenthesis following the number of clock periods and is shown as: (r/w) where r is the number of read cycles and w is the number of write cycles included in the clock period number. Recalling that either a read or write cycle requires four clock periods, a timing number given as 18(3/1) relates to 12 clock periods for the three read cycles, plus 4 clock periods for the one write cycle, plus 2 cycles required for some internal function of the processor.

NOTE
The number of periods includes instruction fetch and all applicable operand fetches and stores.

E.2 OPERAND EFFECTIVE ADDRESS CALCULATION TIMES

Table E-1 lists the number of clock periods required to compute an instruction's effective address. It includes fetching of any extension words, the address computation, and fetching of the memory operand. The number of bus read and write cycles is shown in parenthesis as (r/w). Note there are no write cycles involved in processing the effective address.

Table E-1. Effective Address Calculation Times

	Addressing Mode	Byte	Word	Long
	Register			
Dn	Data Register Direct	0(0/0)	0(0/0)	0(0/0)
An	Address Register Direct	0(0/0)	0(0/0)	0(0/0)
	Memory			
(An)	Address Register Indirect	4(1/0)	8(2/0)	16(4/0)
(An)+	Address Register Indirect with Postincrement	4(1/0)	8(2/0)	16(4/0)
−(An)	Address Register Indirect with Predecrement	6(1/0)	10(2/0)	18(4/0)
d(An)	Address Register Indirect with Displacement	12(3/0)	16(4/0)	24(6/0)
d(An, ix)*	Address Register Indirect with Index	14(3/0)	18(4/0)	26(6/0)
xxx.W	Absolute Short	12(3/0)	16(4/0)	24(6/0)
xxx.L	Absolute Long	20(5/0)	24(6/0)	32(8/0)
d(PC)	Program Counter with Displacement	12(3/0)	16(4/0)	24(6/0)
d(PC, ix)	Program Counter with Index	14(3/0)	18(4/0)	26(6/0)
#xxx	Immediate	8(2/0)	8(2/0)	16(4/0)

*The size of the index register (ix) does not affect execution time.

E.3 MOVE INSTRUCTION EXECUTION TIMES

Tables E-2, E-3, and E-4 indicate the number of clock periods for the move instruction. This data includes instruction fetch, operand reads, and operand writes. The number of bus read and write cycles is shown in parenthesis as: (r/w).

Table E-2. Move Byte Instruction Execution Times

Source	Destination								
	Dn	An	(An)	(An)+	−(An)	d(An)	d(An, ix)*	xxx.W	xxx.L
Dn	8(2/0)	8(2/0)	12(2/1)	12(2/1)	12(2/1)	20(4/1)	22(4/1)	20(4/1)	28(6/1)
An	8(2/0)	8(2/0)	12(2/1)	12(2/1)	12(2/1)	20(4/1)	22(4/1)	20(4/1)	28(6/1)
(An)	12(3/0)	12(3/0)	16(3/1)	16(3/1)	16(3/1)	24(5/1)	26(5/1)	24(5/1)	32(7/1)
(An)+	12(3/0)	12(3/0)	16(3/1)	16(3/1)	16(3/1)	24(5/1)	26(5/1)	24(5/1)	32(7/1)
−(An)	14(3/0)	14(3/0)	18(3/1)	18(3/1)	18(3/1)	26(5/1)	28(5/1)	26(5/1)	34(7/1)
d(An)	20(5/0)	20(5/0)	24(5/1)	24(5/1)	24(5/1)	32(7/1)	34(7/1)	32(7/1)	40(9/1)
d(An, ix)*	22(5/0)	22(5/0)	26(5/1)	26(5/1)	26(5/1)	34(7/1)	36(7/1)	34(7/1)	42(9/1)
xxx.W	20(5/0)	20(5/0)	24(5/1)	24(5/1)	24(5/1)	32(7/1)	34(7/1)	32(7/1)	40(9/1)
xxx.L	28(7/0)	28(7/0)	32(7/1)	32(7/1)	32(7/1)	40(9/1)	42(9/1)	40(9/1)	48(11/1)
d(PC)	20(5/0)	20(5/0)	24(5/1)	24(5/1)	24(5/1)	32(7/1)	34(7/1)	32(7/1)	40(9/1)
d(PC, ix)*	22(5/0)	22(5/0)	26(5/1)	26(5/1)	26(5/1)	34(7/1)	36(7/1)	34(7/1)	42(9/1)
#xxx	16(4/0)	16(4/0)	20(4/1)	20(4/1)	20(4/1)	28(6/1)	30(6/1)	28(6/1)	36(8/1)

*The size of the index register (ix) does not affect execution time.

Table E-3. Move Word Instruction Execution Times

Source	Destination								
	Dn	An	(An)	(An)+	−(An)	d(An)	d(An, ix)*	xxx.W	xxx.L
Dn	8(2/0)	8(2/0)	16(2/2)	16(2/2)	16(2/2)	24(4/2)	26(4/2)	20(4/2)	32(6/2)
An	8(2/0)	8(2/0)	16(2/2)	16(2/2)	16(2/2)	24(4/2)	26(4/2)	20(4/2)	32(6/2)
(An)	16(4/0)	16(4/0)	24(4/2)	24(4/2)	24(4/2)	32(6/2)	34(6/2)	32(6/2)	40(8/2)
(An)+	16(4/0)	16(4/0)	24(4/2)	24(4/2)	24(4/2)	32(6/2)	34(6/2)	32(6/2)	40(8/2)
−(An)	18(4/0)	18(4/0)	26(4/2)	26(4/2)	26(4/2)	34(6/2)	32(6/2)	34(6/2)	42(8/2)
d(An)	24(6/0)	24(6/0)	32(6/2)	32(6/2)	32(6/2)	40(8/2)	42(8/2)	40(8/2)	48(10/2)
d(An, ix)*	26(6/0)	26(6/0)	34(6/2)	34(6/2)	34(6/2)	42(8/2)	44(8/2)	42(8/2)	50(10/2)
xxx.W	24(6/0)	24(6/0)	32(6/2)	32(6/2)	32(6/2)	40(8/2)	42(8/2)	40(8/2)	48(10/2)
xxx.L	32(8/0)	32(8/0)	40(8/2)	40(8/2)	40(8/2)	48(10/2)	50(10/2)	48(10/2)	56(12/2)
d(PC)	24(6/0)	24(6/0)	32(6/2)	32(6/2)	32(6/2)	40(8/2)	42(8/2)	40(8/2)	48(10/2)
d(PC, ix)*	26(6/0)	26(6/0)	34(6/2)	34(6/2)	34(6/2)	42(8/2)	44(8/2)	42(8/2)	50(10/2)
#xxx	16(4/0)	16(4/0)	24(4/2)	24(4/2)	24(4/2)	32(6/2)	34(6/2)	32(6/2)	40(8/2)

*The size of the index register (ix) does not affect execution time.

Table E-4. Move Long Instruction Execution Times

Source	Destination								
	Dn	An	(An)	(An)+	−(An)	d(An)	d(An, ix)*	xxx.W	xxx.L
Dn	8(2/0)	8(2/0)	24(2/4)	24(2/4)	24(2/4)	32(4/4)	34(4/4)	32(4/4)	40(6/4)
An	8(2/0)	8(2/0)	24(2/4)	24(2/4)	24(2/4)	32(4/4)	34(4/4)	32(4/4)	40(6/4)
(An)	24(6/0)	24(6/0)	40(6/4)	40(6/4)	40(6/4)	48(8/4)	50(8/4)	48(8/4)	56(10/4)
(An)+	24(6/0)	24(6/0)	40(6/4)	40(6/4)	40(6/4)	48(8/4)	50(8/4)	48(8/4)	56(10/4)
−(An)	26(6/0)	26(6/0)	42(6/4)	42(6/4)	42(6/4)	50(8/4)	52(8/4)	50(8/4)	58(10/4)
d(An)	32(8/0)	32(8/0)	48(8/4)	48(8/4)	48(8/4)	56(10/4)	58(10/4)	56(10/4)	64(12/4)
d(An, ix)*	34(8/0)	34(8/0)	50(8/4)	50(8/4)	50(8/4)	58(10/4)	60(10/4)	58(10/4)	66(12/4)
xxx.W	32(8/0)	32(8/0)	48(8/4)	48(8/4)	48(8/4)	56(10/4)	58(10/4)	56(10/4)	64(12/4)
xxx.L	40(10/0)	40(10/0)	56(10/4)	56(10/4)	53(10/4)	64(12/4)	66(12/4)	64(12/4)	72(14/4)
d(PC)	32(8/0)	32(8/0)	48(8/4)	48(8/4)	48(8/4)	56(10/4)	58(10/4)	56(10/4)	64(12/4)
d(PC, ix)*	34(8/0)	34(8/0)	50(8/4)	50(8/4)	50(8/4)	58(10/4)	60(10/4)	58(10/4)	66(12/4)
#xxx	24(6/0)	24(6/0)	40(6/4)	40(6/4)	40(6/4)	48(8/4)	50(8/4)	48(8/4)	56(10/4)

*The size of the index register (ix) does not affect execution time.

E.4 STANDARD INSTRUCTION EXECUTION TIMES

The number of clock periods shown in Table E-5 indicates the time required to perform the operations, store the results, and read the next instruction. The number of bus read and write cycles is shown in parenthesis as: (r/w). The number of clock periods and the number of read and write cycles must be added respectively to those of the effective address calculation where indicated. In Table E-5 the headings have the following meanings: An = address register operand, Dn = data register operand, ea = an operand specified by an effective address, and M = memory effective address operand.

Table E-5. Standard Instruction Execution Times

Instruction	Size	op <ea>, An	op <ea>, Dn	op Dn, <M>
ADD	Byte	—	8(2/0)+	12(2/1)+
	Word	12(2/0)+	8(2/0)+	16(2/2)+
	Long	10(2/0)+**	10(2/0)+**	24(2/4)+
AND	Byte	—	8(2/0)+	12(2/1)+
	Word	—	8(2/0)+	16(2/2)+
	Long	—	10(2/0)+**	24(2/4)+
CMP	Byte	—	8(2/0)+	—
	Word	10(2/0)+	8(2/0)+	—
	Long	10(2/0)+	10(2/0)+	—
DIVS		—	162(2/0)+*	—
DIVU		—	144(2/0)+*	—
EOR	Byte	—	8(2/0)+***	12(2/1)+
	Word	—	8(2/0)+***	16(2/2)+
	Long	—	12(2/0)+***	24(2/4)+
MULS		—	74(2/0)+*	—
MULU		—	74(2/0)+*	—
OR	Byte	—	8(2/0)+	12(2/1)+
	Word	—	8(2/0)+	16(2/2)+
	Long	—	10(2/0)+**	24(2/4)+
SUB	Byte	—	8(2/0)+	12(2/1)+
	Word	12(2/0)+	8(2/0)+	16(2/2)+
	Long	10(2/0)+**	10(2/0)+**	24(2/4)+

NOTES:
+ Add effective address calculation time
* Indicates maximum value
** The base time of 10 clock periods is increased to 12 if the effective address mode is register direct or immediate (effective address time should also be added).
*** Only available effective address mode is data register direct
DIVS, DIVU — The divide algorithm used by the MC68008 provides less than 10% difference between the best and worst case timings.
MULS, MULU — The multiply algorithm requires 42 + 2n clocks where n is defined as:
  MULS: n = tag the <ea> with a zero as the MSB; n is the resultant number of 10 or 01 patterns in the 17-bit source, i.e., worst case happens when the source is $5555.
  MULU: n = the number of ones in the <ea>

E.5 IMMEDIATE INSTRUCTION EXECUTION TIMES

The number of clock periods shown in Table E-6 includes the time to fetch immediate operands, perform the operations, store the results, and read the next operation. The number of bus read and write cycles is shown in parenthesis as: (r/w). The number of clock periods and the number of read and write cycles must be added respectively to those of the effective address calculation where indicated. In Table E-6, the headings have the following meanings: # = immediate operand, Dn = data register operand, An = address register operand, and M = memory operand.

Table E-6. Immediate Instruction Clock Periods

Instruction	Size	op#, Dn	op#, An	op#, M
ADDI	Byte Word Long	16(4/0) 16(4/0) 28(6/0)	— — —	20(4/1)+ 24(4/2)+ 40(6/4)+
ADDQ	Byte Word Long	8(2/0) 8(2/0) 12(2/0)	— 12(2/0) 12(2/0)	12(2/1)+ 16(2/2)+ 24(2/4)+
ANDI	Byte Word Long	16(4/0) 16(4/0) 28(6/0)	— — —	20(4/1)+ 24(4/2)+ 40(6/4)+
CMPI	Byte Word Long	16(4/0) 16(4/0) 26(6/0)	— — —	16(4/0)+ 16(4/0)+ 24(6/0)+
EORI	Byte Word Long	16(4/0) 16(4/0) 28(6/0)	— — —	20(4/1)+ 24(4/2)+ 40(6/4)+
MOVEQ	Long	8(2/0)	—	—
ORI	Byte Word Long	16(4/0) 16(4/0) 28(6/0)	— — —	20(4/1)+ 24(4/2)+ 40(6/4)+
SUBI	Byte Word Long	16(4/0) 16(4/0) 28(6/0)	— — —	12(2/1)+ 16(2/2)+ 24(2/4)+
SUBQ	Byte Word Long	8(2/0) 8(2/0) 12(2/0)	— 12(2/0) 12(2/0)	20(4/1)+ 24(4/2)+ 40(6/4)+

+ add effective address calculation time

E.6 SINGLE OPERAND INSTRUCTION EXECUTION TIMES

Table E-7 indicates the number of clock periods for the single operand instructions. The number of bus read and write cycles is shown in parenthesis as (r/w). The number of clock periods and the number of read and write cycles must be added respectively to those of the effective address calculation where indicated.

Table E-7. Single Operand Instruction Execution Times

Instruction	Size	Register	Memory
CLR	Byte	8(2/0)	12(2/1) +
	Word	8(2/0)	16(2/2) +
	Long	10(2/0)	24(2/4) +
NBCD	Byte	10(2/0)	12(2/1) +
NEG	Byte	8(2/0)	12(2/1) +
	Word	8(2/0)	16(2/2) +
	Long	10(2/0)	24(2/4) +
NEGX	Byte	8(2/0)	12(2/1) +
	Word	8(2/0)	16(2/2) +
	Long	10(2/0)	24(2/4) +
NOT	Byte	8(2/0)	12(2/1) +
	Word	8(2/0)	16(2/2) +
	Long	10(2/0)	24(2/4) +
S_{CC}	Byte, False	8(2/0)	12(2/1) +
	Byte, True	10(2/0)	12(2/1) +
TAS	Byte	8(2/0)	14(2/1) +
TST	Byte	8(2/0)	8(2/0) +
	Word	8(2/0)	8(2/0) +
	Long	8(2/0)	8(2/0) +

\+ add effective address calculation time.

E.7 SHIFT/ROTATE INSTRUCTION EXECUTION TIMES

Table E-8 indicates the number of clock periods for the shift and rotate instructions. The number of bus read and write cycles is shown in parenthesis as: (r/w). The number of clock periods and the number of read and write cycles must be added respectively to those of the effective address calculation where indicated.

Table E-8. Shift/Rotate Instruction Clock Periods

Instruction	Size	Register	Memory
ASR, ASL	Byte	10 + 2n(2/0)	—
	Word	10 + 2n(2/0)	16(2/2) +
	Long	12 + 2n(2/0)	—
LSR, LSL	Byte	10 + 2n(2/0)	—
	Word	10 + 2n(2/0)	16(2/2) +
	Long	12 + 2n(2/0)	—
ROR, ROL	Byte	10 + 2n(2/0)	—
	Word	10 + 2n(2/0)	16(2/2) +
	Long	12 + 2n(2/0)	—
ROXR, ROXL	Byte	10 + 2n(2/0)	—
	Word	10 + 2n(2/0)	16(2/2) +
	Long	12 + 2n(2/0)	—

\+ add effective address calculation time
n is the shift count

E.8 BIT MANIPULATION INSTRUCTION EXECUTION TIMES

Table E-9 indicates the number of clock periods required for the bit manipulation instructions. The number of bus read and write cycles is shown in parenthesis as: (r/w). The number of clock periods and the number of read and write cycles must be added respectively to those of the effective address calculation where indicated.

Table E-9. Bit Manipulation Instruction Execution Times

Instruction	Size	Dynamic		Static	
		Register	Memory	Register	Memory
BCHG	Byte Long	— 12(2/0)*	12(2/1) + —	— 20(4/0)*	20(4/1) + —
BCLR	Byte Long	— 14(2/0)*	12(2/1) + —	— 22(4/0)*	20(4/1) + —
BSET	Byte Long	— 12(2/0)*	12(2/1) + —	— 20(4/0)*	20(4/1) + —
BTST	Byte Long	— 10(2/0)	8(2/0) + —	— 18(4/0)	16(4/0) + —

+ add effective address calculation time
* indicates maximum value

E.9 CONDITIONAL INSTRUCTION EXECUTION TIMES

Table E-10 indicates the number of clock periods required for the conditional instructions. The number of bus read and write cycles is indicated in parenthesis as: (r/w). The number of clock periods and the number of read and write cycles must be added respectively to those of the effective address calculation where indicated.

Table E-10. Conditional Instruction Execution Times

Instruction	Displacement	Trap or Branch Taken	Trap or Branch Not Taken
B$_{CC}$	Byte Word	18(4/0) 18(4/0)	12(2/0) 20(4/0)
BRA	Byte Word	18(4/0) 18(4/0)	— —
BSR	Byte Word	34(4/4) 34(4/4)	— —
DBCC	CC True CC False	— 18(4/0)	20(4/0) 26(6/0)
CHK	—	68(8/6) + *	14(2/0) +
TRAP	—	62(8/6)	—
TRAPV	—	66(10/6)	8(2/0)

+ add effective address calculation time
* indicates maximum value

E.10 JMP, JSR, LEA, PEA, AND MOVEM INSTRUCTION EXECUTION TIMES

Table E-11 indicates the number of clock periods required for the jump, jump-to-subroutine, load effective address, push effective address, and move multiple registers instructions. The number of bus read and write cycles is shown in parenthesis as: (r/w).

Table E-11. JMP, JSR, LEA, PEA, and MOVEM Instruction Execution Times

Instruction	Size	(An)	(An)+	−(An)	d(An)	d(An, ix)*	xxx.W	xxx.L
JMP	−	16(4/0)	−	−	18(4/0)	22(4/0)	18(4/0)	24(6/0)
JSR	−	32(4/4)	−	−	34(4/4)	38(4/4)	34(4/4)	40(6/4)
LEA	−	8(2/0)	−	−	16(4/0)	20(4/0)	16(4/0)	24(6/0)
PEA	−	24(2/4)	−	−	32(4/4)	36(4/4)	32(4/4)	40(6/4)
MOVEM M → R	Word	24+8n (6+2n/0)	24+8n (6+2n/0)	−	32+8n (8+2n/0)	34+8n (8+2n/0)	32+8n (10+n/0)	40+8n (10+2n/0)
	Long	24+16n (6+4n/0)	24+16n (6+4n/0)	−	32+16n (8+4n/0)	32+16n (8+4n/0)	32+16n (8+4n/0)	40+16n (8+4n/0)
MOVEM R → M	Word	16+8n (4/2n)	−	16+8n (4/2n)	24+8n (6/2n)	26+8n (6/2n)	24+8n (6/2n)	32+8n (8/2n)
	Long	16+16n (4/4n)	−	16+16n (4/4n)	24+16n (6/4n)	26+16n (6/4n)	24+16n (8/4n)	32+16n (6/4n)

n is the number of registers to move
* is the size of the index register (ix) does not affect the instruction's execution time

E.11 MULTI-PRECISION INSTRUCTION EXECUTION TIMES

Table E-12 indicates the number of clock periods for the multi-precision instructions. The number of clock periods includes the time to fetch both operands, perform the operations, store the results, and read the next instructions. The number of read and write cycles is shown in parenthesis as: (r/w).

In Table E-12, the headings have the following meanings: Dn = data register operand and M = memory operand.

Table E-12. Multi-Precision Instruction Execution Times

Instruction	Size	op Dn, Dn	op M, M
ADDX	Byte	8(2/0)	22(4/1)
	Word	8(2/0)	50(6/2)
	Long	12(2/0)	58(10/4)
CMPM	Byte	−	16(4/0)
	Word	−	24(6/0)
	Long	−	40(10/0)
SUBX	Byte	8(2/0)	22(4/1)
	Word	8(2/0)	50(6/2)
	Long	12(2/0)	58(10/4)
ABCD	Byte	10(2/0)	20(4/1)
SBCD	Byte	10(2/0)	20(4/1)

E.12 MISCELLANEOUS INSTRUCTION EXECUTION TIMES

Tables E-13 and E-14 indicate the number of clock periods for the following miscellaneous instructions. The number of bus read and write cycles is shown in parenthesis as: (r/w). The number of clock periods plus the number of read and write cycles must be added to those of the effective address calculation where indicated.

Table E-13. Miscellaneous Instruction Execution Times

Instruction	Register	Memory
ANDI to CCR	32(6/0)	—
ANDI to SR	32(6/0)	—
EORI to CCR	32(6/0)	—
EORI to SR	32(6/0)	—
EXG	10(2/0)	—
EXT	8(2/0)	—
LINK	32(4/4)	—
MOVE to CCR	18(4/0)	18(4/0)+
MOVE to SR	18(4/0)	18(4/0)+
MOVE from SR	10(2/0)	16(2/2)+
MOVE to USP	8(2/0)	—
MOVE from USP	8(2/0)	—
NOP	8(2/0)	—
ORI to CCR	32(6/0)	—
ORI to SR	32(6/0)	—
RESET	136(2/0)	—
RTE	40(10/0)	—
RTR	40(10/0)	—
RTS	32(8/0)	—
STOP	4(0/0)	—
SWAP	8(2/0)	—
UNLK	24(6/0)	—

+ add effective address calculation time

Table E-14. Move Peripheral Instruction Execution Times

Instruction	Size	Register → Memory	Memory → Register
MOVEP	Word	24(4/2)	24(6/0)
	Long	32(4/4)	32(8/0)

+ add effective address calculation time

E.13 EXCEPTION PROCESSING EXECUTION TIMES

Table E-15 indicates the number of clock periods for exception processing. The number of clock periods includes the time for all stacking, the vector fetch, and the fetch of the first instruction of the handler routine. The number of bus read and write cycles is shown in parenthesis as: (r/w).

Table E-15. Exception Processing Execution Times

Exception	Periods
Address Error	94(8/14)
Bus Error	94(8/14)
Interrupt	72(9/6)*
Illegal Instruction	62(8/6)
Privileged Instruction	62(8/6)
Trace	62(8/6)

*The interrupt acknowledge bus cycle is assumed to take four external clock periods.

Index

Index

Abort function, 97
Accumulator, 17
Addition
  accommodated by all computers, 54
  effect on zero flag, 56
  See also Instructions: Data Processing, Arithmetic
  instead of shifting, 74
  instructions in MC68000
    ABCD, 59
    ADD, 55, 56
    ADDA, 55, 73, 75
    ADDI, 55
    ADDQ, 55
    ADDX, 56, 74
    examples, 55–57
    part of data processing instructions, 53
  operation in 68000, 2
  use of extend flag, 56
Address block, 120
Address bus
  in eight-bit devices, 3, 4–5
  in MC68000
    buffering, 22
    effect of data strobe, 10
    not multiplexed, 10
    pins for, 9, 10
Address error, 42
  as causing exception state, 77, 78, 124
  exception vector number for, 80
Addresses
  address-fetching circuits, 4–5
  addition of offset to, 5
  alteration through address register, 74
  as part of data strobe signal, 10
  assignment in breakpoint command, 120
  calculation with arithmetic-logic unit, 5
  column address, 22
  decoding in VU68K, 116, 118
  during bit manipulation, 66
  during compare instructions, 58
  during data transfer, 11
  during MOVEP instruction, 68
  during TAS instruction, 66
  exception vector address, 78, 80
  exclusion from NOT instruction, 60
  fault address, 79
  in loops, 69
  in memory segmentation, 4
  input/output address, 108
  limitation on instructions affecting, 73
  refresh address, 22
  reset address, 103
  return address, 77, 148
  row address, 22
  starting address, 120, 144, 145, 148
  terminating address, 120, 144, 145
  user-vector address, 84
  See also Effective address
Addressing modes
  as design consideration, 2, 3
  effect on condition codes, 55
  in eight- versus 16-bit devices, 1–2, 3
  inherent (implied) mode, 43, 52
  memory address modes in MC68000, 42, 47, 52
    address register indirect, 43, 45, 47–48, 52
    with displacement (offset), 43, 45, 49–50, 53, 75
    with index and displacement (offset), 43, 45, 50–51, 53, 75
    with postincrement, 43, 45, 48–49, 53, 58, 70, 74
    with predecrement, 43, 45, 49, 53, 56, 59, 70, 74
  examples, 48–51
  mode bits as defining, 44
  use with logical instructions, 60
  orthogonality in MC68000, 54
  program control modes in MC68000, 42, 53, 70
  program counter with displacement (offset), 52, 53, 74, 75
  program counter with index, 43, 52, 53, 75
  use with logical instructions, 60
  register direct modes in MC68000, 42, 45, 52

314 INDEX

register direct modes (continued)
  address register direct, 43, 45, 47, 74
  data register direct, 43, 45–47
  examples, 45–47
  status register direct, 43
  use with logical instructions, 60
special address modes in MC68000, 42, 51
  absolute long, 43, 44, 45, 51, 52, 70
  absolute short, 43, 44, 45, 51, 52, 70, 74
  immediate mode, 43, 44, 45, 51–52, 62
  quick immediate mode, 52, 55, 67
  use with logical instructions, 60
Address lines
  address strobe defining validity of, 10
  buffering of, 22, 23
  during interrupt, 83–84, 85, 99
  for linear addressing, 4
  gates for decoding, 34
  in MC68000, 4, 9, 10, 15, 22
  in VU68K, 114
Address range
  in eight-bit devices, 3
  in MC68000, 3, 10, 69, 73
  in MC68230, 108, 110
Address register
  as destination, 58
  as frame pointer, 71
  as index register, 50, 53
  cycles to create, 74
  during halted state in VU68K, 121
  examination and modification of, 122
  in arithmetic instructions, 55, 56, 58, 74
  in data transfer instructions, 67, 70, 74
  in MC68000, 3, 17
  in register direct addressing mode, 45, 47
  in register indirect addressing mode, 47–51, 53
  orthogonality with addressing modes in MC68000, 54
Address strobe ($\overline{AS}$)
  assertion of peripheral devices, 10
  buffering of, 22
  defining validity of address and function code lines, 10
  during Test-and-Set instruction, 10
  effect on NAND gates, 14
  effect on read/write line, 12
  for assertion of latching input, 22
  in interrupt acknowledge bus cycle, 83–84, 87, 88, 99
  for clearing watchdog timer, 34
  for read cycle, 11
  in MC68000, 10, 12, 14, 22
  in reset, 26, 29
  in VU68K, 114, 123
  in write cycle, 11, 12
AND
  gate, 99
  instruction, 60, 61, 62, 77, 99, 104
    See also Instructions: Data processing, Logical operation code of 6800, 2
Arbitration circuits, 37
Arithmetic-logic unit (ALU), 5
Array, 47, 50, 51, 82
ASCII codes, 6, 7–8, 107, 112, 130, 144, 146
Assembler in MC68000
  directives of, 70, 102–103, 126
  location counter of, 126
  signaling error, 55
Assert, definition of, 10
Asynchronous Communications Interface Adapter (ACIA). *See* 6850
Asynchronous versus synchronous operation, 114
Audio cassette, 19, 21, 92, 98

Baud rate with ASCII, 112
Baud rate generator, 21, 93, 114. *See also* MC14411
Binary-coded decimal (BCD)
  bytes as, 6
  during arithmetic instructions in MC68000, 59
  in 4004, 1
  notation, 9
  use of data processing instructions in, 53
  use of nibbles to represent, 6
Bit (binary digit). *See also* bytes; nibbles
  address bits in VU68K, 116, 118
  as flag, 6
  as logical data types, 6
  as string, 6
  bit pattern of 6850, 99, 101
  block-selection bits, 116, 118
  data bit, 101
  data entry rate as ratio of bits and bytes, 101
  definition of, 6
  high-order bit, 63, 65, 118
  in longword, 3
  in word, 3
  instructions
    during various instructions in MC68000, 60, 61, 63, 64–65
    for manipulation of
      BCLR, 65
      BGHG, 65
      BSET, 65
      BTST, 65, 104
      TAS, 10, 15, 65, 66

low-order bit, 63, 65
manipulation singly and otherwise, 53
mask bit, 78, 91
mode bit as defining addressing mode, 44
most significant bit (msb), 60
number, 66
operation code of 6800, 2
page bits, 4
parity bit, 94, 101
register bit, 44
sign bit, 64
start bit, 94, 101
stop bit, 94, 101
stream bit, 94
values of, 6
word-selection bits in VU68K, 116, 118
Block, 6, 47, 48, 70
Block diagram to define system, 19
Bonds, A. B., 114
Boundary, 42, 44, 82, 120, 145
Branches
    instructions, 53
        Bcc, 69
        BEQ, 69, 73
        BGT, 69
        BHI, 69
        BLT, 69
        BNE, 73, 104
        BRA, 53, 69, 104
        BRS, 53
        DBcc, 69–70, 73
        DBEQ, 73
        DBNE, 70
        DBRA, 70
        JMP, 53, 69
        JSR, 53, 69, 71, 72
        RTS, 69, 71, 72
        Scc, 74
        in VU68K, 119, 130
    in program counter mode with index, 52
    to exception vector, 78
    use of flag in, 6
Breakpoint in VU68K
    constants for, 124
    effect of ORG directive on, 124
    effect with G command, 121
    location of breakpoint table in memory area, 126
    purpose of, 120
    removal of, 122, 142, 147
    setting, 120, 142
    table, 126, 128
    with single-step mode, 120
    with tracing, 120, 123

Buffer. *See* memory
Buffering
    double buffering defined, 107
    effect on speed, 28
    in exception handling, 79
    in small 68000-based system, 19, 22, 23
    See also 8T97, 74LS245, 74LS373
Bus control
    asynchronous control in MC68000, 9, 10–12, 28
        See also Address strobe, Data acknowledge, Data strobe, Read/write
    synchronous control in MC68000, 14–15
        See Enable, valid memory address, valid peripheral address
    for termination of bus cycle, 11, 14, 15, 34, 91
    pins in MC68000 for, 9
Bus cycle in MC68000, 11, 14, 15
Bus exception (error)
    as causing entry into supervisor mode, 18
    as causing exception state, 77, 78, 124
    as causing halted state, 76
    check for during reset, 25
    exception vector number for, 80
    in interrupt control signals, 99
    in memory accessing, 13
    line ($\overline{\text{BERR}}$) in MC68000, 9, 15, 91
    parity error, 91
    spurious interrupt, 91
Bus fault, 15, 25
Bus grant ($\overline{\text{BG}}$), 15, 37
Bus grant acknowledge ($\overline{\text{BGACK}}$), 15, 37
Busicomp, 1
Bus latency, 29, 33, 34
Bus multiplexing, 10
Bus request ($\overline{\text{BR}}$) line, 15, 37
Bus timeout, 34
Bus-wait technique, 119
Byte
    accessing to avoid address error, 42
    as binary-coded decimal value, 6, 59
    as character, 6
    in bit manipulation instructions, 66
    as measure of memory buffer, 119
    as number, 6
    as semaphore, 66
    as word, 6
    checksumming of, 74
    data byte, 22
    data entry rate as ratio of bits and bytes, 101
    data register in MC68000, 17
    data strobe for transfer, 11, 12
    definition of, 6, 46
    for exception vectors, 78

Byte (continued)
  fetching in VU68K, 134
  for reading ROM, 19
  in monitor of VU68K, 123
  operands, 11, 48, 55, 59
  operation of instructions on, 3
  output from VU68K, 129
  reset of byte count, 146

Carter, Edward M., 114, 124
Characters
  as causing interrupt, 118
  byte as, 6
  echoing of, 119
  effect of monitor in VU68K, 118, 119
  from queue, 132
  input characters to VU68K, 123, 131
  representation by codes, 7–8
  string, 8, 127
Checksum, 74, 112
Chip enable, 22
Chip select, 14, 94
Clear (CLR) instruction, 45, 49, 50–51, 55, 74
Clear to Send (CTS) signal, 94, 95
Clock
  baud rate generator, 21
  circuit, 23, 29
  cycle during reset, 24
  E clock in MC68000, 34
  frequencies for peripheral devices, 28
  in MC14411, 101
  in 6850, 94
  in VU68K, 114
  interrupts, 83, 98
  oscillator, 28
  pins in MC68000 for, 9
Clock-stretching cycle, 32
Codes, 7, 51, 52. *See also* ASCII
Column, 40
Compare (CMP)
  instructions
    CMP, 55
    CMPA, 58, 75
    CMPI, 58
    CMPM, 58, 70
  operation code in 6800, 2
Compiler, 54
Computer Terminal Corp. (Datapoint), 1
Condition code
  effect of instructions in MC68000 on, 55, 64, 73, 81
  in conditional branch instructions, 69
  initialization of, 73

register in MC68000, 17, 53
unaffected by address operations, 73
See also Flags
Control lines, 28, 39–40
Control registers in 6850, 94–95
Control signals in MC68000, 22
Control unit, 5
Cost, 32
Counter, *See* 74161
Cycle stealing, 36–41

Data. *See also* Bits; Exception, Vector; Lists; Stacks; Strings;
  boundaries, 42, 44, 82, 120
  data-fetching circuits, 4–5
  entry rate, 101
  input/output buffer, 79
  processing by arithmetic-logic unit, 5
  protection of, 11
  retrieval from memory buffer, 119
  stream, 104
  Tables; Variables
  treatment by 6850, 94
  types, 6–8
Data acknowledge (DTACK) line
  as design consideration, 11
  asynchronous characteristics, 12, 28
  bus cycle termination in MC68000, 11
  bus error, 13
  DTACK RAM signal, 40
  generation circuit for, 26, 35, 37
  in clock stretching, 32
  intentional versus unintentional delays, 12
  in read cycle, 11–12
  mentioned, 15, 17
  spurious interrupts, 91
  synthesis in VU68K, 114
  termination of interrupt acknowledge bus cycle, 84, 86–87
Data block, 120
Data bus
  bidirectional, 22
  buffers, 11, 22, 94, 100
  control by data strobe in MC68000, 10, 11
  during interrupt acknowledge bus cycle, 85
  effect of data acknowledge line, 11
  in eight-bit devices, 4–5
  in read cycle in MC68000, 11
  pins in MC68000 for, 9, 10
  6850 in eight- versus 16-bit bus, 68
  size affecting representation of ordinals, 6
  word as measure of, 6

Data carrier detect ($\overline{DCD}$) signal in 6850, 94, 95
Data lines
  during user-defined vectored interrupt, 84–85
  in system clock, 28
Datapoint (Computer Terminal Corp.), 1
Data memory, definition of, 13
Data register
  accessing by data register direct addressing, 45
  as index register, 50, 53
  as working register in VU68K, 123
  during halted state in VU68K, 121
  examination and modification of, 122
  for loops, 69–70, 73
  in MC68000, 3, 17, 54
  in quick immediate mode, 52
  receiver/transmit registers in 6850, 94, 95
  use in data processing instructions, 56, 59, 62, 65
  use in data transfer instructions, 67, 68–69
Data strobe signals
  for byte, longword, and word transfers, 11
  for MC68230, 106
  for read cycle, 11
  for write cycle, 11, 12
  lower and upper data strobe ($\overline{LDS/UDS}$), 10, 11, 118
Data transfer
  in MC68000, 10–11
  instructions for
    EXCHANGE, 53
    LEA, 70, 71, 72, 74
    MOVE, 42, 46, 47, 48, 49, 51, 56, 66, 70, 74, 77, 103, 104, 107
    MOVEA, 67, 70, 73, 75
    MOVEM, 66, 67, 74, 75, 79
    MOVEP, 68
    MOVEQ, 66, 67, 75
    PEA, 70, 71
    SWAP, 53
  in VU68K, 121
Debounced switch, 97
Debugging, 70, 81, 82
Decoder, See also 74LS138
  in VU68K, 118
Decoding
  addresses, 116
  circuit, 34
Default value of MC68000, 42
Delay line, 12
Delimiter, 145
Design considerations, 1–6
  data acknowledge line, 11
  modular programming, 70

speed in executing instructions, 28
Direction-enable pin, 22
Discrete gates, 118
Displacement (offset)
  in branch instructions, 69, 119
  in indexed addressing, 5
  in LINK instructions, 71–72
  in MOVEP instruction, 68
  positive-negative technique for, 50
Division, 53
  exception vectors for, 80, 82
  instructions
    DIV, 74, 78
    DIVS, 57
    DIVU, 57
  limitation on operands, 57
  limitation on use of LSR instruction, 64, 67
  zero divide, 80, 82, 124, 125

Effective address
  as causing exception state, 78
  calculation by address arithmetic-logic unit, 5
  definition of, 42
  destination effective address, 45, 67
  extension of, 44
  formation of, 41, 45
  in address register indirect addressing mode, 53
  in direct addressing mode, 45, 47
  in instruction format of 16-bit device, 2
  in shifting instructions, 64
  lines in MC68000, 10
  mode, 42
  movement by MOVEA instruction, 67
  register as part of, 42
  single versus double addresses, 45
  source effective address, 45
Eight-bit devices
  address bus, 3
  addressing modes, 1
  arithmetic logic unit, 5
  comparison with 16- and 32-bit devices, 1–2, 3
  8008, 1
  8080, 1
  hardwired logic unit, 5
  history, 1
  instructions
    as defining operand, 17
    fetching, 4–5
    format, 1, 2
  memory accessing, 3–4
  numbers, 6

318 INDEX

Eight-bit devices (continued)
  peripheral devices, 5–6
  registers, 1
  word width, 3
  Z80, 1
  See also 6800
8T97, 22
8008, 1
8080, 1
8086/8088 16-bit Microprocessor Primer, 6
Emulator, 80
Enable signal (E) in MC68000, 14–15, 22
Encode, 85
EOR instruction, 2, 60, 61–62, 77
Error, 124
Even addresses in MC68000, 11
Exception
  definition of, 76
  exception (error) handling
    effect of monitor in VU68K on, 118
    flowchart of, 76–77, 78
    format of subroutine for, 79
  exception state, 76–77
  external versus internal exceptions, 78
  intentional exception, 81
  vector
    data memory, 13
    effect of ORG directive on, 124
    in autovectored interrupt system, 16–17
    in vectored interrupt system, 16
    interrupt, 21
    offset, 79
    number, 16–17, 78, 80
    placement in memory map of MC68000, 21, 78, 124
    reset, 21, 24–25
    size of, 78
    stack pointer, 21
    table, 13, 22, 25, 124
    trap, 21
  supervisor mode, 77
  See Interrupt; Trap
EXCHANGE instruction, 53
EXT instruction, 75

Factor, 34
Fault address, 79
Fixed-point numbers, definition of, 54
Flags
  breakpoint flag in monitor of VU68K, 127, 147
  condition code flags
    carry (C), 18, 56, 58, 62, 63, 65, 66
    extend (X), 18, 56, 58, 65, 66
    generally, 58, 64
    negative (N), 18, 58
    overflow (V), 18, 58, 81, 82
    zero (Z), 18, 56, 58
  definition of, 6
  importance of, 55
  in arithmetic instructions, 56, 58
  interrupt mask, 24
  logical bit as, 6
  single-trace flag in monitor of VU68K, 147
  status flags of MC68000
    interrupt (I0 - I2), 18, 77, 89
    supervisor (S), 18, 24, 76, 77, 127
    trace (T), 18, 24, 77, 78, 81, 82, 83
    user (U), 76, 77
  status flags of 6850
    RDRF, 95, 104
    TDRA, 104
  testing by conditional branch instruction, 53
  unaffected by address operations in MC68000, 73
  use of, 6
Flip-flops in reducing wait states, 32. *See also* 74LS175
Four-bit devices, 1
4004 (MCS-4), 1
4116, 19
Frame pointer, 71–72
Function control (FC) in MC68000
  code lines, 10, 13–14, 83, 87, 88, 89
  interrupt acknowledge bus cycle, 99
  pins for, 9

Gates
  AND gate, 99
  controlling direction of buffers, 22
  decoding address lines, 34
  effect on speed, 28
  for function control line, 14
  logic gates in hardwired logic units, 5
  NAND gate, 14, 86, 99
  NOR gate, 88
  OR gate, 26, 118
Ground, 22

Halt ($\overline{\text{HLT}}$)
  circuit, 19, 23–28
  line in MC68000, 9, 15
  signal, 26
Halted state, 76, 120, 121
Hardwired logic units, 5
Hexadecimal
  address, 44, 126
  conversion of characters to, 123

INDEX 319

conversion of characters from, 130
notation, 22
High-level languages, 54, 70–72

Indexed addressing, 5. *See also* Addressing modes
Index register in MC68000
   in address register indirect with index and displacement, 50, 53
   in program counter with index, 52, 53
   mentioned, 17
Information, 3, 6, 15
Input/output (I/O)
   address register indirect with displacement for accessing, 50
   audio cassette circuit, 19
   buffering, 118
   circuit, 76
   exception from request for service of, 76, 118
   in MC68230, 104, 105
   memory-mapped in MC68000, 10n, 92
   mentioned, 41, 53
   parallel versus serial, 92
   ports of VU68K, 114, 118
   6850 as both, 94
Instructions
   addressing mode of, 44
   as causing internal exceptions, 78
   example formats of double and single effective address, 45–47
   exceptions from illegal instructions, 76
   execution during Normal State, 76
   execution times, 73
   fetching, 4–5
   in eight- and 16-bit devices, 1, 4–5
   in MC68000
      data processing (manipulation) instructions, 53, 54
         arithmetic instructions, 52
            in MC68000, 55–59, 67
         bit manipulation instructions, 65–66
         logic (logical) instructions, 55, 60–62
         shifting instructions, 63–63, 74
      data transfer (movement) instructions, 53, 66
      emulator lines, 80, 82
      exception vector number, 80
      for quick immediate mode, 55
      illegal instructions, 82, 124
      in program counter with index mode, 52
      input buffer, 79
      interrupt request lines, 83
      operation of, 3
      orthogonality of, 54
      position independence instructions, 70
      program control instructions, 53
         conditional branch instructions, 53, 69–70
         unconditional branch instructions, 69
      system control instructions, 53
   mentioned, 13
   trap, 123
   variations among registers, 55
Instruction cycle time, 29
Instruction format of MC68000, 44
Instruction set
   as design consideration, 2
   for arithmetic operations, 54
   of MC68000, 54, 102
Integer
   as subset of fixed-point numbers, 54–55
   definition of, 6, 54
   radix point of, 54
   representation in two's complement form, 6–7
Intel Corp., 1
Interfacing
   as design consideration, 2
   audio cassette, 92
   centronix parallel printer interface, 92, 106
   in MC68000, 9, 19
   input/output, 92
   RAM and ROM, 34
   See also 6850
Internal organization as design consideration, 2
Interrupt
   abort function, 99
   and exception state, 76, 78, 83
   bus-wait technique to disable, 119
   circuit, 41, 85
   control, 9, 16–18
   error, 42, 124
   in cycle stealing, 36
   in MC68000
      and supervisor mode, 77, 81
      comparison of mask and request levels, 83
      daisy chain, 88, 90
      during single-step mode in VU68K, 122
      exception vectors, 21, 80, 84–85, 124
      for communication serial-port interrupts, 116, 118, 128
      for keyboard serial-port interrupts, 116
      function control lines, 13
      interrupt acknowledge bus cycle (IACK), 83–86, 88, 89–91, 99
      interrupt-handling routines in VU68K, 118, 148

320 INDEX

Interrupt (continued)
    interrupt request ($\overline{\text{IRQ}}$), 88–89
    levels of, 83, 87, 88, 89–91, 116, 118
    lines for (IPLO-IPL2), 9, 16–17, 83, 85, 86, 89, 91, 98, 116
    logic in 6850, 94
    mask bits, 78, 91, 128
    masking interrupt level, 77, 78
    nonmaskable interrupts, 83, 89–90
    pins for, 9
    priority interrupt system, 87
    offset, 86
    software interrupt, 81
    74LS273, 97, 98
    spurious interrupt, 91, 124
    synchronizer, 97
    termination of, 119
    user (intentional) interrupts
        autovectored, 16, 80, 83, 87, 116, 119
        exception vectors for, 80, 119
        vectored, 12, 83, 84–85
    with MC68230, 105
    logic in 6850, 94

Jumper wire, 22

Label, definition of, 70
Latch
    after data acknowledge signal, 35
    for demultiplexing, 10
    for interrupts, 85, 98
    in MC68230, 107
    See also 74LS373
Link instruction, 71
Lists, 13
Load command, 2, 121, 139
Logical shift instructions (LSL/LSR), 63, 64
Longword
    accessing to avoid address errors, 42
    address operations, 74
    address register, 17
    data register, 17
    data strobe for transfer, 11
    extension of word, 74
    fetching in VU68K, 134
    for instructions affecting addresses, 73
    formation in MC68000, 42
    number of bits in, 3, 46
    operands, 47, 55
    operation of instruction on, 3
    output from VU68K, 129
Loops, 69, 73, 146
Low-power Schottky (LS), 29

Macro, 82

MC14411, 99, 100, 101
MCS-4 (4004), 1
MC68A364, 19, 34, 35
MC68000L4, 19
MC68020, 88
MC68230 (Parallel Interface/Timer (PI/T))
    acknowledge signal, 107
    addresses, 106
    audio cassette interface, 21, 92, 111–112
    bit pattern, 109
    bit stream, 110
    block diagram of, 105
    bus trap error, 106
    byte operation, 106
    comparator, 112–113
    control register, 109
    data acknowledge ($\overline{\text{DTACK}}$) line, 106
    data bus, 106
    data in/out lines, 112
    data-direction register, 105
    $\overline{\text{DATA STROBE}}$, 107
    direct memory access, 105
    double buffering of, 107
    handshake lines (H1-H4), 104, 105–106, 107
    input/output pins for, 104, 105
    instructions, 109
    interrupts, 98, 105, 106, 107
    parallel interface function of, 21
    parallel interface ports
        Port A, 104–105, 107, 109
        Port B, 104–105, 107
        Port C, 104, 106
    printer interface, 92
    programming, 108–110, 111–112
    read, 106
    registers, 106
    selection of memory area for, 34, 92, 93
    serial data rate, 110
    signals, 106
    S record, 111, 112, Appendix
    system bus, 106
    timer, 104, 105, 106, 110
    write, 106
MC3456, 25
Mask bits. *See* Interrupts
Memory
    as location of operands in arithmetic instruction, 56
    block, 70, 116, 120
    buffer, 118–119, 128, 131
    circuits to interface RAM and ROM, 34–41
    data memory, 13
    decoding, 22
    effect of monitor of VU68K, 118
    enable signals, 34–35, 118

INDEX

even and odd memory, 12
fetching instructions from, 4–5
in VU68K system, 114, 118
intentional delay of data acknowledge signal for, 12
location of exception vectors of VU68K, 124
nonresident memory, 91
overlapping of RAM and ROM, 34
pointer, 120, 121
RAM
  access times, 29
  bytewide, 19
  connection with word-selection bits in VU68K, 118
  dynamic RAM (DRAM), 10, 19, 22, 28, 41
  refresh, 22, 35–36
  select line for, 118
  timer circuit for, 35
  use with Low-power Schottky and Schottky, 32
  See also 4116
Read-only (ROM), 19, 21, 22. See also MC68A364
  connection with word-selection bits in VU68K, 118
  effect of DTACK generation circuit, 35, 37
  watchdog timer if write tried, 34
scratchpad, 22
shift register memory, 1
shifting operands in, 64, 65
static memory, 11
supervisor memory, 14
user memory, 14, 22
word as measure of memory area, 6
  See Stack
Memory accessing
  accessing times, 32, 33
  bus error, 13
  direct memory access (DMA)
    control, 9, 15
    with MC68230, 105
  in eight-bit device, 3
  in MC68000, 4, 9
  linear accessing, 4
  memory segmentation, 4
  paging, 3–4
Memory controller in MC68000, 10
Memory handling
  as design consideration, 2
  intentional delay in data acknowledge line, 12
Memory location
  affected by data transfer instructions, 53
  affected by shifting instructions, 63
  as trap, 77
  comparison in compare memory instruction, 58
  during bit manipulation instructions, 65, 67
  examination and modification of, 121, 135
  use during arithmetic instructions, 59
Memory management unit, 91
Memory map
  exception vectors in, 78
  for MC68000, 10n, 21–22, 34
  for VU68K, 114, 118
  in 6850, 74
Memory range
  in eight versus 16-bit devices, 1
  in MC68000, 10
  input-output locations in, 50
Microprogramming, 5
Mnemonics, 47
Modem, 19, 21, 98, 99, 114
Monitor for VU68K (VUBUG)
  branch, 130
  breakpoint
    flag, 127
    mode, 146
    remove, 142, 147
    set, 142
    table in memory area, 126, 128
  buffered input/output for ports, 118
  carriage return, 133, 142, 144, 146, 148
  Carter, Edward M., 124
  command
    character, 144, 147
    mode, 119, 120, 121, 128
    processor, 130
  commands, 134
    b command, 120
    c command, 120
    CONTROL-C (ctrl-c), 119, 133
    CONTROL-L (ctrl-l), 121, 140
    CONTROL-Q (ctrl-q), 119, 127
    CONTROL-S (ctrl-s), 119, 127, 129
    CONTROL-X (ctrl-x), 121, 140
    D command, 120, 144, 145
    E command, 120–121, 140
    Go (g) command, 120, 121, 122, 123, 148
    L command, 121
    M command, 121, 122
    Prototype (P) command, 122, 141
    R command, 121, 122, 124
    S command, 122
    T command, 122, 123
  control variables, 128
  conversion from hexadecimal to ASCII, 130
  emulator mode, 120–121, 140
  error, 142
  exception vector table, 124, 125

Monitor for VU68K (continued)
  header, 147
  input character, 131
  interrupt handling, 124, 125, 148
  interrupt mask, 128
  interrupts for ports,
  linefeed, 133, 146
  loading, 139, 148
  memory buffer, 128, 131
  memory dump, 142, 144–145
  memory examination, 127, 135
  memory mode, 121
  object code, 152
  ORG directive, 124, 125
  output from, 129
  program counter, 133, 148
  prototype table in memory area, 126
  queue, 124, 128, 132, 133
  register mode, 122
  register examination, 127, 136
  register save area, 124, 126, 128
  reset of byte count, 146
  restart, 133
  return address, 148
  serial communication port, 129, 132, 139
  S-format, 139
  single-step mode, 120, 121, 122, 147, 148
  6850, 127, 128, 129
  stack, 126, 128, 133
  stack pointer, 128
  status register, 133, 147, 148
  system mode, 122, 141
  system stack in memory, 126
  temporary storage areas, 127, 134
  terminal buffer, 127
  trace mode, 146, 147
  traps, 123–124, 148
  United States Air Force, Computer Science Department, 124
  user stack, 127
  Vanderbilt University, Computer Science Department, 124
  write, 145
Morgan, Christopher, 6
Most significant bit (msb), 7, 60
Motorola, 1, 2, 3, 5–6, 10, 92, 121
Multiplexing
  74LS153, 22, 40–41
  in MC68000, 10, 22, 24
  signal (Column/Row), 40
Multiplication, instructions for
  as part of data processing instructions, 53
  limited in MC6800 to 16-bit operands, 57
  MUL, 74

MULS, 57
MULU, 57
use of LSL instruction for, 64, 74

NAND flip flop, 26
National Semiconductors, 1
Negate
  definition of, 10
  instructions for
    NBCD, 59
    NEG, 58
    NEGX, 59
Nibbles
  as defining operation word, 45
  definition of, 6
Normal state, 76
NOT instruction, 60
Numbers. *See* Integer; Ordinal

Object code, 121, 152
Odd addresses in MC68000, 11
Opcode. *See* Operation word
Open-collector inverter, 26
Operand
  absence in inherent mode, 52
  as part of data strobe signal, 10
  data register, 17
  decimal operands, 59
  destination operand, 52, 56, 57, 58
  effect on condition codes, 55
  fixed operand, 13
  in data processing instructions, 55, 56, 57, 58, 59, 60, 61, 64–65, 74
  in data transfer instructions, 67
  in effective address, 42, 44
  in instruction format of 16-bit devices, 2, 44
  in memory addressing mode, 47, 49, 50
  in register direct addressing, 45, 47
  in special addressing modes, 51–52
  multiplication of, 74
  size affecting choice of instructions, 74
  size limitation, 55, 57
  source operand, 56, 58
  unaffected in various divisions, 82
Operating system program, 19
Operation word (opcode or op word)
  accessing to avoid address error, 42
  bit instruction, 65
  conditional branch instructions, 69
  effective address, as part of, 42, 43, 44, 45, 46–47
  for emulator line, 82
  in arithmetic instructions, 58
  in immediate mode, 51

INDEX

in inherent mode, 52
in instruction formats, 2, 44
nibbles as defining, 45
OR instruction, 2, 60, 62, 77
Ordinal, 6–7
Orthogonality, 54
Overflow, 82

Page, 3–4, 92
Paging, 3–4
Parallel circuits, 19, 21
Parallel Interface/Timer (PI/T). See MC68230
Parameters, 71
Parity, 91, 94
Peripheral devices
  as design consideration, 2, 5
  clock frequencies for, 14, 28
  effect of Request to Send signal, 99
  for MC68000 family
    assertion by address strobe, 10
    autovector device, 17
    compatability among MC68000 family, 88
    compatability with 6800 family, 5, 22
    interfacing with enable signal, 14
    interrupt acknowledge bus cycle, 87, 89
    interrupt request output (IRQ), 87, 89
    limitation on exception vectors used for, 80n
    memory map for, 10n, 22, 92
  for VU68K, 118
  intentional delay in data acknowledge line, 12
  interfacing, 34, 68. See also MC68230
  interrupts, 17
  of 6800, 5, 22, 34, 68
  programming for, 19
  6850 as, 118
Pins in MC68000, 9–10
Power On Reset ($\overline{POR}$) signal, 26
Power supply
  for 74LS148, 98
  in disabling latching input, 22
  in negating address strobe in MC68000, 10
  pins in MC68000 for, 9
Prefetch queue, 5
Printing, 19, 92, 97, 106–107
Privilege violation, 80, 124
Procedural calls, 71
Program counter (PC)
  addressing modes, 42, 43, 52, 53
  distinguished from assembler location counter, 126
  during exception state, 77–78, 79, 121
  during trace service routine, 82–83
  during unconditional branch instructions, 69
  effect of various return instructions on, 79–81
  in MC68000, 3, 15, 17, 21
  in paging, 3–4
  in reset vector, 79, 80
  in VU68K, 121, 122, 123, 126, 133
  return address for, 148
  user program counter, 121, 122
Program execution
  halted state, 76, 120
  instruction-by-instruction, 122
Programming
  design considerations for, 1–2, 3, 55
  designation of frame pointer, 71
  effect of instructions on status register flags, 55
  in MC68000, 3, 4, 19, 54, 55, 73–75
  modular programming, 70
  object code, 121
  of 6850, 102–103
  of MC68230, 108–110, 111
  of traps, 77
  position-independent programs, 52, 70
  prototype command in monitor of VU68K, 141
  registers for, 3
  trace routines, 82
  use of emulator instructions, 82
  use of proper instructions, 73
  use of supervisor versus user mode, 76
Pull-up resistor, 10, 22, 26, 98

Queue, 13, 128, 132, 133

Radix point, 54
RAM. See Memory
RDA signal, 95
Read
  data transfer, 22
  during clear instruction, 74
  during MOVE instruction, 74
  during supervisor versus user mode, 77
  during Scc instruction, 74
  effect of data strobe on cycle, 10
  in bit manipulation, 66
  in MC68000, 11, 22
  initiation of, 11
  multiplexing for, 22
  of semaphore byte, 66
  registers of 6850, 94
  timing of, 11, 29
  zero-padding of values for, 123
Read-modify-write cycle (R-M-W) in MC68000, 10, 15, 66

Read-write
  control of data-bus buffers, 11
  line (R/$\overline{\text{W}}$)
    in MC68000, 10, 11, 12, 15, 22
    in 6800, 11
    in 6850, 94
  signal (RAW), 40
Receiver-transmitter, 94
Refresh, 36
Registers. *See also* Address, condition code, data, index, shift, source, or status register; Program counter; Trap instructions: CHK
  affected by data processing instructions, 61, 63
  affected by data transfer instructions, 53, 67
  as design consideration, 3
  and instructions, 73
  comparison in eight- versus 16-bit devices, 1–2, 3
  effect on condition codes, 55
  examination and modification of, 122, 136
  for paging, 3–4
  in bit manipulation, 65
  in effective address, 42, 43, 44
  in MC68000, 3, 17–18
  in rotate instructions, 65
  in stacking operation, 67, 74
  in VU68K, 121, 126
  multiplication of, 74
  pointer, 122
  register bit in defining addressing mode, 44
  register save area, 124, 126, 128
Request to Send ($\overline{\text{RTS}}$) signal from 6850, 94, 95
Rerun cycle in MC68000, 15, 91
Reset
  address, 103
  and supervisor mode, 77
  as distinguished from abort function, 97
  byte count, 146
  circuit, 19, 22, 23–28
  effect on buffers in VU68K, 119
  effect on posts in VU68K, 119
  effect on stack in VU68K, 119
  exception state, 24, 53
    exception vectors, 13, 21, 22, 79, 80, 119
    interrupt lines, 78
    reset as causing, 77, 78, 79
  flags during initiation of, 24
  flowchart of, 25
  input, 26
  instruction, 53, 77
  line in MC68000, 9, 15

manual reset, 76n
master reset, 103–104
pin in MC68000 for, 26
signal, 24
trace service routine, 83
Return instructions
  RTE, 77, 79–81, 83, 119, 123
  RTS, 81, 122
  RTR, 81
Rotate instructions
  ROL, 63, 64–65
  ROR, 63, 64–65
  ROXL, 63, 74
  ROXR, 63
Row, 144, 145
Row address signal (RAS), 28, 29, 36, 40
RS-232 protocol, 99

Scratchpad, 22
Segmentation. *See* Memory segmentation
Semaphore, 66
74LS14, 107
74LS138
  during interrupt, 87–88
  for function control lines of MC68000, 13
  selection of memory area for 6850, 34
74LS148, 87, 97, 98
74LS153. *See* multiplexing
74LS175 in watchdog timer, 34
74LS245, 22, 24
74LS273, 97, 98
74LS373, 22
74161, 114
Serial circuits, 19
Serial communication, 21
Serial ports. *See also* VU68K
  circuits for, 99, 100
  protocol for, 99
S-format, 121, 139, 153–157
Shift
  instructions, 63–65
  register
    for intentional delay of data acknowledge signal, 12
    in 6850, 94
    in watchdog timer, 34
Sign bit, 7, 64, 67
Signals, 10, 19
Single-step circuit, 26, 27
Single-step mode in VU68K, 120, 121, 122
16-bit devices
  comparison with eight-bit devices, 1–2
  hardwired logic unit, 5
  instruction format of, 1, 2

INDEX 325

integers, 7
memory accessing, 3–4
memory addressing modes, 1
memory addressing range, 1
numbers, 7
peripherals, 5–6
registers, 1
word in, 6
word width of, 3
6800 (prefix MC for Motorola devices)
  interrupts, 16
  mentioned, 1
  operation code (op code), 2
  peripheral devices of, 5, 14–15, 22, 34, 68
  read/write line, 11
  status register, 17–18
  valid memory address ($\overline{VMA}$), 14
  with 6850, 92
6850 (Asynchronous Communications Interface Adapter (ACIA))
  address line, 97
  addresses, 97, 102, 127
  as audio-cassette interface, 92
  as peripheral device, 118
  baud rate, 99–101, 112
  bit pattern, 99, 101
  block diagram of, 94
  break condition, 96
  buffering, 101
  bus, 96
  bytes, 96
  chip select lines (CS0-2), 95
  clear to send ($\overline{CTS}$) line, 95, 99
  data carrier detect ($\overline{DCD}$) line, 95, 96
  data set ready (DSR) signal, 99
  data stream, 96
  double device, 94
  E clock, 97
  error flag, 96
  framing error (FE), 96
  in VU68K, 114, 118
  initializing, 128
  internal counter, 101
  interrupt, 101
  interrupt request bit ($\overline{IRQ}$), 95, 96, 104
  loop, 104
  master reset, 96
  MC68000 data bus, 96
  memory location in MC68000, 22
  memory-mapped ports in eight- versus 16-bit devices, 68
  modem, 95, 96, 98, 99
  output to, 129
  parity error, 96
  priority interrupt levels, 98
  programming, 102–103
  read, 96, 97
  read/write line, 95
  receive data (RX DATA) signal, 99
  receiver-data register flag, 104
  receiver overrun (OVRN), 96
  register select (RS) lines, 95
  registers of
    control, 94–95, 99, 101
    data register, 102
    receiver-data register (RDR), 95, 96, 102
    status (Read only) register, 94, 95, 96, 101, 102, 104
    transmit-data register, 95, 96, 101, 102
    write only, 94
  request to send (RTS) signal, 99, 104
  reset, 95, 96
  serial communication, 21
  start bit, 96, 101
  status bits, 95–96
  stop bit, 96, 101, 104
  synchronization error, 96
  synchronous, 97
  transmit data (TX DATA) signal, 99
  treatment of data by, 94
  write, 96, 97
6116, 118
Size of MC68000, 9
Source register, 62
Speed
  as design consideration, 2, 5, 28
  clock of VU68K, 114
  effect of buffers on, 28
  effect of gates on, 28
  effect of hardwired logic unit on, 5
  effect of word width on, 3
  for 6850, 99
  of execution, 74
  of MC68000L4, 19
  mentioned, 29
  use of multiple arithmetic-logic units for, 5
Stack (System stack)
  access by return instruction, 81
  check on bounds, 82
  clear, 128
  data memory, 13
  during exception state, 77
  during external reset, 79, 119
  in address register indirect, 48, 49, 50
  in branch instruction, 69
  in LINK instruction, 71
  in MOVEM instructions, 74

Stack (continued)
  in position-independence instructions, 70
  loading operations, 49
  location in memory area of VU68K, 126
  storing of frame pointer, 71
  supervisor stack, 82–83
  unloading operation, 48
  user stack, 133
Stacking operation, 47, 67
Stack pointer (SP)
  during activation of 6850, 103
  during reset, 24, 79
  effect of return instructions on, 79–81, 82
  in address register indirect with
      postincrement, 48
  in MC68000, 3, 17, 21
  supervisor stack pointer (SSP), 3
  use in exception state, 77, 79
  use in LINK/UNLNK instructions, 71
  user stack pointer (USP), 3, 77, 128
  vector, 21, 80
Static memory, 11
Status bits, supervisor versus user mode, 77
Status register (SR)
  affected by data processing instructions, 58, 62
  affected by data transfer instructions, 53
  affected by system control instructions, 53
  bit pattern for user-interrupt vectors, 127
  during exception state, 76–78, 79, 121
  during supervisor versus user mode, 77
  during trace service routine, 82–83
  effect of various return instructions on, 79–81
  interrupt masks of, 83
  in MC6800, 17–18, 24
  in MC68000, 17
  in monitor of VU68K, 133
  in 6850, 94, 95
  return pattern, 148
  save area for, 126
  trace bit of, 122, 123, 147
  user status register, 121
String
  check on bounds of, 82
  comparison of, 70
  data memory, 13
  definition of, 8
  in monitor of VU68K, 123, 129
  manipulation of, 70
  significance of, 6
  use of, 8
STOP instruction, 77
Subtraction
  accommodated by all computers, 54
  in compare instructions, 58

instructions for
  SBCD, 59
  SUB, 55, 57, 74
  SUBA, 57, 75
  SUBI, 57
  SUBQ, 57
  SUBX, 57
  Part of data processing instructions, 53
  operation code of 6800, 2
Supervisor mode in MC68000
  exception vector number for privilege
      violation, 80
  function control lines as indicating, 13, 14
  use in exception-handling routines, 77
Supervisor mode in MC68000
  privileges of, 76, 77
    instructions available during, 77, 79
    status bits during, 77
  status of S/U flags, 18, 76
  trace, 82
  trap exception, 81
  use of stack pointer, 17
Supervisory memory, 14
System control See also Bus error line; Halt
      line; Reset line
  instructions, 53
  lines in MC68000, 15
  pins in MC68000 for, 9
  use of supervisor mode by programs for, 76

Tables, 13, 48
TDRA signal, 95
Temporary register, during exception state, 76
Terminal
  connection to VU68K, 114, 118
  8008, 1
  emulator mode, 121
  interface with 6850, 102
  interrupts from, 98, 119
  notation for keys on, 120
  operation of VU68K as, 120–121, 140
  protocol for, 99
  serial connection to, 19, 21, 92
Test-and-Set instruction, 10, 15, 65, 66
Texas Instruments (TI), 1
32-bit devices
  comparison with eight-bit devices, 1–2
  hardwired logic unit, 5
  numbers, 7
  word in, 6
Timer, 35
  control signals of circuit for, 37–38
  for reset, 25
  in MC68230, 104, 105
  See MC3456

INDEX 327

Tracing
    and exception state, 76, 77, 78, 80, 82–83
    instruction-by-instruction, 123
    with breakpoints in VU68K, 120
Trap
    address trap error, 42
    and supervisor mode, 77
    definition of, 77
    exception state, 76, 77, 78, 80, 82–83
    exception vector, 21
    for tracing, 82
    handling routine, 148
    in VU68K, 118, 119, 123–124
    instructions
        CHK, 78, 80, 81–82, 124
        tracing of, 123
        TRAP, 78, 80, 81
        TRAPV, 78, 80, 81, 82, 124
    single-step trap, 122
TST instruction, 55, 58
TTL logic, 1, 33
Two's complement form, 6–7, 69

United States Air Force Academy, Computer
    Science Department, 114, 124
User mode in MC68000
    function control lines as indicating, 13, 14
    privilege of, 76–77
    status of S/U flag, 76
        instructions available during, 77
        status bits during, 77
    privilege violation exception, 79, 80
Unconditional branch instructions, 53
UNLNK instruction, 71, 72

Valid memory address ($\overline{\text{VMA}}$), 14–15
Valid peripheral address ($\overline{\text{VPA}}$), 14–15, 17, 34
    in VU68K, 114
    interrupt acknowledge signal for, 98, 99
    spurious interrupts, 91
    terminating interrupt acknowledge bus cycle,
        87
Values, comparison during logical state, 6
Vanderbilt University, Computer Science
    Department, 114, 124
Variables
    areas, 71
    in data memory, 13
    in stack, 50, 71
Vector. *See* Exception: Vector
VUBUG. *See* Monitor for VU68K
VU68K
    acknowledge signal, synthesis of, 114
    address bits
        memory-block selection bits, 116, 118

        word-selection bits, 116, 118
    address decoding, 116, 118
    address lines, 114
    address strobe, 114
    asynchronous versus synchronous operation,
        114
    baud-rate generator, 114
    Bonds, A. B., 114
    branch instruction, 119
    bus-wait technique in, 119
    Carter, Edward M., 114, 124
    clock speed, 114
    connection to modem, 114
    connection to terminal, 114, 118
    data acknowledge line and signal, 114
    decoder, 118
    effect of reset, 119
    input/output ports, 114, 118, 119–120
    interrupts, 115, 116, 118, 119
    limitation on return instructions, 119
    loading, 121
    memory, 114, 116, 118
    memory map, 114, 118
    mode-select line, 118
    registers, 121
    schematic of, 114, 115–117
    6850, 114
    United States Air Force Academy, Computer
        Science Department, 114
    Vanderbilt University, Computer Science
        Department, 114
    valid peripheral address ($\overline{\text{VPA}}$) line, 114
    See also Monitor of VU68K
Wait states, 12, 28, 32, 35, 119
Waite, Mitchell, 6
Watchdog timer circuit
    diagram of, 34–35
    interrupt acknowledge signal for, 98
    signaling bus error, 13, 91
Word
    address register, 17
    addressing to avoid error, 42
    as block, 6
    bits in, 3, 46
    as default value in MC68000, 42
    boundary, 48, 78
    data register, 17
    data strobe for transfer, 11
    definition of, 6
    extension word, 51, 52
    extension of word-address, 74
    extension of word-data, 74
    fetching, 134
    for instructions affecting addresses, 73
    for reading ROM, 19

Word (continued)
  in bit manipulation, 66
  in MC68000, 10
  operands, 47, 55
  operation of instructions on, 3
  output from VU68K, 129
  selection in VU68K, 116
  special status word, 79
  storage during exception-handling subroutines, 77
  width, 3, 46
  word-address operations, 74
Write, 32
  data transfer, 11, 22
  during supervisor versus user mode, 77
  initiation of, 11
  limitation on clear instruction, 74
  limitation on MOVE instruction, 74
  limitation on Scc instruction, 74
  multiplexing for, 22
  protection of ROM against, 19
  registers of 6850, 94
  speed, 29
  to ports in VU68K, 119, 145
  timing of, 11, 12
  zero-padding of values, 123

Z80, 1
Zilog, 1